WITHDRAWN

Core Topics in Endocrinology in Anaesthesia and Critical Care

Core Topics in Endocrinology in Anaesthesia and Critical Care

Editors

George M. Hall
Professor of Anaesthesia at St George's, University of London, UK

Jennifer M. Hunter
Professor of Anaesthesia at the University of Liverpool, UK

Mark S. Cooper
Clinical Senior Lecturer in Endocrinology and Diabetes at the Centre for Endocrinology, Diabetes and Metabolism, University of Birmingham, UK

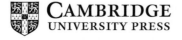
CAMBRIDGE
UNIVERSITY PRESS

CAMBRIDGE UNIVERSITY PRESS
Cambridge, New York, Melbourne, Madrid, Cape Town, Singapore,
São Paulo, Delhi, Dubai, Tokyo

Cambridge University Press
The Edinburgh Building, Cambridge CB2 8RU, UK

Published in the United States of America by Cambridge University Press, New York

www.cambridge.org
Information on this title: www.cambridge.org/9780521509992

First published 2010

Printed in the United Kingdom at the University Press, Cambridge

A catalogue record for this publication is available from the British Library

Library of Congress Cataloguing in Publication data
  Core topics in endocrinology in anaesthesia and critical care / [edited by]
  George M. Hall, Jennifer M. Hunter, Mark S. Cooper.
      p. ; cm.
  Includes bibliographical references and index.
  ISBN-13: 978-0-521-50999-2 (hardback)
  ISBN-10: 0-521-50999-8 (hardback)
  1. Endocrine glands–Diseases–Patients–Hospital care.   2. Critical care medicine.
  3. Anesthesia.   I. Hall, George M. (George Martin)   II. Hunter, Jennifer M.   III. Cooper, Mark S.
  [DNLM: 1. Endocrine System Diseases–surgery.   2. Critical Illness–therapy.   3. Diabetes Mellitus–drug
  therapy.   4. Diabetes Mellitus–physiopathology.   5. Diabetes Mellitus–surgery.
  6. Perioperative Care–methods. WK 148 C797 2010]
  RC649.C53   2010
  616.4′028–dc22   2009050378

ISBN 978-0-521-50999-2 Hardback

Contents

Contributors

Steven Ball
Newcastle University, UK
Royal Victoria Infirmary, Newcastle upon
Tyne, UK

Simon V. Baudouin
Newcastle University, UK
Royal Victoria Infirmary, Newcastle upon
Tyne, UK

Jane K. Beattie
Royal Liverpool University Hospital, UK

Ann E. Black
Great Ormond Street Hospital, London, UK
University College London Institute of Child
Health, UK

Mark S. Cooper
Centre for Endocrinology, Diabetes and
Metabolism, University of Birmingham, UK

Peter A. Farling
Royal Victoria Hospital, Belfast, Northern
Ireland, UK

A. B. Johan Groeneveld
Vrije Universiteit Medical Centre, Amsterdam,
The Netherlands

George M. Hall
St George's, University of London, UK

Jennifer M. Hunter
University of Liverpool, UK

Saheed Khan
Vrije Universiteit Medical Centre, Amsterdam,
The Netherlands

Angus McEwan
Great Ormond Street Hospital, London, UK
University College London Institute of Child
Health, UK

Philip R. Michael
Royal Liverpool University Hospital, UK

Brian Mullan
Royal Victoria Hospital, Belfast, Northern
Ireland, UK

Paul G. Murphy
St James University Hospital, Leeds, UK

Grainne Nicholson
St George's, University of London, UK

Pauline M. O'Neil
Royal Alexandra Hospital, Paisley, Scotland, UK

Christopher J. R. Parker
Royal Liverpool University Hospital, UK

Barbara Philips
St George's, University of London, UK

Charles S. Reilly
Royal Hallamshire Hospital, Sheffield, UK

Heidi J. Robertshaw
St George's, University of London, UK

Neville Robinson
Northwick Park & St Mark's Hospitals,
Harrow, UK

Mark E. Seubert
Vrije Universiteit Medical Centre, Amsterdam,
The Netherlands

Martin Smith
University College London Hospitals, UK

David J. Vaughan
Northwick Park & St Mark's Hospitals,
Harrow, UK

Nigel R. Webster
Institute of Medical Sciences, Aberdeen,
Scotland, UK

Saffron Whitehead
St George's, University of London, UK

Foreword

The clinical interface between endocrinologists/diabetologists and anaesthetists/intensive care physicians and the joint management of their patients is more than a marriage of convenience. Endocrinologists are all too aware that patients with underlying endocrine disease bring additional anaesthetic risks and concerns. Examples include patients with acromegaly and hypopituitarism, thyrotoxicosis and phaeochromocytoma. Perhaps one of the most common concerns necessitating cross-referral in hospitals is the patient with established diabetes mellitus. The optimal management of such a patient in terms of metabolic control and insulin therapy across anaesthesia and in an intensive care setting is of paramount importance.

But the area has moved on much further: research advances over the last 5 years have highlighted how careful metabolic control of patients on intensive care units can significantly improve outcome. This is particularly true in the management of hyperglycaemia and hyponatremia and may also now include the concept of relative adrenal insufficiency. For the endocrinologist/ diabetologist, therefore, it is essential that this knowledge now becomes embedded in their evidence-based clinical practice. For the anaesthetist and the intensive care physician, a greater appreciation of the endocrine basis for abnormal biochemical results in patients within intensive care units is equally important if improvements in patient morbidity and mortality are to be realised.In this timely publication, Professors Hall and Hunter and Dr Cooper have solicited and edited 18 topical chapters from experts in the field that will address all of these issues. Section 1 details the perioperative care of patients with endocrine disease; Section 2 – the care of patients with diabetes; and Section 3 – endocrine disorders that arise in the critically ill patient. To have this information under one cover is an admirable achievement and one that will be of immense value to medical practitioners involved in managing sick patients.

Paul M Stewart MD FRCP FMedSci
Professor of Medicine

Preface

Endocrine disorders are a disparate group of diseases of complex pathophysiology. Some of these disorders, such as diabetes mellitus, are increasingly common in the developed world. Diabetic patients can present at any age to anaesthetists of all grades and in every sub-specialty. In this specialist anaesthetic text, there is a detailed discussion of all aspects of an anaesthetist's involvement with diabetes, be it in paediatric, obstetric or intensive care practice, or when these patients undergo routine surgery. For greater understanding, an outline of the pathophysiology of diabetes mellitus is provided.

Thyroid dysfunction is another common endocrine disorder of which all anaesthetists have significant experience. It is essential for anaesthetists to understand the many different diseases that affect this gland, be they malignant or autoimmune, how such diseases are managed medically and how they affect anaesthetic practice.

Other endocrine disorders are far less common than diabetes mellitus and thyroid disease. The challenges for any anaesthetist with the rarer disorders of the adrenal, pituitary and parathyroid glands, or with endocrine disorders of the gut, are very different from managing a diabetic patient. No practitioner will have great experience of anaesthetising such patients. Thus it is apposite to have contributions from well recognised experts in these areas brought together into one text.

Only recently have endocrine disorders in critically ill patients been given detailed consideration. This book considers not only the topical subjects of glucose control in the critically ill and the critically ill diabetic patient, but also the very rare disorders of the thyroid gland that present to intensivists. Fluid and electrolyte imbalance, the effects of critical illness on adrenal physiology and the role of glucocorticoid replacement are considered. Understanding of such disorders is incomplete, but in this text we update all anaesthetists involved in acute medicine in these complex areas.

To increase the understanding of the pathophysiology and medical management of such patients, it has been most advantageous to have a distinguished endocrinologist as a co-editor. We hope that Mark Cooper's significant contributions will enhance anaesthetists' understanding of the multidisciplinary approach that is required in the management of the complex endocrine patient perioperatively.

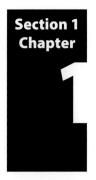
Perioperative care of patients with endocrine disease

Anaesthesia for patients with pituitary disease

Paul G. Murphy

Introduction

The human neuroendocrine system has two components – hormonal secretion that is controlled by the hypothalamo-pituitary axis and the extra-hypothalamic neurohormones, such as somatostatin, atrial natriuretic peptide and the peptide hormones of the gastrointestinal tract. This chapter principally concentrates on the clinically significant disorders of the hypothalamo-pituitary axis, which through their anatomical and physiological complexity can present the anaesthetist with a wide variety of challenging perioperative problems. The most common lesions of this axis are benign adenomas of the anterior lobe of the pituitary gland. While principal attention focuses on the resulting endocrine hypersecretion that may be associated with such disorders, due regard should also be given to the potential 'mass effect' that such lesions may be exerting on neighbouring brain tissue as well as any consequences of the treatment that a patient may have received for their condition.

Clinical anatomy and physiology of the hypothalamo-pituitary-neuroendocrine axis

The hypothalamus is responsible for the maintenance of homeostasis and the integration of nervous and endocrine control mechanisms. It regulates many of the body's autonomic functions, such as temperature, thirst and hunger, blood pressure and volume, sleep and sexual function, and is intimately related, both anatomically and functionally, to the pituitary gland [1]. Anatomically it is regarded as a component of the diencephalon, the most rostral part of the brainstem, and lies within the walls and floor of the third ventricle of the brain. It is a complex collection of nervous and

endocrine tissue, and contains a number of nuclei that have either a direct (neuronal) or indirect (vascular) communication with the pituitary gland.

The pituitary gland is similarly a composite of endocrine and nervous tissue that is located at the base of the brain and connected to the hypothalamus by the pituitary stalk. It weighs less than 1 g under normal circumstances, and lies within the sella turcica, a bony fossa of the skull base. The roof of the pituitary fossa is created by an incomplete fold of dura, the diaphragma sella, through which passes the pituitary stalk. The fossa is limited posteriorly by the clivus and both anteriorly and inferiorly by the bony air sinuses of the sphenoid bone. Important anatomical relationships of the pituitary gland are shown in Figure 1.1 [2]. Laterally on either side lie the cavernous sinuses, various cranial nerves and beyond them the temporal lobes. Superiorly are found the pituitary stalk, the diaphragma sella and the optic nerves/chiasm, and beyond them the hypothalamus and third ventricle.

The gland itself is organised embryologically, anatomically and functionally into two parts (Figure 1.2). The anterior lobe (adenohypophysis) is derived embryologically from Rathke's pouch, an upgrowth from the roof of the pharynx, and consists of cords of endocrine secretory tissue organised around an extensive network of sinusoids which arise from a local vascular network that extends from the hypothalamus to the anterior lobe along the pituitary stalk.

Classically, cell types of the anterior lobe have been categorised histologically according to the presence and staining characteristics of intracellular granules, this being a reflection of a more fundamental functional characteristic of endocrine tissue that has differentiated into one of five secretory cell types (Table 1.1). The secretory functions of the anterior lobe are under indirect (vascular) hypothalamic control, mediated by releasing

Core Topics in Endocrinology in Anaesthesia and Critical Care, eds. George M. Hall, Jennifer M. Hunter and Mark S. Cooper. Published by Cambridge University Press. © Cambridge University Press 2010.

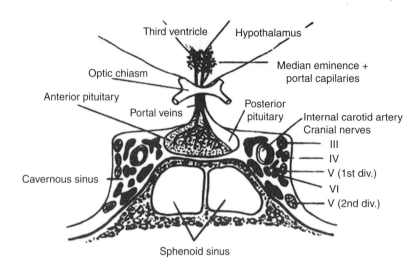

Fig. 1.1 Schematic coronal view of the hypothalamus and pituitary gland, demonstrating their anatomical relationships with neighbouring structures. From Cobb and Jackson [32] with permission.

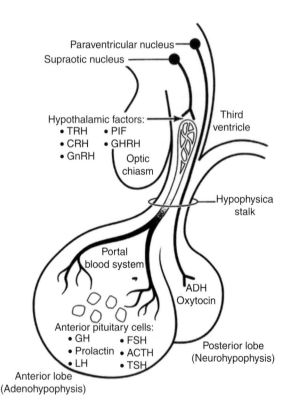

Fig. 1.2 Functional anatomy of the hypothalamo-pituitary axis of neurohormonal secretion. ACTH, adrenocorticotrophic hormone; ADH, antidiuretic hormone; CRH, corticotropin releasing hormone; FSH, follicle stimulating hormone; GH, growth hormone; GHRH, growth hormone releasing hormone; GnRH, gonadotropin releasing hormone; LH, luteinising hormone; PIF, prolactin-inhibiting factor; TRH, thyroid releasing hormone; TSH, thyroid stimulating hormone. From Albin [33] with permission.

hormones which are synthesised within the supra-optic nuclei of the hypothalamus and then delivered to the adenohypophysis via the portal vascular network described above. In contrast, the posterior lobe (neurohypophysis) is true nervous tissue, a caudal extension of nerve fibres that project from cell bodies within the paraventricular and supra-optic nuclei to the posterior lobe via the pituitary stalk. The hormones antidiuretic hormone (ADH, alternatively known as arginine vasopressin or simply vasopressin) and oxytocin are synthesised in these cell bodies prior to neuronal transport to nerve endings within the posterior lobe, their release remaining under direct nervous hypothalamic control.

The synthesis and secretion of the hormonal products of the adenohypophysis is subject to complex, multilevel regulation, as summarised in Figure 1.3. With the exception of the lactotroph, the dominant hypothalamic influence is a stimulatory one, which is in turn regulated by negative feedback control exerted at both the pituitary and hypothalamic level. The classic example of such a self-regulating negative feedback system is the hypothalamo-pituitary-thyroid axis. In contrast, prolactin secretion is under largely inhibitory control that is mediated by dopamine. The synthesis and release of growth hormone (GH) is stimulated by growth hormone releasing hormone (GHRH) and inhibited by somatostatin. Despite such individual variations, the overall 'set point' for the various hypothalamo-pituitary endocrine systems is influenced by a variety of neuro-environmental inputs from higher brain centres (Figure 1.3) that include stress, exercise, sexual activity, environmental temperature, altered day/night patterns and steroid hormone levels.

Table 1.1 Hormone products of the pituitary gland.

Anterior lobe (adenohypophysis)

Hormone	Properties
Growth hormone (GH)	The 191-amino-acid product of the somatotroph cells that amount to as much as 50% of the total secretory capacity of the anterior lobe Widespread anabolic properties, including promotion of bone and muscle development Promotes use of lipid as an energy source by stimulating lipolysis. Impairs glucose utilisation and induces insulin resistance, 'pancreatic burnout' and frank diabetes mellitus Effects largely mediated by the somatomedins, such as insulin-like growth factor (IGF), which are synthesised in the liver in response to GH The hypothalamic peptides somatotropin and somatostatin respectively stimulate and inhibit the secretion of GH. Secretion is increased by starvation (particularly chronic protein deficency), hypoglycaemia, glucagon, exercise, stress trauma and sleep. Excess of GH leads to acromegaly (or gigantism if developing prior to epiphysial fusion), while an absence of it or its peripheral receptors causes pituitary dwarfism
Prolactin (PRL)	Protein product of the lactotroph, the extent of which increases markedly during pregnancy and lactation Promotes lactation and plays a minor role in breast development Synthesis and release of prolactin is largely under hypothalamic inhibitory control mediated by dopamine Secretion is increased by suckling, stress, exercise and sexual intercourse
Thyroid stimulating hormone (TSH)	Glycoprotein product of thyrotroph cells Stimulates all known secretory activities of the thyroid glandular tissue, including the proteolysis of thyroglobulin, and iodide uptake Release is stimulated by thyroid releasing hormone (TRH), a tripeptide synthesised by neurons found throughout the hypothalamus. Negative feedback control is very sensitive, and operates principally at the level of the pituitary rather than the hypothalamus. TRH secretion is increased principally by prolonged exposure to cold environments, and also rises in response to anxiety or excitement. The absence of TRH reduces but does not abolish TSH secretion
Adrenocorticotrophin hormone (ACTH)	Secreted by corticotroph cells that comprise approximately 15% of anterior lobe secretory tissue Synthesised as a large precursor molecule, proopiomelanocortin, which also has within its 240 amino-acid sequence γ-melanocyte stimulating hormone (γ-MSH), β-lipotropin and β-endorphin ACTH itself is a 39-amino-acid polypeptide, which stimulates the synthesis of glucocorticoids and androgens from the zona fasciculata and reticularis of the adrenal cortex. Tissue degradation of ACTH releases α-MSH. Secretion of ACTH is stimulated by corticotrophin releasing hormone (CRH), a 41-amino-acid polypeptide synthesised by neurons arising mainly from the paraventricular nucleus of the hypothalamus Cortisol exerts negative feedback control on the synthesis and release of ACTH at the level of both the hypothalamus and the pituitary CRH production is increased in response to all kinds of stress, including trauma, surgery, pain, infection, extremes of temperature and many debilitating diseases. There is very little ACTH production in the absence of CRH
Gonadotrophins (follicular stimulating hormone, FSH, and luteinising hormone, LH)	Glycoprotein products of the gonadotroph cells In the male, LH stimulates the secretion of testosterone while FSH is responsible for stimulating spermatogenesis In the female, FSH and LH are intimately involved in the production of oestrogen and progesterone, and the regulation of the menstrual and ovulatory cycles Release is controlled by gonadotrophin releasing hormone (GnRH), a 10-amino-acid polypeptide, which is synthesised in neurons concentrated in the arcuate nucleus of the hypothalamus Negative feedback control is largely at the hypothalamic level, and exerted by testosterone in the male, and oestrogen and progesterone in the female. GnRH release is also modulated by higher centres, most notably the limbic system

Posterior lobe (neurohypophysis)

Antidiuretic hormone (ADH)	Nonapeptide, also known as arginine vasopressin or simply vasopressin, that acts upon vasopressin 1 receptors in peripheral vascular smooth muscle and vasopressin 2 receptors in the kidney Its principal physiological action is to promote renal reabsorption of water from distal convoluted tubule and collecting duct; also induces vasoconstriction in hypovolaemia Duration of effect 1–2 hours
Oxytocin	Nonapeptide, chemically very similar to ADH. Promotes contraction of the myometrium during labour of myoepithelial cells in the breast during lactation

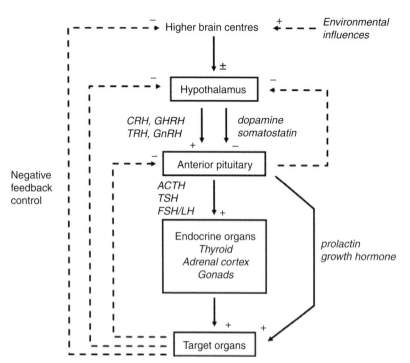

Fig. 1.3 Negative feedback control of the hypothalamo-pituitary axis. ACTH, adrenocorticotrophic hormone; CRH, corticotropin releasing hormone; FSH, follicle stimulating hormone; GHRH, growth hormone releasing hormone; GnRH, gonadotropin releasing hormone; LH, luteinising hormone; TRH, thyroid releasing hormone; TSH, thyroid stimulating hormone.

Clinical features of pituitary disease

The majority of clinically significant pituitary conditions are the result of tumour or tumour-like conditions that arise from either within the gland itself or in surrounding parasellar tissues. Although the differential diagnosis of a mass within or around the pituitary fossa is extensive and a reflection of the diverse histology of this area of the skull base, the majority are adenomas of the anterior lobe that develop from one or other of the differentiated secretory cell types of the adenohypophysis. Although they commonly display a variable degree of local invasiveness they very rarely metastasise, and so cannot be considered to be malignant by the usual definition.

Only a proportion of pituitary tumours declare themselves clinically – indeed incidental pituitary lesions are found in up to 25% of autopsies [3]. In general terms, pituitary adenomas can present in one of three ways: by virtue of the hypersecretion of the hormonal product(s) of the gland, by growing to a size sufficient to exert a mass effect on neighbouring structures, or through a combination of the two. Adenomas that secrete adrenocorticotrophic hormone (ACTH) or thyroid stimulating hormone (TSH) have profound physiological effects and usually present as small tumours (microadenomas) that can be difficult

to locate both radiologically and surgically. The functional consequences of prolactin-secreting tumours in females of childbearing age may similarly present early in their natural history, although this will be less likely in males or postmenopausal females. In contrast, a quarter of adenomas are endocrinologically inert [4]. Such tumours only become clinically significant when they have grown to a size sufficient to elicit a mass effect, and are known as macroadenomas. Tumours of the somatotroph that secrete GH usually present with features of both a mass effect and hormonal hypersecretion: this is because of the insidious pathophysiological consequences of an excess of GH and the extended time interval between onset and clinical diagnosis [5].

The principal clinical features of a sellar mass lesion are headache, visual disturbance and endocrine hyposecretion. Headache results from either stretching of the diaphragma sella, erosion of the bony sella turcica, or, in acromegaly, re-architecturing of the membranous bones of the skull. Very occasionally, headache may be indicative of raised intracranial pressure secondary to obstruction of the third ventricle or foramen of Munro, and it is essential therefore that clinical assessment is supplemented by appropriate imaging to exclude the possibility of obstructive hydrocephalus. The classical visual disturbance of a pituitary mass lesion is a bitemporal haemianopia that results from compression of the optic chiasm by a tumour arising from the pituitary fossa, although this may be further complicated by ophthalmoplegia if the tumour extends laterally. Some degree of hypopituitarism is frequently seen in patients with macroadenomas, and is a result of either direct destruction of secretory tissue by the expanding tumour mass, or by so-called 'stalk compression' in which obstruction of the pituitary stalk by tumour deprives the anterior lobe of the hypothalamic hormones that normally regulate secretion. The hypopituitarism of stalk compression is therefore usually accompanied by modest hyperprolactinaemia, since, as noted above, the lactotrophic cells are under predominantly inhibitory control.

Endocrine hyposecretion syndromes

The endocrine hyposecretion syndromes associated with pituitary disease of relevance to perioperative care include adrenocortical insufficiency, hypothyroidism and diabetes insipidus. Sellar or parasellar lesions rarely present with failure of posterior lobe function [6], although it is a relatively frequent complication of surgical resection. Regardless, it is important to confirm the adequacy of adrenocortical, thyroid and posterior lobe function preoperatively, and to plan perioperative hormone replacement accordingly.

Although frequently asymptomatic, adrenocortical insufficiency can be a life-threatening condition, particularly in patients with acute concurrent illness. Clinical features include nausea and vomiting, anorexia and weight loss, orthostatic hypotension, general malaise, hyponatraemia and hypoglycaemia. The renin-angiotensin-aldosterone axis is preserved, so that in comparison to Addison's disease, fluid and electrolyte abnormalities are less severe. Persistently low levels of plasma cortisol are suggestive of adrenal insufficiency, although dynamic tests of pituitary function, that examine the ability of the hypothalamo-pituitary-adrenal axis to increase cortisol secretion in response to a biochemical stress (e.g., hypoglycaemia or glucagon) are a more sensitive measure of the reserve of this component of the stress response. Diagnosis of adrenocortical insufficiency requires a high index of suspicion, particularly when faced with a patient who is unexpectedly hypotensive, hyponatraemic and hypoglycaemic. In the acute setting, patients require hydrocortisone 100 mg i.v. *statim*, followed by 25–50 mg 6 hourly together with saline resuscitation, and possibly glucose.

Similarly, *pituitary-related hypothyroidism* is usually less severe than primary thyroid failure. Clinical features include reduced metabolic rate, lethargy, voice change, cold intolerance, constipation, bradycardia and heart failure, dry cold skin and myxoedema, memory loss and confusion. Anaesthesia and surgery in patients with untreated hypothyroidism carries a high mortality. Patients show exquisite sensitivity to and reduced metabolism of all classes of anaesthetic drugs, and doses should be reduced accordingly and wherever possible titrated against effect. Emergence from anaesthesia may be very prolonged, necessitating postoperative respiratory support. The normal ventilatory responses to hypercapnia and hypoxia are obtunded and perioperative hypothermia is common. Furthermore, clinical response to thyroid replacement therapy may take 10 days or more and, although more rapid correction can be achieved with liothyronine (triiodothyronine, T_3), there is a significant risk of precipitating myocardial ischaemia and heart failure.

Central diabetes insipidus (DI) is the principal consequence of failure of the posterior pituitary lobe, and is the result of failure of secretion of ADH. The cardinal features of DI are excessive thirst and the excretion of large volumes of dilute urine, sometimes in excess of 1000 ml per hour. It is easily treated with desmopressin (1-deamino-8-D-arginine vasopressin, DDAVP), a synthetic analogue of ADH that has a longer half life and which lacks the vasoconstricting properties of the endogenous hormone. Although desmopressin is usually administered orally or intranasally, postoperatively it can be given as a subcutaneous or intra-muscular injection. Withholding DDAVP in the postoperative period will result in excessive diuresis, hypovolaemia and electrolyte disorders, and clinicians should be particularly aware of the potential to confuse oligo-anuria with urinary retention. Failure to secrete oxytocin only becomes clinically evident during and after childbirth. Although spontaneous labour and vaginal delivery may be possible [7], some have reported a high incidence of failed labour [8], and it is prudent to consider this group of patients as high-risk parturients. Difficulties with breastfeeding may also be encountered, both because of failure of the 'let down' reflex that is mediated by oxytocin and also because of anterior lobe failure and inadequate prolactin secretion.

Hormone hypersecretion syndromes

Whilst prolactinomas are the commonest functional pituitary adenoma, the pathophysiological consequences of hyperprolactinaemia make no specific demands on perioperative care. Thyroid stimulating hormone-secreting tumours are very uncommon, so that in practice it is Cushing's disease and acromegaly that are of greatest significance, although the clinician should also be aware that pituitary tumours occasionally coexist with neoplasias of extra-hypothalamic endocrine tissue (Chapter 6).

Cushing's syndrome/disease

The term Cushing's disease is reserved for an excess of glucocorticoid that is the result of hypersecretion of ACTH from a pituitary corticotroph adenoma, the more generic term Cushing's syndrome being applied to a non-specific state of chronic glucocorticoid excess regardless of cause. Cushing's disease is more common in women, and carries a 50% 5-year mortality if left untreated. Corticotroph adenomas usually present as microadenomas, and inferior petrosal venous blood sampling may be required in order to distinguish between pituitary and ectopic sources of excess ACTH. Although surgical removal is considered to be the definitive treatment for Cushing's disease, many of the adverse physiological features of the condition, listed in Table 1.2, can be promptly checked and indeed reversed with agents such as ketoconazole, metyrapone and trilostane that interfere with the synthesis of cortisol in the adrenal cortex. Such therapies may also be of value in the acute setting.

Table 1.2 Clinical features of Cushing's syndrome.

Type	Clinical features
General	Central obesity with limb wasting ('orange on a stick') Dorsocervical fat pad ('buffalo hump') Supraclavicular fat pads Moon and plethoric facies Exophthalmos
Dermatological	Skin atrophy, with loss of subcutaneous fat and increased fragility, striae Liddle's sign (skin peels off with removal of adhesive tape) Easy bruising Poor wound healing and increased risk of dehiscence Hyperpigmentation (when condition is a result of excess ACTH) Oily facial skin with acne and hirsuitism
Cardiovascular	Refractory systemic hypertension with left ventricular hypertrophy and diastolic failure Na +/− water retention and dependent oedema Congestive cardiac failure Cardiomyopathy and myocardial irritability Increased incidence of venous thromboembolism
Respiratory	Obstructive sleep apnoea Respiratory function may be impaired by obesity, kyphoscoliosis, cortisol-induced myopathy and hypokalaemia
Musculoskeletal	Proximal muscle wasting (aggravated by hypokalaemia); may be unable to rise from the squatting position, and in severe cases are unable to climb stairs Accelerated osteoporosis, vertebral compression fractures, leading to kyphoscoliosis Aseptic necrosis of femoral head Pathological rib fractures
Gastrointestinal	Peptic ulceration Gastro-oesophageal reflux
Metabolic	Hyperinsulinaemia, glucose intolerance and insulin-dependent diabetes mellitus Hypercalcuria secondary to increased bone resportion Polyuria and polydypsia Hypokalaemia and hypochloraemic alkalosis in severe cases
Neurological	Psychiatric disorders
Genito-urinary	Infertility, amenorrhoea, reduced libido, impotence Asymptomatic bacterial colonisation of urinary tract
Immunological	Standard inflammatory response to infection may be masked Increased susceptibility to infection in severe cases
Haematological	Polycythaemia, granulocytosis and lymphopenia

The typical habitus of a patient with Cushing's syndrome is one of truncal obesity, proximal limb myopathy, moon facies and hirsuitism. Despite their outward appearance, patients with Cushing's syndrome are frail and require careful management in all aspects of perioperative care. Exophthalmos secondary to retro-orbital deposits of fat is seen in a third of patients with Cushing's disease, and specific care must be taken to avoid corneal injury, particularly during head and neck surgery. Osteoporotic vertebral collapse may render regional analgesia more difficult and patient handling and positioning more hazardous. Atrophic skin is easily damaged, particularly at pressure points, when applying traction or when removing adhesive tape. Peripheral veins are often small and friable so that peripheral venous access can be difficult to establish and carries a high risk of subsequent extravasation. Although central venous cannulation may appear advantageous, this can be hampered by cervical obesity and supraclavicular fat pads and complicated by an increased risk of blood-borne infection, necessitating placement under ultrasound guidance [9] and strict adherence to asepsis during catheter placement and use [10].

Over 80% of patients with Cushing's disease have systemic hypertension, which may often be refractory to standard treatment. A variety of explanations for cortisol-mediated hypertension have been proposed, including increased cardiac output [11], increased hepatic production of angiotensinogen [12], increased sensitivity to endogenous and exogenous vasopressors [13], reduced levels of vasodilating prostaglandins, and increased Na+ influx into vascular smooth muscle [14]. However, more recent evidence points to cortisol-mediated activation of the mineralocorticoid receptor. Thus, whilst under normal circumstances 11β-hydroxysteroid dehydrogenase type 2 converts cortisol to the inactive cortisone, high levels of cortisol saturate its capacity, allowing cortisol to activate the mineralocorticoid receptor [15]. Long-standing Cushing's disease is associated with eccentric left ventricular hypertrophy and diastolic ventricular failure, changes that usually regress after successful treatment. Haemodynamic instability at the time of induction should be pre-empted, and it may be invaluable to establish invasive intra-arterial pressure monitoring under local anaesthesia beforehand. There is a significantly higher risk of perioperative venous thromboembolic disease, and appropriate antithromboembolic measures must be applied rigorously.

Patients with Cushing's disease should be assumed to have potential airway and respiratory difficulties perioperatively, due to obesity, musculoskeletal changes and an increased incidence of obstructive sleep apnoea (see Acromegaly section below) [16]. A large 'buffalo hump' may interfere with supine positioning on the operating table and impede both airway management and surgical access. Respiratory function may be further impaired in the postoperative period, particularly in patients with proximal muscle wasting, and it is sensible to care for these patients in a high dependency or intensive care environment in the immediate postoperative period. Glucose intolerance is seen in almost two thirds of patients with Cushing's disease, half of whom will have frank diabetes mellitus that will require appropriate perioperative management (Chapter 9). Particular care will be needed in the postoperative period for patients undergoing potentially curative resection of ACTH-secreting tumours, since glucose intolerance may resolve rapidly. In view of the increased incidence of peptic ulceration, it is probably best to avoid non-steroidal anti-inflammatory drugs in this group of patients.

Acromegaly

Acromegaly, derived from the Greek *acron* (extremity) and *megale* (great), is a chronic, progressive, multisystem disease caused by an excess of GH. It almost always results from the hypersecretion of GH from a functioning somatrophic pituitary adenoma, although on rare occasions it can be due to ectopic secretion of GHRH, usually from carcinoid tumours. Growth hormone has widespread anabolic properties on all organs and tissues other than the brain, specifically stimulating the differentiation of bone growth and muscle cells. It promotes lipolysis, increases free fatty acid levels and impairs glucose utilisation and cellular sensitivity to insulin. The effects of GH are mediated largely by the somatomedins, most notably insulin-like growth factor-1 (IGF-1, somatomedin C), which are synthesised in the liver in response to GH.

Although acromegaly can on rare occasions develop prior to puberty and epiphyseal fusion (thereby causing acromegalic gigantism), it is more commonly a disease of middle age. The outward appearances of advanced acromegaly are characteristic, but changes develop so slowly that the patient is usually unaware of their significance. The disease is therefore characteristically well advanced at the time of diagnosis – indeed it has been estimated that the mean time from onset to presentation is over eight years. Tumours are

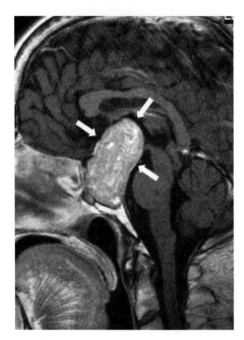

Fig. 1.4 Sagittal MRI image of pituitary macroadenoma (arrowed).

typically macroadenomas (Figure 1.4), and as a consequence patients display not only the specific features of acromegaly but also the visual impairment and endocrine hyposecretion that accompany a pituitary mass lesion. Acromegaly presents the anaesthetist with challenges that are both considerable and varied (Table 1.3). Although attention inevitably focuses upon potentially life-threatening cardiorespiratory complications of the disease, due regard should also be given to some of its more practical problems.

If left untreated, acromegaly is associated with a significant reduction in life expectancy, with the cause of death usually attributable to the cardiovascular complications of the disease [17]. Hypertension occurs in up 40% of acromegalic individuals [18], can be refractory to standard therapy, and on very rare occasions is the result of coexisting phaeochromocytoma or Cushing's disease. However, left ventricular hypertrophy is also seen in 50% of normotensive acromegalics [19], and is associated with an increase in stroke volume and cardiac output. Diastolic ventricular failure is the principal feature of acromegalic cardiomyopathy, and may be the result of interstitial myocardial fibrosis [20]. Systolic function is generally well preserved, although it may be compromised by (small vessel) coronary artery disease. Resolution of some of these cardiovascular features of acromegaly can be anticipated following successful

medical or surgical therapy, although diastolic dysfunction may remain [21].

The acromegalic presents three interrelated potential airway problems – a possibly difficult airway/intubation on induction, sleep apnoea and an increased risk of mechanical airway obstruction in the postoperative period. It is widely recognised that laryngoscopy and tracheal intubation may be more difficult in the acromegalic, this being attributed to a combination of macrognathia, macroglossia and expansion of the soft tissues of the pharynx, larynx and tracheal mucosa. Historically, many have advocated elective tracheostomy, although this rarely seems to be necessary in current practice [22]. Nevertheless, airway problems on the induction of anaesthesia must always be anticipated and planned for. For instance, Schmitt et al. demonstrated that as many as 20% of acromegalic patients assessed as Mallampati class 1 and 2 preoperatively were difficult to intubate [23], whilst Hakala et al. showed that oral fibreoptic intubation following induction of anaesthesia may be just as difficult as direct laryngoscopy [24]. Reassuringly, both these and other studies have revealed that airway maintenance and manual 'bag and mask' ventilation is usually straightforward, and that endotracheal intubation is achievable with standard techniques such as external laryngeal pressure and the use of a gum elastic bougie or airway exchange catheter [25]. Soft tissue enlargement may mean that insertion of bulky devices such as the intubating laryngeal mask airway is difficult [26], whilst experience with disposable optical devices such as the Airtraq® is inevitably limited. Awake fibreoptic intubation is increasingly regarded as the favoured solution for difficult intubation in the acromegalic patient, although whether this should be restricted to those where problems might be anticipated (for instance in patients with obstructive sleep apnoea, poor Mallampati grade or other risk factors) or be the standard approach remains to be defined. Whatever technique is chosen, a full range of airway and intubation equipment must be available, including the means to urgently restore oxygenation via trans-tracheal insufflation. Furthermore, although laryngeal visualisation is widely recognised as the principal obstacle to tracheal intubation, soft tissue infiltration of the tracheal mucosa, and the consequent airway narrowing, may impede the passage of a tracheal tube and increase the risk of postoperative stridor and life-threatening airway obstruction. Finally, whilst attention has focused on airway issues at the induction of anaesthesia, these very same issues may have similar

Table 1.3 Clinical features of acromegaly.

Type	Clinical features
Dermatological	Thickening of skin Profuse perspiration Seborrhoea Acne vulgaris and suppurative hydradenitis Hirsuitism
Musculoskeletal	Acral enlargement (increased glove and shoe size) Arthralgia (increasing cartilage width), progressing to extensive and crippling osteoarthritis Hyperostosis frontalis Macrognathia, prognathism and malocclusion Temporo-mandibular joint dysfunction Cervical spondylosis, kyphoscoliosis Proximal myopathy
Respiratory	Deepening of voice (vocal cord infiltration and expansion of bony air sinuses) Macroglossia Soft tissue infiltration of the pharyngo-larynx Sleep apnoea (both central and obstructive) and consequent respiratory failure Increased lung volumes
Cardiovascular	Hypertension and eccentric left ventricular hypertrophy Ischaemic heart disease Arrhythmias and heart block Cardiomyopathy Bi-ventricular failure
Metabolic	Glucose intolerance and diabetes mellitus Hypercalcuria (secondary to increased gastrointestinal absorption) and renal calculi Hypertriglyceridaemia Goitre and hyperthyroidism Multiple endocrine neoplasia syndrome, type I (parathyroid, pancreas, adrenal tumours) Hyperprolactinaemia, hypogonadism, adrenocortical insufficiency and hypothyroidism (secondary to pituitary mass effect)
Neurological	Lethargy (possibly as a feature of obstructive sleep apnoea and sleep fragmentation) Nerve entrapment syndromes (e.g., carpal tunnel syndrome) Lumbar radiculopathy and spinal stenosis Headache, visual failure and cranial nerve palsies (secondary to pituitary mass effect)

if not greater significance for postoperative care. Thus, significant sleep apnoea is reported to occur in as many as 70% of acromegalic patients, is usually of the obstructive type and is thought to be the result of soft tissue enlargement of the upper airway tissues [27, 28]. The perioperative implications of sleep apnoea for the acromegalic have been well described [29] and deterioration in airway control must be anticipated. Respiratory function may be further exacerbated by kyphoscoliosis and a proximal myopathy.

Preoperative evaluation should include a thorough cardiorespiratory and endocrine assessment; particular attention must be paid to assessment of the airway. It must be emphasised that many of the clinical complications of acromegaly may persist after apparently successful medical or surgical treatment for the condition. Specific enquiry should be made regarding sleep apnoea, since this may indicate patients in whom airway difficulties, cardiac instability and postoperative cardiorespiratory failure is most likely [30]. Features of significant obstructive sleep apnoea include crescendo snoring, choking and apnoeic episodes during sleep, restless and unrefreshed sleep, nocturia, daytime somnolence, poor concentration and memory loss. Polycythaemia and carbon dioxide retention are suggestive of clinically advanced sleep apnoea that will invariably be accompanied by fluid retention, pulmonary hypertension and right-sided heart failure. Preoperative transthoracic echocardiography assesses not only left ventricular size and performance, but also estimates pulmonary pressures. Although the anaesthetic technique is dominated by management of the airway, other implications of acromegaly must also be considered. Haemodynamic instability should be expected, particularly in those patients with hypertension or cardiomyopathy and the anaesthetic management modified accordingly. Careful attention should be paid to positioning – nerve entrapment syndromes may be exacerbated by inadequate attention to potential pressure areas, arthritic problems may be unnecessarily worsened postoperatively and the standard operating table may need extending for the acromegalic giant. Postoperative care for the acromegalic patient should be provided initially in a high dependency or intensive care setting, particularly in patients with established sleep apnoea who will require opioid analgesia. Nasal continuous positive airway pressure (CPAP) is contraindicated in patients who have recently undergone trans-sphenoidal surgery (because of the risk of tension pneumocephalus), and it is this group of patients, together with those with tracheal mucosal infiltration and narrowing, who may benefit from a planned temporary tracheostomy.

Patients with acromegaly have a higher incidence of surgical pathologies such as osteoarthritis of large joints, goitre and malignant tumours of the large bowel. The anaesthetist will occasionally encounter a patient in whom the diagnosis is suspected but not confirmed. While under many circumstances it may be possible to delay surgery for an endocrine diagnosis to be made and an appropriate treatment strategy established, there will be other occasions where clinical urgency dictates that surgical intervention, for instance the resection of an obstructing adenocarcinoma of the large bowel, must take precedence. In such situations, the principal risks to the patient include those specific to acromegaly as described above, but also pituitary apoplexy (see below), postoperative adrenocortical (and thyroid) insufficiency and worsened hydrocephalus from unsuspected obstruction of the third ventricle. A CT (or preferably an MRI) head scan will be useful in both confirming the presence of a pituitary macroadenoma and also to exclude obstructive hydrocephalus. Blood should be taken for baseline endocrine investigations (including GH, IGF-1, prolactin, thyroid function and cortisol), and the integrity or otherwise of the visual fields established. In circumstances where the surgery must proceed, it is recommended that, unless the surgery is life saving, patients with objective evidence of untreated acromegaly are best transferred to a hospital able to provide neurosurgical and neuroendocrine surveillance in the postoperative period. As a minimum, it is recommended that the patient receive perioperative hydrocortisone replacement therapy, that scrupulous

attention is given to the correction of perioperative hypovolaemia, haemodynamic instability and coagulopathy, that the patient is monitored in an environment where sleep-related disorders of airway control can be managed and that any postoperative headache or impairment of conscious level be investigated with an urgent CT head scan.

Pituitary apoplexy

The term pituitary apoplexy refers to the acute presentation of a rapidly expanding pituitary lesion, in which insults such as hypotension, shock or coagulopathy precipitate haemorrhagic infarction of a gland whose blood supply is already jeopardised by tumour or pregnancy [31]. The result is acute failure of anterior lobe function (that of the posterior lobe is usually preserved), and similarly rapid evolution of a pituitary mass lesion. Causes include major surgery (particularly when complicated by hypotension and haemostatic failure) and specifically coronary artery surgery, head trauma, sickle cell crisis, blood dyscrasias, spinal anaesthesia and obstetric haemorrhage (Sheehan's syndrome). The principal clinical features are severe headache (that is frequently mistaken for subarachnoid haemorrhage), nausea and vomiting, acute visual disturbance (particularly diplopia and ocular paresis, but also loss of visual acuity and impairment of the visual fields), ptosis and confusion, and in the parturient, failure of lactation. Successful management requires a strong index of suspicion, management of adrenocortical failure with 0.9% sodium chloride i.v. and hydrocortisone replacement and referral to the local neurosurgical unit for urgent trans-sphenoidal decompression. The short Synacthen test is unreliable in these circumstances since the adrenal cortex remains responsive to exogenous stimulation for some weeks after endogenous ACTH secretion has been lost.

Management of patients undergoing trans-sphenoidal resection of a pituitary adenoma

Not all pituitary tumours are adenomas, and not all pituitary adenomas require surgical treatment – for instance, many prolactinomas and some tumours of the somatotroph can be treated medically, whilst small, non-functioning tumours may require nothing other than surveillance. Indications for surgery include relief of mass effect, correction of endocrine hypersecretory syndromes, such as Cushing's disease, acromegaly and very rarely thyrotoxicosis of pituitary origin, and the pursuit of a tissue diagnosis. There are two principal surgical approaches to the pituitary gland – the extracranial route which gains access to the pituitary fossa via the sphenoid air sinuses, and the transcranial approach which requires a craniotomy. In centres equipped with operating microscopes and video fluoroscopy over 95% of surgical resections of pituitary adenomas are now performed trans-sphenoidally, with transcranial resection being reserved for occasions in which the trans-sphenoidal approach has failed, when the tissue diagnosis of a suprasellar tumour is in some doubt or when there is little or no intrasellar component to the tumour.

The trans-sphenoidal approach confers a number of potential advantages to both patient and clinician. Surgical trauma and blood loss are usually minimal, and the procedure is generally well tolerated. The approach offers direct visualisation of the gland that can be difficult to achieve transcranially, and avoids the generic hazards of a craniotomy. Complications of trans-sphenoidal surgery include persistent cerebrospinal fluid (CSF) rhinorrhoea and the associated risk of postoperative meningitis, and many units advocate the administration of prophylactic antibiotics directed against common nasopharyngeal commensal organisms. Although panhypopituitarism is a rare complication, some disruption of anterior lobe function should be anticipated, and many units initiate perioperative hydrocortisone replacement therapy until such time as the integrity of the hypothalamo-pituitary-adrenal axis can be confirmed. Transient DI may be seen in as many as 50% of patients, although recovery can be expected in the majority. Haemorrhage resulting from injury to the cavernous sinus, or to the carotid artery that lies therein, is uncommon but can be difficult to control and so is on occasion life threatening. Injury to one or more of the cranial nerves associated with the sinus leads to predictable neurological impairment, although this is rare and usually transient. Cerebral ischaemia and stroke may develop as a result of vasospasm, thromboembolism or compression from surgical packs introduced to control haemorrhage.

Uncomplicated trans-sphenoidal surgery represents minimal physiological disruption and is generally well tolerated. However, the patient may present with advanced endocrine disease combined with an intracranial mass lesion, and for these reasons, as well as in anticipation of the potential complications of surgery, patients should be approached and prepared as if they were undergoing transcranial surgery. Preoperative assessment has a number of specific objectives. The extent and functional consequence of a pituitary mass lesion should be evaluated and particular note should be made of any visual field defect or hydrocephalus. The nature of any endocrine dysfunction should be defined and a deliberate enquiry of the relevant complications of any endocrine disorder thoroughly pursued. (Although attention inevitably focuses on the anaesthetic implications of acromegaly and Cushing's disease, due consideration should also be given to the possibility of multiple endocrine neoplasia syndromes, as well as adrenal and thyroid insufficiency.) Current medical therapy should be reviewed, and hormonal and antihypertensive therapy should be continued. Where necessary, patients should be counselled regarding awake intubation and invasive monitoring, and warned of the postoperative nasal obstruction caused by the use of nasal packs and reassured accordingly. Sedative premedication should be modest and care taken to avoid respiratory depression particularly in patients with suspected sleep apnoea or hydrocephalus.

Trans-sphenoidal surgery places a number of demands upon the anaesthetic technique. Inevitably, reliance will be placed upon the anaesthetist to administer prophylactic antibiotics and intravenous hydrocortisone replacement therapy. If difficulties in access to suprasellar components of a tumour are anticipated, the anaesthetist may be asked to insert a lumbar intrathecal catheter (this to allow intraoperative injection of air or saline to promote descent of the tumour into the operative field of view). Access to the airway is shared with the surgeon, and further restricted by an operating microscope, portable X-ray imaging arms and display monitors, together with instrument trolleys and various personnel. The choice and positioning of the endotracheal tube should minimise any interference with surgical access, and many centres use preformed RAE or flexible armoured tubes to avoid the need for angle pieces and catheter mounts. The oropharynx should be packed with saline-soaked gauze to stabilise the tracheal tube and prevent the accumulation of blood and other secretions in the pharynx and stomach. Although various surgical approaches are described, those that involve fracture of the bony nasal septum can be associated with considerable swings in blood pressure that may result in troublesome haemorrhage into both the surgical field and the upper airway.

To combat this, neuroanaesthetists frequently apply a topical vasoconstricting/local anaesthetic solution to the nasal mucosa, although systemic analgesic supplements, and less commonly specific hypotensive agents such as labetalol or hydrallazine, may be required. Both the delivery of intravenous fluids and drugs, and non-invasive blood pressure measurements may be repeatedly interrupted by a surgeon leaning forwards and across a patient's torso towards the operating microscope, and wherever possible vascular cannulae should be sited away from the surgical approach. Many neuroanaesthetists will choose to use invasive arterial pressure monitoring in these circumstances. Emergence from anaesthesia should be both smooth and rapid to enable a clinical neurological examination as soon as possible in the recovery room. An anaesthetic technique based upon a combination of sevoflurane, remifentanil and a short-acting muscle relaxant has considerable merit in this regard; intravenous morphine is frequently required in the recovery room.

Although the specific implications of Cushing's disease or acromegaly for postoperative care have been discussed elsewhere, all patients should be considered to be at risk of potential airway difficulties and therefore monitored in an appropriately nursed and equipped environment. Patients often feel more comfortable sat up, and should be nursed therefore on a bed or trolley that allows the sitting position to be achieved easily and safely (both for patients and staff). Oxygen therapy via a facemask should be provided for the first postoperative night, and all patients receive intravenous 0.9% sodium chloride solution until they are able to take oral fluids adequately. Postoperative neurological observations should match the potential for complications, including visual function (direct injury to the optic pathways, chiasmal prolapse), pupillary light reflex and eye movement (cranial nerve injury) and regular estimation of conscious level as measured by the Glasgow Coma Scale (postoperative intracranial haematoma, hydrocephalus, cerebral vasospasm and other forms of arterial injury). Staff should be alert to the potential for DI (suggested when the patient continues to pass large quantities of urine of inappropriately low osmolality/sodium concentration despite an elevated plasma osmolality/sodium concentration). Furthermore, although an Addisonian crisis is unlikely in patients receiving perioperative hydrocortisone replacement the possibility should nevertheless be considered in a patient with unexplained hypotension or shock, particularly if it is accompanied by hyponatraemia and hypoglycaemia.

References

1. Guyton AC, Hall JE. The pituitary hormones and their control by the hypothalamus. In *Textbook of Medical Physiology*, 11th edn. LosAltos, CA, Lange Medical Publications, 2005, pp. 846–56.

2. Murphy PG. Anaesthesia for pituitary surgery. *Baillières Clin Anaesthesiol* 1999; **13**(4): 575–91.

3. Burrow GN, Wortzman G, Rowcastle NB, et al. Microadenomas of the pituitary and abnormal sellar tomograms in an unselected autopsy series. *N Engl J Med* 1987; **304**: 156–8.

4. Thapar K, Koracs K, Muller PJ. Clinical-pathological correlations of pituitary tumours. *Baillières Clin Endocrinol Metab* 1995; **9**: 243–70.

5. Hennessey JV, Jackson IMD. Clinical features and differential diagnosis of pituitary tumours with emphasis on acromegaly. *Baillières Clin Endocrinol Metab* 1995; **9**: 271–314.

6. Abboud CF. Anterior pituitary failure. In Melmed S. ed. *The Pituitary*, 2nd edn. Oxford, Blackwell Publishing, 2002, pp. 349–404.

7. Ozkan Y, Colak R. Sheehan syndrome: clinical and laboratory evaluation of 20 cases. *Neuro Endocrinol Lett* 2005; **26**: 257–60.

8. Overton CE, Davis CJ, West C, et al. High risk pregnancies in hypopituitary women. *Hum Reprod* 2002; **17**: 1464–7

9. Bodenham AR. Ultrasound imaging by anaesthetists: training and accreditation issues. *Br J Anaesth* 2006; **96**: 414–17.

10. Berenholtz SM, Pronovost PJ, Lipsett PA, et al. Eliminating catheter-related bloodstream infections in the intensive care unit. *Crit Care Med* 2004; **32**: 2014–20.

11. Pirpiris M, Young S, Dewar E, et al. Hydrocortisone-induced hypertension in men: the role of cardiac output. *Am J Hypertens* 1993; **6**: 287–94.

12. Mantereo F, Boscaro M. Glucocorticoid-dependent hypertension. *J Steroid Biochem Mol Biol* 1992; **43**: 409–13.

13. Keegan MT, Atkinison JL, Kasperbauer JL, Lanier WL. Exaggerated hemodynamic responses to nasal injection and awakening from anesthesia in a Cushingoid patient having transsphenoidal hypophysectomy. *J Neurosurg Anesthesiol* 2000; **12**: 225–9.

14. Kornel L, Manisundaram B, Nelson WA. Glucocorticioids regulate Na^+ transport in vascular smooth muscle through the glucocorticoid receptor mediated mechanism. *Am J Hypertens* 1993; **6**: 736–44.

15. Hammer F, Stewart PM. Cortisol metabolism in hypertension. *Best Pract Res Clin Endocrinol Metab* 2006; **20**: 337–53.

16. Nemergut EC, Dumont AS, Barry UT, Laws ER. Perioperative management of patients undergoing transsphenoidal pituitary surgery. *Anesth Analg* 2005; **101**: 1170–81.

17. Coloa A, Marzullo P, Di Somma C, Lombardi G. Growth hormone and the heart. *Clin Endocrinol (Oxf)* 2001; **54**: 137–54.

18. Lopez-Velasco R, Escobar-Morreale HF, Vega B , et al. Cardiac involvement in acromegaly: specific myocardiopathy or consequence of systemic hypertension. *J Clin Endocrinol Metab* 1997; **82**: 1047–53.

19. Ciulla M, Arosio M, Barelli MV, et al. Blood pressure-independent cardiac hypertrophy in acromegalic patients. *J Hypertens* 1999; **17**: 1965–9.

20. Herrmann BL, Bruch C, Saller B, et al. Acromegaly: evidence for a direct relation between disease activity and cardiac dysfunction in patients without ventricular hypertrophy. *Clin Endocrinol (Oxf)* 2002; **56**: 595–602.

21. Rossi E, Zuppi P, Pennestri F, et al. Acromegalic cardiomyopathy: left ventricular filling and hypertrophy in active and surgically treated disease. *Chest* 1992; **102**: 1204–8.

22. Ovaasapian A, Doka JC, Romsa DE. Acromegaly: use of fibreoptic laryngoscopy to avoid tracheostomy. *Anesthesiology* 1981; **54**: 429–30.

23. Schmitt H, Buchfelder M, Radespiel-Troger M, Fahlsbusch R. Difficult intubation in acromegalic patients. *Anesthesiology* 2000; **93**: 110–14.

24. Hakala P, Randell T, Valli H. Laryngoscopy and fibreoptic intubation in acromegalic patients. *Br J Anaesth* 1998; **80**: 345–7.

25. Nemergut EC, Zuo Z. Airway management in patients with pituitary disease. *J Neurosurg Anesthesiol* 2006; **18**: 73–7.

26. Law-Kourne J, Liu N, Szekelly B, Fischler M. Using the intubating laryngeal mask airway for ventilation and endotracheal intubation in anesthetized and unparalysed acromegalic patients. *J Neurosurg Anesthesiol* 2004; **16**: 11–13.

27. Fatti LM, Scacchi M, Pincelli AI, et al. Prevelance and pathogenesis of sleep apnea and lung disease in acromegaly. *Pituitary* 2001; **4**: 259–62.

28. Perks WH, Horrocks PM, Cooper RA, et al. Sleep apnoea in acromegaly. *Br Med J* 1980; **280**: 894–7.

29. Piper JG, Dirks BA, Traynelis VC, VanGilder JC. Perioperative management of and surgical outcome in the acromegalic patient with sleep apnea. *Neurosurgery* 1995; **36**: 70–4.

30. Loadsman JA, Hillman DR. Anaesthesia and sleep apnoea. *Br J Anaesth* 2001; **86**: 254–66.

31. Embil JM, Kramer M, Kinnear S, Light RB. A blinding headache. *Lancet* 1997; **350**: 182.

32. Cobb WE, Jackson IMD. *Emergency Medicine*. Boston, Little, Brown & Co., 1992.

33. Albin MS. *Textbook of Neuroanaesthesia with Neurosurgical and Neuroscience Persepctives*. New York, McGraw-Hill Co., 1997, p. 153.

Chapter

2

Thyroid disease

Peter A. Farling

Introduction

Many patients who require anaesthesia will have coincidental disease of their thyroid gland. The majority of these cases will not present any problems to the anaesthetist or to the patient; however, a small number will exhibit significant difficulties. These difficulties may be due either to the nature of the goitre or, more rarely, to a severe metabolic upset. The anaesthetist should be able to deal with acute airway complications throughout the perioperative phase [1]. This chapter will review thyroid physiology and the anaesthetic management of patients with disease of the thyroid.

Anatomy

The butterfly-shaped thyroid gland is situated in the anterior region of the neck just deep to the strap muscles at the level of the C5 to T1 vertebrae [2]. It normally weighs 10–20 g and is responsible for secreting hormones that control metabolism throughout the body (Figure 2.1).

The thyroid originates from the floor of the pharynx and descends from the foramen caecum, at the base of the tongue, through the thyroglossal duct to its normal position in the neck. Thyroglossal cysts may result if the thyroglossal duct fails to degenerate. An isthmus connects the two lobes and 50% of people have a pyramidal lobe in front of the larynx. There is an abundant blood supply from the superior and inferior thyroid arteries and occasionally the thyroidea ima. These arise from the external carotid artery, the thyrocervical trunk of the subclavian artery and the arch of the aorta respectively. They provide the gland with one of the highest rates of blood flow per gram of tissue, 5 ml min^{-1} g^{-1}. The superior thyroid artery is adjacent to the external laryngeal nerve that supplies the cricothyroid muscle. Ligation of the artery may damage the external laryngeal nerve resulting in dysphonia. The inferior thyroid artery is closely associated with the recurrent laryngeal nerve although the relationship is highly variable. Damage of the recurrent laryngeal nerve will lead to paralysis of the ipsilateral vocal cord.

Physiology

The structural units of the thyroid gland consist of round follicles, or acini, filled with colloid and surrounded by a single layer of epithelial thyroid cells [3]. Thyroxine (T_4) and triiodothyronine (T_3) are synthesised within the colloid by iodination and condensation of tyrosine molecules from thyroglobulin. This glycoprotein is synthesised in the thyroid cells and secreted into the colloid. Iodide is transported actively from the plasma by the thyroid cells and oxidised to iodine by thyroid peroxidase. Iodine is bound to the tyrosine molecule at position three to form mono-iodotyrosine (MIT) which is then iodinated at position five to form diiodotyrosine (DIT). A coupling reaction occurs and two DIT molecules combine to form T_4 with the release of alanine. Triiodothyronine is probably formed by the condensation of MIT and DIT. Lysosomal proteases within the thyroid cells remove thyroid hormones from thyroglobulin and these are secreted into the blood (Figure 2.2).

Approximately 100 nmol of T_4 and 10 nmol of T_3 are secreted by the thyroid gland per day. Plasma proteins bind thyroid hormones and the normal total plasma T_4 is 103 nmol l^{-1}.

Thyroid function is controlled by fluctuations in the amount of thyroid stimulating hormone (TSH) in the blood. Thyroid stimulating hormone is released from the anterior pituitary and is itself controlled by the hypophysiotropic hormone, thyrotropin releasing hormone (TRH). Thyroid stimulating hormone is inhibited by the negative feedback effect of circulating T_4 and T_3. Somatostatin also inhibits the release of

Core Topics in Endocrinology in Anaesthesia and Critical Care, eds. George M. Hall, Jennifer M. Hunter and Mark S. Cooper. Published by Cambridge University Press. © Cambridge University Press 2010.

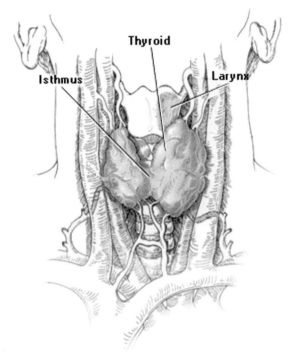

Fig. 2.1 Anatomy of the thyroid gland. From Standring [2] with permission.

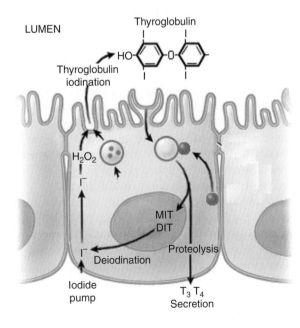

Fig. 2.2 The thyroid cell and synthesis of thyroid hormones. DIT, diiodotyrosine; MIT, monoiodotyrosine.

TSH. Thyroid stimulating hormone stimulates thyroid function by increasing iodide binding and increasing synthesis of iodotyrosines, T_3, T_4 and thyroglobulin.

Thyroid hormones stimulate O_2 consumption, affect growth, regulate lipid metabolism and increase the absorption of carbohydrates from the gut. Thyroxine and T_3 bind to thyroid receptors in the nuclei of cells and this hormone receptor complex causes alterations in the expression of enzymes that regulate cell function, hence the widespread physiological effects of thyroid hormones.

The parafollicular or C (clear) cells of the thyroid gland produce calcitonin, a linear polypeptide hormone, that reduces blood calcium by opposing the effects of parathyroid hormone (PTH) (Chapter 3). Increased levels of calcitonin are found in medullary thyroid carcinoma.

Chapter 17 provides a detailed account of thyroid physiology in relation to critical care patients.

Hypothyroidism

The term 'myxoedema' was first used in 1877 by William Miller Ord [4]. The signs and symptoms of hypothyroidism are predictable consequences of the physiological effects of the lack of thyroid hormones. Iodine 150 μg is the minimal daily intake that is required for normal thyroid function in adults and the incidence of hypothyroidism depends upon the amount of iodine in the diet. The prevalence of hypothyroidism in iodine-sufficient areas is 5:1000 for overt and 15:1000 for the subclinical form [5]. While iodine deficiency remains the most common cause of hypothyroidism globally, it is rare in the developed world. Autoimmune thyroiditis, the commonest cause in the developed world, occurs when an unknown trigger stimulates the immune system to produce autoantibodies that reduce T_4 production. Hypothyroidism may result from treatment of hyperthyroidism or thyroid cancers, e.g., radioiodine therapy. Drugs such as lithium, amiodarone and interferon may also induce hypothyroidism. Underactivity of the pituitary gland (Chapter 1) may result in reduced levels of TSH and hence hypothyroidism. In the developed world, congenital hypothyroidism is usually detected during the neonatal screening process.

Hypothyroidism results in depression of myocardial function, decreased spontaneous ventilation, abnormal baroreceptor function, reduced plasma volume, anaemia, hypoglycaemia, hyponatraemia and impaired hepatic drug metabolism. Psychiatric presentations include cognitive dysfunction, affective disorders and psychosis. Hypothyroid patients should be rendered euthyroid before elective surgery and close communication with the metabolic physicians is advised.

Levothyroxine sodium is the treatment of choice for maintenance therapy. The adult dose is 50–100 µg once daily adjusted in increments of 25–50 µg according to response. The half-life of T_4 is seven days and so its effect will not be immediately apparent. The half life of T_3 is only 1.5 days. As T_3 sodium has a more rapid effect than levothyroxine, it is used in severe hypothyroid states when a rapid response is required. Triiodothyronine 20 µg is equivalent to levothyroxine 100 µg. The decision whether or not to postpone surgery in a patient with hypothyroidism will depend on a number of factors, not least the urgency of the procedure. Pre-assessment clinics should detect clinical or poorly controlled hypothyroidism and T_4 treatment should be optimised prior to elective surgery. There is no evidence to suggest that surgery should be delayed for patients with sub-clinical hypothyroidism.

It is logical to avoid premedication in hypothyroid patients and to employ regional anaesthesia wherever possible. Thyroxine may be omitted on the morning of surgery but it is advisable to give the patient's usual morning dose of T_3. Careful perioperative cardiovascular monitoring and judicious use of anaesthetic drugs due to the hypometabolic state is essential.

Preventative measures should be adopted to protect against hypothermia. Due to an increased incidence of adrenocortical insufficiency and a reduced adrenocorticotropic hormone response to stress, it has been recommended that hypothyroid patients should receive hydrocortisone cover during periods of increased surgical stress [6].

Hashimoto's disease

First described in 1912 by a Japanese physician, this was the first autoimmune disease to be recognised. Antibodies against thyroid peroxidase and thyroglobulin produce inflammation, a reduction in follicular cells and hence hypothyroidism. Goitre may arise and there is an occasional association with non-Hodgkin's lymphoma.

Myxoedema coma

A number of events may precipitate decompensation in an unsuspected or poorly treated hypothyroid patient. These include infection, trauma and cardiorespiratory failure. The combination of intravenous T_3 and T_4 is recommended in the management of preoperative myxoedematous coma. Careful administration is essential, particularly in the elderly, as angina may

be precipitated [7]. The intensive care management of myxoedematous coma is discussed in Chapter 17.

Hyperthyroidism

Thyrotoxicosis affects approximately 2% of women and 0.2% of men in the general population. The prevalence of hyperthyroidism in iodine-sufficient areas is 2:1000 for overt and 6:1000 for sub-clinical hyperthyroidism [5]. Pre-assessment clinics should detect clinical or poorly controlled hyperthyroidism and antithyroid treatment should be optimised prior to elective surgery. There is no evidence to suggest that surgery should be delayed for patients with sub-clinical hyperthyroidism. Cases have been reported where unexplained tachycardia during anaesthesia has subsequently been shown to be due to sub-clinical hyperthyroidism [8].

The causes of hyperthyroidism include the autoimmune condition Graves' disease, toxic nodular goitre, thyroiditis and drug-induced hyperthyroidism, for example, during amiodarone therapy (Table 17.2).

Graves' disease

First described in 1835 by an Irish doctor, Robert James Graves, this is the combination of a diffuse goitre, hyperthyroidism and eye signs. A German, von Basedow, independently described the same combination of symptoms and so in Europe the term Basedow's disease may be more common [4].

The classical features of thyrotoxicosis include heat intolerance, hyperactivity, weight loss, tremor and eye signs. Of importance to the anaesthetist are the cardiovascular effects of hyperthyroidism including atrial fibrillation, congestive cardiac failure and ischaemic heart disease. Thrombocytopaenia may be associated with thyrotoxicosis. In an attempt to prevent the dreaded complication of 'thyroid storm', patients should be rendered euthyroid prior to surgery [9]. This is achieved by the use of antithyroid drugs.

Carbimazole is the commonest antithyroid drug used in the UK. It is converted to methimazole after absorption from the small intestine and it decreases the uptake and concentration of iodine by the thyroid. It reduces the formation of DIT, and hence T_3 and T_4, by preventing the peroxidase enzyme from coupling and iodinating the tyrosine residues on thyroglobulin. The dose of carbimazole in adults is 15–40 mg daily until the patient is rendered euthyroid. After 4–8 weeks, this is reduced to a maintenance dose of 5–15 mg.

Propylthiouracil may be used when patients suffer reactions to carbimazole, which are not infrequent. It also inhibits thyroperoxidase but, in addition, blocks

5'-deiodinase, which converts T_4 to T_3. The initial dose of propylthiouracil in adults is 200–400 mg daily and the maintenance dose is 50–150 mg. Side effects of carbimazole and propylthiouracil include rashes and pruritis that are usually treated by antihistamines. Nausea, headache, arthralgia, alopecia and jaundice may also occur. Doctors should be aware of the rare complication of bone marrow suppression, leading to agranulocytosis and aplastic anaemia.

Beta-blockers, particularly propranolol, are used to ameliorate the effects of thyrotoxicosis and are effective in the acute preoperative phase. Longer acting beta-blockers such as atenolol may achieve better control of symptoms. While iodine has been used in conjunction with antithyroid drugs and beta-blockers for preoperative preparation to shrink the gland, there is no benefit in using it as a long-term treatment.

The effect of anaesthetic drugs may be altered by the hypermetabolic state of hyperthyroidism. For example, clearance and distribution volumes of propofol are increased in hyperthyroid patients. When total intravenous anaesthesia is used, propofol infusion rates should be increased to reach appropriate anaesthetic blood concentrations.

Thyroid eye disease

Ophthalmopathy associated with hyperthyroidism affects orbital tissues including the extraocular muscles. It is the commonest cause of proptosis in adults and features include diplopia, photophobia and corneal abrasion. Steroids are used to decrease inflammation but surgical decompression may be required to relieve pressure on the optic nerve. Retrobulbar irradiation has been used and current evidence on safety and efficacy support its use when other treatments have failed [10].

General anaesthesia should be considered as the method of choice for patients with exophthalmos requiring eye surgery.

De Quervain's thyroiditis

This painful inflammation of the thyroid usually occurs in females aged 30–50 years. It may develop following a viral illness, an upper respiratory tract infection or post partum. Treatment is with non-steroidal anti-inflammatory drugs or steroids.

Thyroid crisis

The intensive care management of thyroid crisis is discussed in Chapter 17. The hypermetabolic crisis known as 'thyroid storm' is now rarely seen due to the widespread use of beta-blockers and antithyroid drugs, such as carbimazole. However, thyroid crisis still occurs in uncontrolled hyperthyroid patients as a result of a trigger such as surgery, infection or trauma. Supportive management of thyroid crisis includes hydration, cooling and inotropes. Beta blockade, using propranolol or esmolol, and antithyroid drugs are used as the first line of treatment. However, it should be noted that a thyroid crisis has been reported during beta blockade. An acute thyroid crisis on induction of anaesthesia, which was mistakenly diagnosed as malignant hyperthermia, was successfully treated by dantrolene in 1 mg kg^{-1} boluses. Conversely, a case of malignant hyperthermia occurred during subtotal thyroidectomy in a patient with Graves' disease [11]. Since dantrolene is efficacious in thyroid crisis and malignant hyperthermia, immediate intravenous administration of dantrolene should be considered when a hypermetabolic state occurs during anaesthesia for a patient with Graves' disease. As thyroid hormones sensitise the adrenergic receptors to endogenous catecholamines, the stabilising effect of magnesium sulphate may also be considered in the management of thyroid crisis.

Thyroidectomy

Indications

The indications for thyroidectomy include thyroid malignancy, obstructive symptoms, retrosternal goitre, Graves' disease unresponsive to medical treatment, recurrent hyperthyroidism, occasionally Hashimoto's disease and for cosmetic reasons.

Preoperative assessment

General history taking and examination of patients scheduled for thyroidectomy should include identification of abnormalities of thyroid function. As well as symptoms and signs of hypo- and hyperthyroidism, evidence should be sought of other medical conditions, particularly cardiorespiratory disease and associated endocrine disorders. For example, patients who require thyroidectomy for medullary cancer may have an associated phaeochromocytoma (Chapter 4). The social history is important as singers, teachers and other 'voice professionals' should be warned of the risk of postoperative hoarseness. Problems with airway management will be the main concern of the anaesthetist when confronted by a patient with goitre. The patient may give a history of respiratory difficulties, for example positional dyspnoea, and this may be associated with a degree of dysphagia. Patients with retrosternal goitre may exhibit signs of vena caval obstruction. Pemberton's sign [12] is the development of facial cyanosis, distension of neck veins, stridor and elevation of the jugular venous pressure as the patient raises their arms above their head (Figure 2.3). Some patients refuse to perform this manoeuvre as they experience a suffocating feeling due to caval compression.

Routine investigations include thyroid function tests, full blood screen, urea and electrolytes including serum calcium, chest X-ray and indirect laryngoscopy. Patients may also have had fine needle aspiration of their goitre as a diagnostic test in the outpatient clinic. The usefulness of respiratory function tests is debatable. Respiratory flow volume loops may show evidence of upper airway obstruction in patients presenting with thyroid enlargement but this is usually evident during preoperative clinical assessment.

An ear, nose and throat (ENT) colleague routinely performs the indirect laryngoscopy in order to document any preoperative vocal cord dysfunction. This investigation is useful to the anaesthetist. The use of a fibreoptic instrument to view the vocal cords, if indirect laryngoscopy is unsuccessful, will alert the anaesthetist to the probability of a difficult intubation. However, the ability of an ENT surgeon to visualise the larynx does not equate with the ability of an anaesthetist to intubate the trachea.

Imaging

A chest X-ray is requested to seek evidence of tracheal compression and deviation. Lateral thoracic inlet

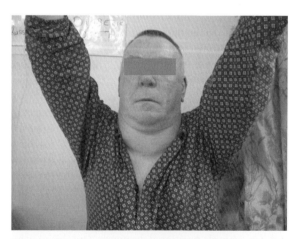

Fig. 2.3 Pemberton's sign – with evidence of significant retrosternal compression.

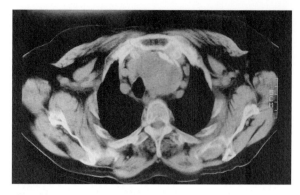

Fig. 2.4 A CT scan of a retrosernal goitre.

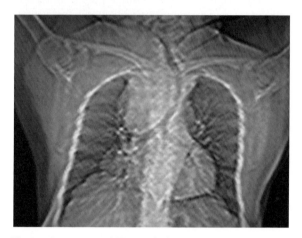

Fig. 2.5 Reconstructed CT scan of a thoracic goitre.

views have traditionally been used to show tracheal compression in the antero-posterior plane.

Other investigations, while not routine, will be of value in certain cases. A CT scan may provide excellent views of retrosternal goitres (Figure 2.4). Reconstructed CT images may improve the information acquired from standard chest X-rays (Figure 2.5).

An MRI scan has the advantage of providing images in the sagittal and coronal planes, as well as transverse views (Figure 2.6).

Helical CT has the ability to reconstruct a 'virtual' airway (Figure 2.7), providing excellent preoperative information [13]. The use of modern imaging techniques for airway assessment will require an assessment of the risk of radiation compared to the potential benefits to the patient. Detailed non-invasive imaging is considered to be valid when it provides information that influences the preoperative decision-making process [14].

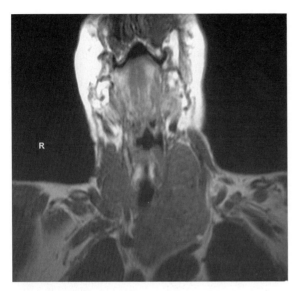

Fig. 2.6 An MRI scan showing enlarged lobe of thyroid.

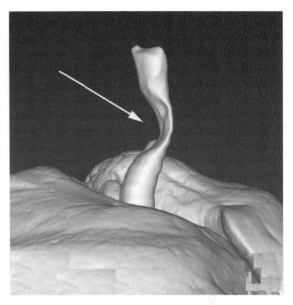

Fig. 2.7 Helical CT virtual airway. Reproduced with kind permission of Assistant Professor Kosaku Toyota.

Following a careful history and examination and with the assistance of a number of investigations, the anaesthetist will be in a position to discuss, with the patient, the various options for airway management. These options will include straightforward intravenous induction with tracheal intubation, inhalational induction or fibreoptic intubation. The patient should be warned what to expect postoperatively and the anxiolytic premedication prescribed.

Anaesthetic technique

Regional anaesthesia

Although thyroidectomy under regional anaesthesia is not routinely practised in the UK, it is possible to perform thyroidectomy under bilateral deep or superficial cervical plexus blocks [15]. There are, however, a number of complications of this technique including vertebral artery puncture, epidural subarachnoid spread and bilateral phrenic nerve block. While regional anaesthesia has been recommended during thyroidectomy for amiodarone-induced hyperthyroidism, there are those who feel that general anaesthesia is just as safe [16].

General anaesthesia

General anaesthesia with tracheal intubation and muscle relaxation is the most popular anaesthetic technique for thyroidectomy. Induction of anaesthesia for a routine thyroidectomy, when no difficulty with intubation is expected, is straightforward. Routine monitoring, including ECG, pulse oximetry and non-invasive blood pressure, is attached to the patient and intravenous access secured. Intravenous induction of anaesthesia is combined with a narcotic analgesic, such as remifentanil, and a non-depolarising muscle relaxant, for example, vecuronium. Oxygen, air and an inhalational anaesthetic, such as sevoflurane, maintain anaesthesia. The increasing utilisation of remifentanil by infusion has reduced the need for nitrous oxide (N_2O). The move away from maintenance of anaesthesia with fentanyl, N_2O and isoflurane has been a result of the quest for a more rapid recovery of patients. Intravenous paracetamol 1 g and morphine 5–10 mg, combined with infiltration of local anaesthetic into the incision by the surgeon, provide postoperative analgesia. Morphine should be given at least 30 minutes before the end of the procedure in order to have a sufficient effect during emergence.

Tracheal intubation

The trachea is usually intubated directly using conventional laryngoscopy. The endotracheal tube should not kink when it attains body temperature during prolonged surgery and so a reinforced tube should be considered. North polar oral endotracheal tubes (Figure 2.8) are an alternative as they keep the respiratory filter away from the surgical field [1]. Nasal endotracheal tubes may also be used, although a vasoconstrictor will be required to prevent epistaxis. It is wise to select a small,

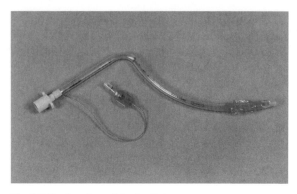

Fig. 2.8 North polar endotracheal tube.

reinforced endotracheal tube if there is any degree of tracheal compression.

The laryngeal mask airway (LMA) has been used with spontaneous respiration and intermittent positive pressure ventilation in thyroid surgery [17]. Contraindications to the use of the LMA include tracheal narrowing and deviation. In order to monitor recurrent laryngeal nerve function, the LMA has been used to facilitate visualisation of vocal cord movement via a fibreoptic laryngoscope [18]. However, there is a risk that the LMA will be displaced during surgery and obstruction may occur due to laryngospasm following surgical manipulation.

Anticipated difficult intubation

If preoperative airway assessment and/or the inability of the ENT surgeon to visualise the cords by indirect laryngoscopy have predicted any difficulty with intubation, then the anaesthetist must have a clear intubation strategy. The anaesthetist should expect that 6% of tracheal intubations for thyroid surgery will be difficult [19]. Whenever there is concern that the airway will be lost if anaesthesia is induced, an awake fibreoptic intubation is the method of choice. This is an example of the overriding philosophy that one must not progress past a point unless it is possible to retrieve the situation. '*Don't burn your bridges*' was taught when, prior to the availability of fibreoptic equipment, inhalation induction was the method of choice. If respiratory obstruction occurred during inhalational induction then the patient should, theoretically, wake up without serious consequences. If inhalational induction was successful then anaesthesia was deepened so that gentle laryngoscopy could be performed prior to the administration of a muscle relaxant. If the larynx was visualised then the muscle relaxant could be given and tracheal intubation performed. However, the possibility to withdraw existed at any point in this strategy. This traditional

technique has regained acceptability due to the introduction of sevoflurane. It can be adopted when the patient is extremely anxious about awake intubation and the anaesthetist believes that the size of the goitre will not cause the airway to be lost after induction of anaesthesia.

Other extreme techniques, such as cardiopulmonary bypass, to manage airway difficulties are mentioned in the Thyroid cancer section, below.

Awake fibreoptic intubation

This may be performed after carefully applying topical anaesthesia to the nose, pharynx and larynx. Cocaine is favoured by some anaesthetists but considered too toxic by others. If lidocaine (lignocaine) is used, a vasoconstrictor should be instilled into the nose to prevent epistaxis.

The nasal route is usually easier than the oral route. This is because the fibrescope is held in the midline and there is a gentler angle to negotiate when approaching the larynx. If the oral route is selected, the gag reflex is a problem when the patient is awake. An antisialogogue is used to reduce secretions. Four per cent topical lidocaine is injected via the laryngoscope when the larynx is visualised. Transtracheal and laryngeal nerve blocks are not easy to perform in patients with large goitres. Small increments of midazolam will make the experience more acceptable and remifentanil has been suggested as a sedative during awake fibreoptic intubation that will reduce the requirement for topical anaesthesia [20]. The dose of remifentanil must be carefully titrated in order to maintain an adequate respiratory rate. With practice, this technique provides ideal conditions; a co-operative patient who is able to tolerate the fibrescope and the lack of irritation to the larynx by local anaesthetic.

Fibreoptic intubation under anaesthesia

Propofol by infusion may be added to the above regimen when fibreoptic intubation is to be performed under anaesthesia. This is indicated when difficult intubation is predicted but the patient prefers to be asleep and the airway is not at risk during induction of anaesthesia. While various connectors make it possible to perform fibreoptic intubation under inhalational anaesthesia, the intravenous technique more effectively prevents pollution. Furthermore, the intravenous technique allows a longer time for the purposes of training.

Unexpected difficult intubation

Occasionally, even though no difficulty has been predicted, the larynx is not easily visualised. The anaesthetic team must be experienced and prepared to cope with the unexpected difficult intubation. Equipment that must be available to deal with such a situation should be in accordance with the recommendations of the Difficult Airway Society [21]. This will include various sizes of endotracheal tubes, gum elastic bougies, an alternative to the Macintosh laryngoscope, usually the McCoy levering laryngoscope, and LMAs. There should be ready access to an intubating fibrescope, some means of transtracheal ventilation, for example a cricothyroid cannula with high-pressure jet ventilation system, and a surgical cricothyroidotomy kit. While the surgeon should be prepared to perform a tracheostomy, even surgical access to the airway will not be an easy option in these extreme circumstances.

The introduction of sugammadex will allow the rapid reversal from any depth of neuromuscular blockade induced by vecuronium or rocuronium, which may prove useful in such circumstances [22].

Positioning the patient

After tracheal intubation, the position of the endotracheal tube is checked, the tube is secured and the patient's eyes are protected. Particular care should be taken when the patient suffers from exophthalmos. The use of head towels prevents the anaesthetist from inspecting the patient's face during the procedure. The patient is positioned with a sandbag below the shoulder blades and the head resting on a padded 'horseshoe'. As the surgeon will need to stand on both sides of the patient during the procedure, the patient's arms are tucked into their sides and a long connector for the intravenous infusion allows access from the foot of the bed. A 25-degree head-up tilt will assist venous drainage, although this should be performed with careful attention to the blood pressure, particularly in patients who have been receiving beta-blockers. Finally, slight head extension will allow the surgeon excellent access to the thyroid gland.

Surgical technique

Pre-incision infiltration with local anaesthetic, for example 10 ml of bupivacaine 0.5%, produces better postoperative analgesia without an increased risk of bruising [23]. The addition of epinephrine (adrenaline) 1:200 000 aids wound haemostasis. Skin flaps are raised and the strap muscles separated in the midline. The upper pole is mobilised and the superior thyroid vessels ligated. Mobilisation of the lobe is completed and the parathyroid glands and recurrent laryngeal nerve are routinely identified and protected during dissection of the thyroid from the trachea. Haemostasis is secured and the strap muscles and platysmal layers apposed. The skin is closed with staples or subcutaneous sutures.

Monitoring of the recurrent laryngeal nerve

Intraoperative nerve monitoring requires placement of electrodes close to the vocal cords. Special endotracheal tubes with surface electrodes may be used or electrodes may be placed directly into the muscles of the larynx. When the recurrent laryngeal nerve is identified, it is stimulated with a current of 0.1 mA, increasing in 0.05 mA increments, until an evoked electromyographic trace (EMG) is obtained. The anaesthetist must choose an appropriate muscle relaxant for endotracheal intubation, and a suitable anaesthetic technique to facilitate this process. Communication between the anaesthetist and clinical physiologist prior to induction of anaesthesia is essential. The surgeon is alerted if an instrument comes close to the recurrent laryngeal nerve. The evidence for the use of intraoperative nerve monitoring during thyroid surgery raises no major safety concerns [24]. Some surgeons find it useful during complex re-operative procedures or operations on large goitres. However, others believe that false negative or false positive readings may lead to misidentification of the nerve and that it may give false reassurance to inexperienced surgeons. It may be used with the patient's consent and the usual arrangements for audit and clinical governance should apply. The evidence that was considered in arriving at this guidance is available [25].

Postoperative care

Any residual neuromuscular block is reversed and the patient is allowed to recover from anaesthesia. If there has been any concern during dissection of the recurrent laryngeal nerve, the vocal cords are visualised and the surgeon reassured. A fibreoptic endoscope may be used to view the vocal cords atraumatically. When adequate spontaneous respiration and laryngeal reflexes have returned, the patient is extubated. Every attempt should be made to prevent coughing, although a recent chest infection or history of cigarette smoking may make this difficult. If there is no immediate respiratory obstruction, the patient is transferred to the recovery ward. The patient is carefully observed for the development of a cervical haematoma and returns to the ward after attaining the appropriate discharge criteria. Signs of hypocalcaemia are treated by calcium supplements and, following total thyroidectomy, T_4 50–100 μg is prescribed daily. Postoperative vocal cord function is examined by indirect laryngoscopy prior to hospital discharge.

Special situations

Graves' disease

Thyroidectomy is offered to patients with autoimmune hyperthyroidism when medical treatment proves inadequate. Patients should be euthyroid prior to surgery. Approximately 3:1000 patients are unable to take antithyroid drugs due to serious adverse reactions, the most severe of which include agranulocytosis, hepatitis, aplastic anaemia and lupus-like syndromes [26]. The clinical manifestations of thyrotoxicosis are usually controlled by beta-blockers, and it has been suggested that beta-blockers alone may be adequate preparation for thyroidectomy. Few surgeons today use Lugol's iodine, which was traditionally given for 10 days preoperatively to reduce bleeding from the thyroid.

Thyroid cancer

There are 20 000 new cases of thyroid cancer each year in the USA with a female to male ratio of 3:1. When thyroidectomy is performed for removal of a thyroid carcinoma there is potentially a greater risk of damage to the recurrent laryngeal nerve. There are various types of thyroid cancers: papillary (78%), follicular (17%), medullary (4%), anaplastic (1%), insular and lymphoma. Patients with differentiated thyroid cancer may be prescribed suppressive doses of T_4 since TSH is considered to be a growth factor in thyroid cancer [27].

Medullary thyroid carcinoma arises from parafollicular or calcitonin-producing C cells. It may be sporadic, familial or associated with phaeochromocytoma in patients with multiple endocrine neoplasia (MEN) type 2A and 2B. The genetic abnormality that produces medullary carcinoma has been determined [28]. If mutations of the rearranged during transfection (RET) proto-oncogene are found on the tenth chromosome then the patient has a high probability of progressing from C-cell hyperplasia to medullary carcinoma. Individuals whose siblings have had medullary carcinoma are offered chromosomal analysis and guidelines exist for the timing of prophylactic thyroidectomy [29].

Papillary carcinoma is the commonest variety and the prognosis depends on the size of the tumour at diagnosis. There is a high cure rate with a 10-year survival of 80–90%. It spreads to local lymph nodes and may require block dissection of the neck. These tumours may involve surrounding tissue and severe obstruction due to tracheal invasion may occur. Extracorporeal oxygenation and cardiopulmonary bypass during tumour resection have been used to manage this difficult situation [30].

Follicular carcinoma is more aggressive than papillary and spreads via the blood to lungs, bone, liver and brain and the metastases can produce T_4. Hürthle cell tumours are thought to be variants of follicular neoplasms. The metastases are more difficult to treat than those of follicular carcinoma as they are far less likely to concentrate radioiodine [31].

Anaplastic carcinoma is extremely malignant and usually only palliative surgery or radiotherapy is indicated.

Insular carcinoma is a rare form of poorly differentiated thyroid cancer that spreads to local lymph nodes and may have pulmonary metastases.

Lymphoma is diagnosed by fine needle aspiration and is usually treated by radiotherapy.

Multiple endocrine neoplasia

As discussed in Chapter 6, patients with MEN type 2 will inevitably develop medullary thyroid cancer. Prophylactic thyroidectomy is advocated in children of MEN type 2 families, who are shown by genetic screening to carry a mutation of the ret-proto-oncogene. Children with MEN type 2B should have thyroidectomy in the first year of life [28].

Large goitres

Endemic goitre still exists in many parts of the world and huge nodular goitres can occur (Figure 2.9). The specimen from the patient in Figure 2.10 weighed 700 g. While these goitres may have a dramatic appearance they often present less of a problem than smaller retrosternal goitres.

Difficult intubation has been associated with huge goitres, although having an experienced assistant lift the goitre anteriorly usually relieves airway obstruction. Other potential problems include excessive blood loss, prolonged operating time and postoperative tracheomalacia. Blood loss is less of a problem when the surgeon dissects the thyroid without transecting it as shown in Figure 2.10.

Use of a small armoured endotracheal tube is recommended to negotiate the compressed and deviated trachea. An armoured endotracheal tube is less

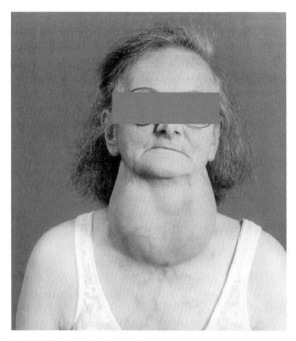

Fig. 2.9 Patient with a large goitre.

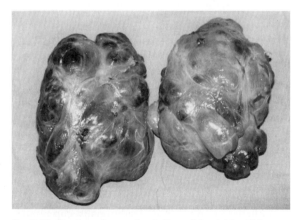

Fig. 2.10 Specimen from patient in Figure 2.9 weighing 700 g.

likely to kink during surgical manipulation while unarmoured tubes may soften during these prolonged procedures.

Lingual thyroid

Embryologically the thyroid grows from the third and fourth branchial arch and descends from the foramen caecum towards the neck. If its development is arrested, a lingual thyroid may result. This can be diagnosed by a thallium or technetium scan and it should be handled carefully, as it may be the patient's only thyroid tissue. Furthermore, it may bleed excessively if biopsy is attempted. The presence of a lingual thyroid should alert the anaesthetist to a potential difficult intubation [32].

Retrosternal goitre

Retrosternal enlargement of the thyroid can be asymptomatic but usually causes compression of mediastinal structures (Figure 2.4). Dyspnoea, choking and hoarseness may occur. Dysphagia is the most common oesophageal symptom but a case has been reported where bleeding from varices was the first presentation of a retrosternal goitre. Superior vena cava syndrome can occur and may be complicated by thrombosis. Retrosternal goitres may also cause cerebral hypoperfusion due to arterial compression and thyrocervical steal, and phrenic and recurrent laryngeal nerve palsies, Horner's syndrome, pleural effusions, chylothorax or pericardial effusions [33].

Despite some retrosternal goitres being large, the cervical incision is often sufficient for removal. This is particularly true if the isthmus of the thyroid lies above the suprasternal notch. As the surgeon manipulates the retrosternal gland, compression of the trachea can be worsened. Tracheal deviation and compression may resolve immediately after excision of the goitre, but tracheomalacia should be anticipated when the patient has complained of a longstanding goitre.

Thoracic goitre

True intrathoracic goitres may first present to the thoracic surgeons as a mediastinal mass. Close co-operation between the anaesthetic team, the endocrine surgeon and the thoracic surgeon will be required to formulate the best anaesthetic management plan. The safest route to the goitre will dictate the choice of either a cervical incision, a median sternotomy or a thoracotomy. Clearly the placement of a double lumen tube would be extremely difficult in these patients (Figure 2.5). The use of bronchial blockers should be considered if the surgeons choose to try the cervical route initially but anticipate a high chance of converting to a thoracotomy. Dissection in the neck may stimulate the carotid sinus and this, coupled with median sternotomy, can produce profound vagal stimulation leading to bradycardia and even sinus arrest. A number of series of thoracic goitres have been published [34]. Since parathyroid surgery also occasionally requires mediastinal exploration, the endocrine theatre team should always have the capability to perform a sternotomy.

Pregnancy

The thyroid normally enlarges slightly during pregnancy and pre-existing goitres may also increase in size [35]. It is important to understand that pregnancy induces metabolic changes that alter thyroid hormone regulation. There is an increase in serum thyroxine-binding globulin (TBG) due to the effects of oestrogen. These effects increase TBG production in the liver and reduce its clearance. The concentration of total serum T_3 and T_4 increases, although measures of total thyroid hormone concentration have generally been replaced by free hormone assays that are unaffected by changes in binding hormone levels. Human chorionic gonadotropin (HCG) has weak thyroid stimulating activity and this causes a slight rise in serum free T_3 and T_4 and a slight fall in serum TSH, usually within the normal range. In the third trimester, the level of free T_3 and T_4 decreases, and TSH rises, due to an increased demand by the fetus. The diagnosis of hyperthyroidism during pregnancy relies on very high levels of T_3 and T_4 and a low TSH. Uncontrolled hyperthyroidism during pregnancy may result in higher incidences of spontaneous abortion, premature labour, low birth-weight babies and still-births. There is also an increase in pre-eclampsia and cardiac complications. Antithyroid drugs cross the placenta but propylthiouracil is preferred to carbimazole as the latter has been associated with aplasia cutis, a rare scalp condition in the fetus. Beta-blockers are not considered teratogenic but growth retardation, low blood sugars and respiratory problems in the neonates have been reported. Radioactive iodine is contraindicated during pregnancy so thyroidectomy may be required in those who cannot tolerate medical therapy. Surgery is best left until the second trimester to avoid teratogenicity, but the patient should be warned of the possibility of spontaneous abortion and premature labour. Appropriate obstetric anaesthetic precautions should be practised depending upon the gestation period.

Trophoblastic disease

Very high levels of HCG may be secreted by molar pregnancies. Plasmapheresis has been used as an alternative to antithyroid medication for the rapid control of severe hyperthyroidism caused by molar pregnancy [36].

Radioiodine treatment

Treatment with radioactive iodine is used for hyperthyroidism, some thyroid carcinomas and for the reduction of goitres in those patients who refuse surgery. It should be remembered that the thyroid might swell and cause airway compression following radioiodine therapy. This situation was predicted and elective awake intubation performed in a patient with massive multi-nodular goitre prior to radioiodine treatment [37].

Postoperative complications

As complications often occur during procedures for recurrent goitre it is important to eliminate the former practice of 'partial thyroidectomy'. When total thyroidectomy is not indicated then at least a total thyroid lobectomy should be performed.

Extubation problems

Coughing at extubation should be avoided but this is often difficult to achieve, particularly if the patient has irritable airways due to smoking or a recent respiratory tract infection. There is a decrease in upper airway reflex sensitivity with increasing age. Possible preventive interventions include extubation during relatively deep anaesthesia and administration of intravenous narcotics or lidocaine. The latter may be administered intravenously, topically, or even placed in the cuff of the endotracheal tube. The rapid emergence from remifentanil reduces the frequency of coughing during emergence from anaesthesia [38].

Haematoma

Meticulous haemostasis is essential when operating in the neck as postoperative haemorrhage is potentially catastrophic. The anaesthetist may be asked to perform a Valsalva manoeuvre (maintain a positive intrathoracic pressure for 10–20 seconds) in order to assess haemostasis prior to wound closure. Recovery ward staff should be experienced at observing the early signs of haematoma formation so that both the surgeon and anaesthetist can be alerted. Traditionally, clip removers were kept at the bedside to enable rapid relief of a haematoma. If it is necessary to re-open the incision to relieve compression of the airway, then it is essential to open all layers. Repeat surgery for haemorrhage is rare and prompt decision making is important. Early re-intubation is recommended so the anaesthetic team should be aware of the problems involved at induction of anaesthesia in a patient for cervical re-exploration. Obviously, the later the intubation is performed the more difficult it becomes as the haematoma expands and compresses the airway. Respiratory obstruction may be due to laryngeal and pharyngeal oedema as a result of venous and lymphatic obstruction by the haematoma, rather than direct tracheal compression. Early re-intubation, rather than precipitous re-opening of the incision, is the best way to manage this complication.

Recurrent laryngeal nerve damage

Good operating technique with routine identification of the recurrent laryngeal nerve greatly minimises accidental nerve injury. Injury to the recurrent laryngeal nerve can occur by a number of mechanisms including ischaemia, contusion, traction, entrapment and actual transection. The incidence of temporary unilateral vocal cord paralysis due to damage to the recurrent laryngeal nerve is 3–4%. Permanent unilateral vocal cord paralysis remains less than 1% of patients and bilateral vocal cord paralysis should be extremely rare [19]. There is a greater risk of nerve damage during surgery for malignancy, Graves' disease and secondary operations [39]. Anatomical variability and distortions will increase the risk of nerve injury, particularly when the surgeon is inexperienced.

Bilateral vocal cord paralysis will lead to stridor at tracheal extubation. Re-intubation will be required and tracheostomy should be considered. Unilateral vocal cord paralysis leads to glottic incompetence, hoarseness, breathlessness, ineffective cough and aspiration. Investigation of nerve injury will include videostroboscopy and laryngeal electromyography (LEMG).

Treatment of laryngeal sensory-motor nerve paralysis can be conservative, with the help of speech therapy. However, early surgical treatment is indicated in cases with severe functional problems. Surgical therapy at 6–9 months after injury is indicated in patients who demonstrate evidence of denervation or little activity on LEMG and have a poor response to a reasonable trial of speech therapy. Many surgical procedures are available including injection laryngoplasty, medialisation thyroplasty, arytenoid adduction, arytenoidopexy, crico-thyroid approximation, endoscopic laser cordotomy and re-innervation procedures [40].

Tracheomalacia

Reports of this rare complication of thyroidectomy are more common in the developing world [41]. Softening of the tracheal rings results from prolonged compression of the trachea by a large goitre. Collapse of the trachea following extubation may lead to life-threatening airway obstruction. The incidence of tracheomalacia will depend on the frequency of this type of goitre but it should be anticipated prior to extubation. The absence of a leak around the deflated cuff of the endotracheal tube should alert the anaesthetist to the possibility of tracheomalacia. Management of tracheomalacia will require urgent re-intubation, a period of artificial ventilation, and possibly tracheostomy or some form of tracheal support with, for example, ceramic rings or tracheopexy.

Laryngeal oedema

Generalised myxoedema of hypothyroidism may include the larynx giving the characteristic hoarse voice and laryngeal oedema has also been reported as an unusual presentation of thyroid lymphoma. Laryngeal complications due to tracheal intubation can be seen during the postoperative indirect laryngoscopy, which is performed to identify recurrent laryngeal nerve damage. Oedema and traumatic lesions have been noted in 4.6% of patients [19]. While trauma to the larynx from the endotracheal tube will cause minor swelling, laryngeal oedema is a rare cause of post-thyroidectomy respiratory obstruction.

Hypocalcaemia

The incidence of hypocalcaemia will depend on the type of surgery performed. After thyroidectomy for large multinodular goitre, temporary hypocalcaemia requiring calcium replacement can occur in 20% of patients [42]. This usually occurs about 36 hours postoperatively. Only 3.1% of patients remained permanently hypocalcaemic and required oral alphacalcidol or calcitriol regularly. Unintentional parathyroidectomy occurred in 11% of one series of 414 thyroidectomies [43]. The identification, recovery and autotransplantation of a parathyroid gland will reduce postoperative hypocalcaemia [44].

Wound complications

Wound infection should be a rare complication and a well-positioned incision should provide a good cosmetic result. Care should be taken during elevation of skin flaps to avoid damage to the anterior cutaneous nerve of the neck. Damage to this structure produces numbness that could prove inconvenient to men when shaving.

Postoperative pain

Patients usually tolerate thyroidectomy very well and require minimal postoperative analgesia. The patient often complains of a stiff neck due to the position during surgery, rather than pain at the site of the incision.

Future developments

As with other endocrine procedures, minimally invasive techniques have been developed for thyroidectomy. Day-procedure thyroidectomies have been performed in some centres, but patient selection, anaesthetic technique, careful observation before discharge and community support are key factors in the success of this approach. The risk of postoperative bleeding should not be underestimated. Laser-induced reduction of thyroid tissue and embolisation by interventional radiologists have been described but are not yet routine procedures.

There are an increasing number of web-based resources that provide updated information on all aspects of thyroid disease for clinicians and patients [45].

Conclusions

Disease of the thyroid gland is common and anaesthetists will be required to manage patients with hypothyroidism and hyperthyroidism as well as patients scheduled for thyroidectomy. Since anaesthesia for thyroidectomy provides many challenges of airway management, the anaesthetist should pay particular attention to preoperative assessment of the airway and should be able to deal with acute airway complications in the perioperative phase.

References

1. Farling PA. Thyroid disease. *Br J Anaesth* 2000; **85**: 15–28.

2. Standring S (Editor in Chief). *Gray's Anatomy,* 39th edn. Edinburgh, Elsevier Churchill Livingstone, 2008, p. 560.

3. Ganong WF. *Review of Medical Physiology, 22nd edn.* New York, McGraw-Hill Professional, 2005, pp. 317–22.

4. Medvei VC. *The History of Clinical Endocrinology.* Carnforth, Lancashire, Parthenon Publishing, 1993, pp. 135–45.

5. Lind P, Langsteger W, Molnar M, Gallowitsch HJ, Mikosch P, Gomez I. Epidemiology of thyroid diseases in iodine sufficiency. *Thyroid* 1998; **8**: 1179–83.

6. Murkin JM. Anesthesia and hypothyroidism: A review of thyroxine physiology, pharmacology and anesthetic implications. *Anesth Analg* 1982; **61**: 371–83.

7. Mathes DD. Treatment of myxedema coma for emergency surgery. *Anesth Analg* 1998; **6**: 450–1.

8. So PC. Unmasking of thyrotoxicosis during anaesthesia. *Hong Kong Med J* 2001; 7: 311–14.

9. Stehling LC. Anesthetic management of the patient with hyperthyroidism. *Anesthesiology* 1974; **41**: 585–95.

10. National Institute for Health and Clinical Excellence (NICE). *Retrobulbar Irradiation for Thyroid Eye Disease.*

Interventional Procedure Guidance 148. London, NICE, 2005.

11. Nishiyama K, Kitahara A, Natsume H, et al. Malignant hyperthermia in a patient with Graves' disease during subtotal thyroidectomy. *Endocr J* 2001; **48**: 227–32.

12. Pemberton HS. Sign of submerged goitre. *Lancet* 1946; **251**: 509.

13. Toyota K, Uchida H, Ozasa H , et al. Preoperative airway evaluation using multi-slice 3D CT for a patient with severe tracheal stenosis. *Br J Anaesth* 2004; **93**: 865–7.

14. Gillespie S, Farling PA. Preoperative assessment of the airway: should anaesthetists be making use of modern imaging techniques? *Br J Anaesth* 2004; **93**: 758–60.

15. Kulkarni RS, Braverman LE. Patwardhan NA. Bilateral cervical plexus block for thyroidectomy and parathyroidectomy in healthy and high risk patients. *J Endocrinol Invest* 1996; **19**: 714–18.

16. Gough J, Gough JR. Total thyroidectomy for amiodarone-associated thyrotoxicosis in patients with severe cardiac disease. *World J Surg* 2006; **30**: 1957–61.

17. Hobbiger HE, Allen JG, Greatorex RG, Denny NM. The laryngeal mask airway for thyroid and parathyroid surgery. *Anaesthesia* 1996; **51**: 972–4.

18. Greatorex RA, Denny NM. Application of the laryngeal mask airway to thyroid surgery and the preservation of the recurrent laryngeal nerve. *Ann R Coll Surg Engl* 1991; **73**: 352–4.

19. Lacoste L, Gineste D, Karayan J, et al. Airway complications in thyroid surgery. *Ann Otol Rhinol Laryngol* 1993; **102**: 441–6.

20. Mingo OH, Ashpole KJ, Irving CJ, Rucklidge MW. Remifentanil sedation for awake fibreoptic intubation with limited application of local anaesthetic in patients for elective head and neck surgery. *Anaesthesia* 2008; **63**: 1065–9.

21. http://www.das.uk.com/equipmentlistjuly2005/htm, accessed 14 September 2009.

22. Nicholson WT, Sprung J, Janowsski CJ. Sugammadex: a novel agent for the reversal of neuromuscular blockade. *Pharmacotherapy* 2007; **27**: 1181–8.

23. Bagul A, Taha R, Metcalfe MS, Brook NR, Nicholson ML. Pre-incision infiltration of local anesthetic reduces postoperative pain with no effects on bruising and wound cosmesis after thyroid surgery. *Thyroid* 2005; **15**: 1245–8.

24. National Institute for Health and Clinical Excellence (NICE). *Intraoperative Nerve Monitoring During Thyroid Surgery. Interventional Procedure Guidance 255.* London, NICE, 2008.

25. http://www.nice.org.uk/nicemedia/pdf/654_overview_for_web191107.pdf, accessed 14 September 2009.

26. Franklyn J. Thyrotoxicosis. *Prescr J* 1999; **39**: 1–8.

27. Biondi B, Filetti S, Schlumberger M. Thyroid-hormone therapy and thyroid cancer: a reassessment. *Nat Clin Pract Endocrinol Metab* 2005; **1**: 32–40.

28. Marsh DJ, Mulligan LM, Eng C. RET proto-oncogene mutations in multiple endocrine neoplasia type 2 and medullary thyroid carcinoma. *Horm Res* 1997; **47**: 168–78.

29. Frilling A, Weber F, Tecklenborg C, Broelsch CE. Prophylactic thyroidectomy in multiple endocrine neoplasia: the impact of molecular mechanisms of RET proto-oncogene. *Langenbecks Arch Surg* 2003; **388**: 17–26.

30. Jeon HK, So YK, Yang JH, Jeong HS. Extracorporeal oxygenation support for curative surgery in a patient with papillary thyroid carcinoma invading the trachea. *J Laryngol Otol* 2008; **23**: 1–4.

31. Yutan E, Clarke OH. Hürthle cell carcinoma. *Curr Treat Options Oncol* 2001; **2**: 331–5.

32. Fogarty D. Lingual thyroid and difficult intubation. *Anaesthesia* 1990; **45**: 251.

33. Anders HJ. Compression syndromes caused by substernal goitres. *Postgrad Med J* 1998; **74**: 327–9.

34. Mussi A, Ambroqi MC, Iacconi P, Spinelli C, Miccoli P, Angeletti CA. Mediastinal goitres: when the transthoracic approach? *Acta Chir Belg* 2000; **100**: 259–63.

35. Collis RE, Plaat F, Urquhart J. *Textbook of Obstetric Anaesthesia*. Cambridge, Cambridge University Press, 2002, pp. 31.

36. Erbil Y, Tihan D, Azezli A , et al. Severe hyperthyroidism requiring therapeutic plasmapheresis in a patient with hydatidiform mole. *Gynecol Endocrinol* 2006; **22**: 402–4.

37. Chakera A, van Heerden PV, van der Schaaf A. Elective awake intubation in a patient with massive multinodular goitre presenting for radioiodine treatment. *Anaesth Intensive Care* 2002; **30**: 236–9.

38. Hohlrieder M, Tiefenthaler W, Klaus H, et al. Effect of total intravenous anaesthesia and balanced anaesthesia on the frequency of coughing during emergence from the anaesthesia. *Br J Anaesth.* 2007; **99**: 587–91.

39. Chiang FY, Wang LF, Huang YF, Lee KW, Kuo WR. Recurrent laryngeal nerve palsy after thyroidectomy with routine identification of the recurrent laryngeal nerve. *Surgery* 2005; **137**: 342–7.

40. Finck C. Laryngeal dysfunction after thyroid surgery: diagnosis, evaluation and treatment. *Acta Chir Belg* 2006; **106**: 378–87.

41. Agarwal A, Mishra AK, Gupta SK, et al. High incidence of tracheomalacia in longstanding goitres: experience from an endemic goitre region. *World J Surg* 2007; **31**: 832–7.

42. Gardiner KR, Russell CFJ. Thyroidectomy for large multinodular goitre. *J R Coll Surg Edinb* 1995; **40**: 367–70.

43. Lee NJ, Blakey JD, Bhuta S, Calcaterra TC. Unintentional parathyroidectomy during thyroidectomy. *Laryngoscope* 1999; **109**: 1238–40.

44. Testini M, Rosato L, Avenia N, et al. The impact of single parathyroid gland autotransplantation during thyroid surgery on postoperative hypoparathyroidism: a multicenter study. *Transplant Proc* 2007; **39**: 225–30.

45. http://www.thyroidmanager.org, accessed 14 September 2009.

Parathyroid disease

Philip R. Michael, Jane K. Beattie and Jennifer M. Hunter

In 1850, Richard Owen first reported the existence of parathyroid glands in mammals, describing to the Zoological Society of London his findings in the Indian rhinoceros. Several other workers also noticed these small structures in the neck at that time [1]. However, it was not until 1877 that Ivar Sandström described the 'new' *glandulae parathyroideae*, having studied them in animals and then in humans [2]. In this chapter, we will consider the basic anatomy and physiology of the parathyroid gland, followed by its pathologies and their implications for anaesthesia.

Anatomy and embryology of the parathyroid gland

There are usually two pairs of parathyroid gland, superior and inferior, each measuring 4 × 2 × 6 mm, surrounded by fat and each weighing approximately 25–40 mg: 80–90% of patients have four parathyroids. They are found on the posterior aspect of the upper and lower poles of the thyroid gland. Cadaveric studies show that the site, size, shape and number of parathyroid glands vary between patients. More than five or fewer than three glands is uncommon [3, 4]. The superior pair are less variable in their position. They develop from the dorsal part of the fourth pharyngeal pouch in the embryo. Over 90% [4] are located in close proximity to the inferior thyroid artery and the recurrent laryngeal nerve at the level of the cricothyroid junction [3], although they can remain at the level of the submandibular gland (Figure 3.1).

The inferior parathyroid glands take origin, along with the thymus, from the third pharyngeal pouch. They descend beyond the superior glands and normally lie at the lower pole of the thyroid. However, they can be carried with the thymus during its migration into the mediastinum. This accounts for the variability: less than 70% of inferior glands are located at the 'normal' anatomical site [4].

There is some disagreement as to whether the parathyroid glands are entirely endodermal in origin, as suggested by conventional embryology [5], or whether there is involvement of the ectoderm and cells from the neural crest [6]. The latter hypothesis has been proposed as the explanation for the involvement of the parathyroid gland in the multiple endocrine neoplasia (MEN) syndromes (Chapter 6) [7]. More recently, studies have demonstrated that the neural crest is not required for the production of pharyngeal pouch structures, including the thyroid, parathyroids and thymus [8, 9].

Histologically, the parathyroid gland consists of solid and follicular parenchyma. The solid parenchyma contains chief cells, oxyphil cells and transitional oxyphil cells, as well as large clear cells. The chief cells are responsible for the production, storage and secretion of parathyroid hormone (PTH), but only some are in an active secretory phase at any given time, with a prominent secretory apparatus. Those chief cells not in active secretion remain in a resting state, and are rich in glycogen [10]. The oxyphil cells have an abundance of mitochondria, but their function is not fully described. It may be that oxyphil cells exist to support the chief cells (Figure 3.2).

Physiology

Parathyroid hormone is secreted by the parathyroid chief cells in response to a fall in the level of circulating, free calcium. Parathyroid hormone is a polypeptide consisting of 84 amino acids. The sequence of the 34 amino acids at the amino-terminal was reported in 1972 [11]. It is this segment which confers the biological activity of PTH.

The PTH precursor, *pre-pro-parathyroid hormone*, is a polypeptide chain of 115 amino acids which is first cleaved within the endoplasmic reticulum of the chief

Core Topics in Endocrinology in Anaesthesia and Critical Care, eds. George M. Hall, Jennifer M. Hunter and Mark S. Cooper. Published by Cambridge University Press. © Cambridge University Press 2010.

cell to produce the 90 amino acid pro-parathyroid hormone. Six more amino acids are then removed within the Golgi apparatus to produce PTH [12]. This occurs shortly before the hormone is released from the secretory granules, since there is little storage of PTH in the gland.

Calcium-sensing receptor and secretion of parathyroid hormone

A fall in the level of circulating calcium is detected by a membrane-bound calcium-sensing receptor which has some interesting features. A slight reduction in serum calcium brings about an almost immediate and measurable increase in the level of PTH, even on a background of a relatively high concentration of circulating calcium. Thus the calcium receptor must have a low affinity for calcium or it would be constantly saturated. Conversely, in order to respond to miniscule changes in serum calcium concentration, it must be particularly sensitive to its ligand [13]. The calcium receptor structure was elucidated and its gene cloned in the early 1990s (Figure 3.3). It is a G-protein coupled receptor of subfamily C. As with the other members of this receptor class, such as the $GABA_B$ receptors and the metabotropic glutamate receptors, it consists of an extracellular domain containing the receptor, seven transmembrane domains and an intracellular portion. Binding of the ligand to the receptor causes a conformational change affecting the intracellular domain which then interacts with the G-protein. This gives rise to an exchange of guanosine triphosphate (GTP) for guanosine diphosphate (GDP) on the G-protein which activates it, thus stimulating the various second messenger cascades,

such as the adenylate cyclase system, the phospholipase system, and the calcium-calmodulin system. The G-proteins identified in the calcium receptor so far include G_{11}, G_q and possibly G_i.

Several different intracellular second messenger systems have been identified within the chief cells

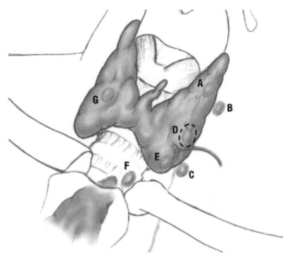

Fig. 3.1 Usual locations of parathyroid adenomata. These positions apply to left- or right-sided glands. A. Superior gland on the posterior surface of the thyroid capsule; may be confined within the thyroid capsule. B. Superior gland in the tracheoesophageal groove lying between the cranial and caudal boundaries of the thyroid gland. C. Superior gland in the tracheoesophageal groove caudal and inferior to the thyroid gland and with no contact with the thyroid gland. D. Superior or inferior gland near the junction of the recurrent laryngeal nerve and the inferior thyroid artery. E. Inferior gland that lies anterior to the trachea and just inferior to the thyroid parenchyma. F. Inferior gland descended into the thyrothymic ligament. G. Superior or inferior parathyroid gland located within the thyroid gland. From Suliburk and Perrier [83] with permission.

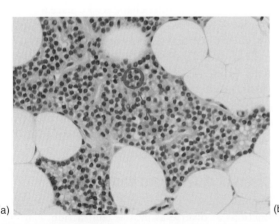

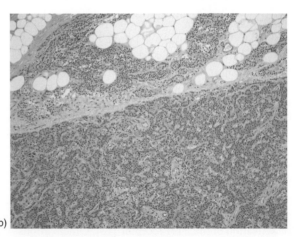

(a) (b)

Fig. 3.2 (a) Histological anatomy of normal parathyroid tissue. The oxyphil cells, marked O, are rich in mitochondria and stain more darkly than the chief cells. (b) Medium power histology of a parathyroid adenoma. There is a clear demarcation between the adenoma and the surrounding normal tissue. Images courtesy of Dr T. Helliwell, Royal Liverpool University Hospital, Department of Histopathology.

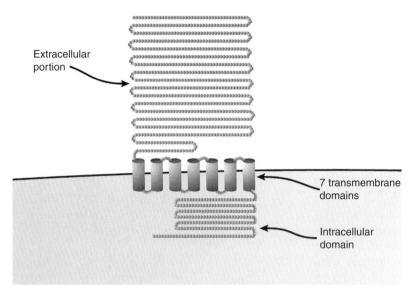

Extracellular portion

7 transmembrane domains

Intracellular domain

Fig. 3.3 The calcium-sensing receptor is a G-protein coupled receptor (subfamily C). The receptor was first cloned in 1993 from DNA extracted from bovine parathyroid tissue. The extracellular domain consists of over 600 amino acids, and includes the binding sites for Ca^{2+} and other polyvalent cations. After Brown et al. [19] with permission.

including the phosphatidylinositol-phospholipase C complex, phospholipase A_2 and phospholipase D. It is thought likely that inhibition of the secondary messenger adenylate cyclase is also involved in the mechanism, given the inverse relationship between calcium concentration and the release of PTH. As yet it remains uncertain which of these second messenger cascades is responsible for the reduction in PTH release associated with an increase in serum calcium [14].

The calcium receptors on the parathyroid chief cells are distributed mainly within structures known as caveolae. These are flask-shaped arrangements of the cell membrane proteins which appear to function as scaffolding. They assist in the binding of calcium ions to the receptor [15].

Calcium receptor function is modulated by a number of other factors. First, production and expression of the receptor protein itself can be regulated. For instance, vitamin D response elements exist within the promoter regions of the calcium receptor gene so that its expression is amplified by dihydroxy-vitamin D. This in part explains the effect of vitamin D upon calcium homeostasis and PTH release. Second, other cations can act as direct agonists at the calcium receptor including magnesium [16]. Release of PTH is inhibited by the action of magnesium on the parathyroid calcium receptor [17]. To complicate matters, magnesium is also a cofactor required for the release of PTH and for activation of the PTH receptor [18]. Other cations that can trigger a second messenger cascade from the calcium receptor include trivalent gadolinium (Gd^{3+}),

which is used as a contrast agent in MRI, and the polyvalent compound neomycin [19].

The relationship between extracellular calcium and release of PTH can be represented by an inverse sigmoidal curve. This suggests that the binding of calcium to the receptor is co-operative, allowing for small variations in serum calcium concentration to give rise to large changes in PTH level over the steep, linear portion of the curve [15]. It is not simply the concentration of extracellular calcium which governs the release of PTH. The calcium receptor is sensitive to the rate of change of calcium so that a rapid fall in calcium gives rise to a greater release of PTH. This effect also appears to exhibit hysteresis so that, at a given serum calcium concentration, the PTH level is greater when extracellular calcium concentration is falling than when it is increasing. Several other changes take place within the parathyroid chief cell to further modulate the response to prolonged hypocalcaemia, beginning with reduction in the breakdown of PTH. This is followed after several hours by increased mRNA transcription of the gene which encodes pre-pro-parathyroid hormone, and the chief cell further develops and enhances its biosynthetic organelles. Finally, the release of PTH is up-regulated in prolonged hypocalcaemia by the proliferation of the parathyroid chief cells themselves [20].

Effects of parathyroid hormone

Calcium plays a pivotal role in many physiological functions as diverse as muscle contraction, neuronal excitation and coagulation, and failure of its homeostasis can have serious consequences. The main function of PTH is to increase the availability within the plasma of free, extracellular calcium. The corollary is that PTH also acts to decrease serum phosphate. The mechanisms for its actions are both direct and indirect. The former depend on the availability of the PTH receptor and its second messengers, whereas the indirect actions largely relate to the increased activation of vitamin D. This latter effect is mediated by cyclic adenosine monophosphate (cAMP) [21].

Action of parathyroid hormone on bone

The primary calcium store is in bone and this, after the kidney, is the predominant target of PTH. Osteoblasts and osteoclasts have been shown to carry the PTH receptor [22]. Calcium in the extracellular fluid is in equilibrium with calcium in the bone matrix. Calcium influx and efflux from bone takes place continuously across the bone surface, with or without the presence of PTH. The presence of PTH alters the set-point of the equilibrium, shifting more calcium from the bone into the extracellular fluid [23]. Calcium efflux also occurs at sites of bone remodelling where osteoclasts chew up bone. Parathyroid hormone promotes increased influx into focal areas of bone where osteoid has been recently laid down by osteoblasts. Unrestrained, the increase in extracellular calcium concentration would cause an increased calcium load to reach the kidneys and to be excreted. There would be continual loss of calcium from bone with resulting impairment in structural integrity. However, the kidneys reabsorb approximately 95% of filtered calcium, and this is affected by several mechanisms including PTH.

The net effect of continuous exposure to high levels of PTH, as in hyperparathyroidism, will be bone resorption. Recent work has shown that with intermittent dosage, once a day, PTH analogues with their short half life may have anabolic effects by increasing the longevity of osteoblasts and encouraging bone remodelling at quiescent bone surfaces. This may be of benefit in the treatment of osteoporosis and recombinant PTH is now available for this purpose [24].

Renal effects

Normally, up to 60% of filtered calcium is reabsorbed by the proximal convoluted tubule of the nephron. This is mainly a passive process along an electrochemical gradient, through calcium channels. These channels may be regulated under certain conditions by G-proteins [25]. In addition, it seems that there is a component of calcium reabsorption in the proximal tubule which is active and dependent on sodium [26]. Another 20% of the filtered calcium is reabsorbed in the loop of Henle. Five per cent is lost in the urine, and the remaining fifteen per cent is reabsorbed by the distal convoluted tubule. It is in the distal nephron that the predominant effects of PTH on the kidney occur.

Parathyroid hormone exerts its renal actions by a mechanism involving G-protein second messenger systems linked to both protein kinase A and protein kinase C [27]. Through these mechanisms, PTH increases the conductance of the tight junctions between the cells to calcium, enhancing calcium diffusion through the paracellular pathway [28]. The transcellular pathway is also affected. Parathyroid hormone causes the insertion of Ca^{2+} channels into the luminal cell membrane. These channels are sensitive to blockade by the dihydropyridine group of calcium channel antagonists, such as nifedipine [29]. The net effect is that reabsorption of calcium by the kidneys is enhanced, reducing the effect of an increased calcium load on renal calcium loss.

Intestinal effects

By increasing the activation of vitamin D in the kidney [21], PTH indirectly increases the absorption of dietary calcium. Activated vitamin D up-regulates the expression of calbindin-D9k. This is an ubiquitous calcium-binding protein which was thought to have a role in the transcellular passage of calcium across many cell types including enterocytes. More recently, however, studies have shown that enterocytes from knockout mice without calbindin-D9k have no differences in their capability to transport calcium from their basal to apical cell membranes [30]. Compensatory mechanisms have been implicated in this ability to transport calcium without calbindin-D9k [31]. Evidence has been found of a direct effect of PTH on cellular calcium uptake and also on calcium transport across the enterocyte, where a PTH receptor has been identified [32].

Effect on phosphate

Serum inorganic phosphate concentration is regulated in a number of ways, and the kidneys play an important role. Several types of sodium phosphate cotransporters (Npt) have been identified in the kidney. Subtypes Npt2a and Npt2c in the brush-border membrane of the proximal convoluted tubule are inhibited by both PTH and by high dietary intake of inorganic phosphate [33]. Parathyroid hormone therefore increases renal clearance of phosphate. Somewhat paradoxically, it also increases intestinal phosphate uptake [32], but the phosphaturic effect is much greater than the absorptive one. However, regulation of phosphate

31

involves a highly complex network of gene expressions. Parathyroid hormone effects on intestinal phosphate absorption may be biphasic, enhancing phosphate uptake at an intermediate plateau of PTH concentration and suppressing uptake at very low or very high levels [34].

Vitamin D

Vitamin D is intricately involved in calcium homeostasis and has a close relationship to parathyroid function. Its functions are widespread and not fully understood, but its main role is to increase dietary absorption of calcium and phosphate. It is important in bone mineralisation processes, and involved in bone remodelling [21].

The two primary sources of vitamin D are from the conversion of 7-dehydrocholesterol to vitamin D3 (cholecalciferol) in the skin and from dietary intake. Synthesis of vitamin D3 in the skin requires the absorption of ultraviolet light. Production is positively correlated with ambient sunlight and inversely with enhanced skin pigmentation, as melanocytes in darker skin absorb more of the ultraviolet light. Vitamin D production in plants is also light dependent, and gives rise to vitamin D2 (ergocalciferol). Vitamin D3 is ingested from animal sources, and D2 is ingested from plants. The difference between cholecalciferol and ergocalciferol occurs only in the side-chains of its structure and not in the active moiety.

Activation of vitamin D is a two-step process. The first stage is hydroxylation, principally in the liver by mitochondrial CYP27A, to 25-hydroxyvitamin D. This is the most stable form of vitamin D in the circulation especially when bound to vitamin D-binding protein. It is this metabolite which is most frequently measured as an indication of vitamin D status. The more active form of vitamin D (by a factor of 1000) than D2 or D3 is 1,25-dihydroxyvitamin D or calcitriol, and its production requires 1-hydroxylation of 25-hydroxyvitamin D by CYP27B1. The latter is primarily a renal enzyme, though it has been identified in a number of extrarenal sites including skin, intestine, brain, placenta and bone [21]. Parathyroid hormone stimulates expression and activity of CYP27B1 and this enhances the activation of vitamin D. There is a negative feedback mechanism by which 1,25-dihydroxyvitamin D suppresses CYP27B1, and there is thought to be direct suppression of the enzyme by calcium. Suppression of production of 1,25-dihydroxyvitamin D, as in an abundance of circulating activated vitamin D or hypercalcaemia, allows an alternative synthetic pathway to produce the water-soluble 24,25-dihydroxyvitamin D and other compounds, which are then excreted in the urine. The responsible enzyme, renal CYP24, is up-regulated by 1,25-dihydroxyvitamin D and calcitonin and suppressed by PTH.

Parathyroid hormone-related peptide (PTHrP)

This is a peptide that is produced in a variety of tissues, such as long bones, the lactating mammary gland and the placenta, and it acts locally in an autocrine or paracrine fashion at the type 1 PTH receptor. It has a similar effect on the receptor to that of PTH, as they have similar amino-acid sequences at their amino-terminals. Its roles are mainly in the regulation of chondrocytes and the growth plates of long bones, but it is also involved in lactation and in placental calcium transport [35]. The production of PTHrP by tumours is the commonest cause of malignancy-associated hypercalcaemia. Conventional PTH assays do not detect it.

Pathological disorders of the parathyroid glands

Hypoparathyroidism

This is either congenital or acquired and can be due to under-functioning of the gland, aberrant production of PTH or a reduced response to PTH.

Causes

Genetic defects and congenital hypoparathyroidism

Congenital absence of the gland occurs most commonly in the DiGeorge sequence, which involves micro-deletion of chromosome 22q11 and is part of the spectrum of velocardiofacial syndrome [36, 37]. Other inherited conditions produce an aberrant form of PTH and inherited mutations in the calcium-sensing receptor can inhibit PTH [38]. This can reduce renal calcium reabsorption, resulting in hypercalcuric hypocalcaemia. Treatment is not indicated as the hypocalcaemia is usually mild, and these patients are at risk of nephrocalcinosis.

Autoimmune polyglandular syndrome type 1 is an autosomal recessive condition which can give rise to hypoparathyroidism, hypoadrenalism and intestinal malabsorption in childhood.

In *pseudohypoparathyroidism (types 1a and 1b)* the structure of PTH is unaffected and its level may be normal or even raised. However, there is a genetic mutation affecting the structure of the alpha subunit of the G_s protein (Gs) in type 1a and affecting the promoter region for G_s in type 1b [35]. Pseudohypoparathyroidism type 1a gives rise to the phenotype known as Albright's hereditary osteodystrophy, which is also seen in pseudopseudohypoparathyroidism [18][38].

Acquired hypoparathyroidism

The most common cause of hypoparathyroidism is iatrogenic. It is due to damage or removal of the parathyroid glands or their blood supply during thyroidectomy or other surgery to the neck. The incidence is dependent on a number of factors including: the extent of resection, the experience of the surgeon, retrosternal extension of the thyroid, malignancy, failure to identify one of the parathyroids intraoperatively and the presence of Graves' disease [18]. A retrospective case study of over 3000 thyroidectomy patients showed an increased likelihood of hypoparathyroidism after extensive or repeat thyroid surgery, and with increasing patient age over 50 years [39]. However, in a prospective study of 170 patients, there was no statistical difference dependent upon surgical experience, central lymph node dissection, parathyroid autotransplantation, or whether the thyroid disease was malignant, in the development of post-thyroidectomy hypoparathyroidism [40].

Other acquired causes of hypoparathyroidism include severe hypomagnesaemia, possibly due to gastrointestinal disease [41], and deposition of heavy metals within the parathyroid tissue, such as iron in haemochromatosis and copper in Wilson's disease.

Clinical features of hypoparathyroidism

These can be divided into those of the underlying condition causing the hypoparathyroidism, such as the velocardiofacial syndrome and the features of the resulting electrolyte imbalance. Hypocalcaemia can be well tolerated, depending upon its severity and duration of onset. Marked hypocalcaemia can be asymptomatic if the disease process has been sufficiently gradual. Presenting features can be vague and non-specific, including generalised tiredness, anxiety and depression, and polyuria. Symptoms may pertain to the neuromuscular excitability that occurs as the extracellular concentration of free, ionised, calcium falls. These begin with numbness and tingling particularly periorally and in the hands and feet, and progress to muscular contraction with carpopedal spasm. As the severity or rapidity of onset of hypocalcaemia increases, central nervous system effects can ensue, such as confusion or even seizures. Alternatively, smooth muscle constriction can predominate, with abdominal pain, bronchospasm and laryngospasm [42]. Generalised skeletal muscle contraction gives rise to tetany, which can be fatal if inadequately treated. The cardiovascular effects of chronic hypocalcaemia may extend to heart failure [18].

The traditional physical signs of hypocalcaemia can be elicited, namely Chvostek's sign and Trousseau's sign. In the former, tapping of the facial nerve gives rise to facial twitching. Trousseau's sign is positive when inflating a sphygmomanometer cuff on the arm to greater than systolic blood pressure for three minutes gives rise to painful carpal spasm. There can also be skin manifestations of hypocalcaemia, especially if the disease process has been prolonged, including rough, dry skin with coarse hair and nails [43].

Diagnosis

The diagnosis of hypoparathyroidism is based on the clinical history and measurement of serum calcium and phosphate, as well as PTH assays. Hyperphosphataemia may accompany the hypocalcaemia. Parathyroid hormone levels will be raised in hypocalcaemia from other causes such as pseudohypoparathyroidism, but will be low in true hypoparathyroidism. Magnesium levels may be depleted. The ECG in hypocalcaemia may show the classic changes of a prolonged ST segment and QT interval.

The history gives clues as to the underlying pathology. A patient may have a history of neck surgery or trauma, which may have other implications for the anaesthetist. Similarly, there may be a positive family history of hypocalcaemia suggesting a hereditary cause.

Treatment

This is aimed at the underlying pathology and correction of the resulting metabolic disturbance. The urgency of the restoration of serum calcium levels is dictated by the severity of symptoms. Mild, chronic hypocalcaemia can be treated with oral calcium supplements. Conversely, severe or life-threatening symptoms with heart failure and cardiovascular collapse, convulsions or tetanic contractions, may require intravenous administration of calcium by infusion in addition to the supportive measures provided by a level two or three dependency unit. Artificially elevating the serum calcium over many years in the absence of the renal protection offered by PTH can give rise to nephrolithiasis and renal failure [38, 44], but this is very unlikely in the acute phase.

Many treatment regimes involve high doses of vitamin D in order to increase gastrointestinal absorption of calcium and make up for the deficit in renal activation of vitamin D. It can be administered as inactive vitamin D, alphacalcidol (1α hydroxyvitamin D), or calcitriol (1,25-dihydroxyvitamin D – the active form). Thiazide diuretics increase renal calcium reabsorption and are also used.

Until recently, the option of utilising replacement hormone therapy in hypoparathyroidism has proved ineffective. As a peptide hormone, oral administration of PTH is limited by its breakdown by intestinal peptidases. Marketing such a drug for intravenous use would be unattractive, because of the availability of alternative treatment with oral calcium and vitamin D analogues, and the relatively small potential user base. However, in recent years injectable PTH (in the form of the amino terminal residues 1–34) has become available in a user-friendly pen, primarily for the treatment of osteoporosis [44]. Several studies by Winer et al. have compared its use favourably with traditional treatments for parathyroid deficiency [45–47], so it may become routine treatment in the near future.

Primary hyperparathyroidism

An excessive production of PTH in a patient who would otherwise have a normal serum calcium is termed primary hyperparathyroidism. The excess circulating PTH gives rise to a hypercalcaemic state, secondary to the increased activation of vitamin D, enhanced renal reabsorption and intestinal absorption of calcium, and excessive bone demineralisation. There is an associated hypophosphataemia as urinary excretion of phosphate is increased.

Causes

A solitary parathyroid adenoma is the causative factor in at least 80% of cases of primary hyperparathyroidism [38]. The remaining 15–20% are largely due to hyperplasia in several parathyroid glands. The very rare causes of primary hyperparathyroidism encompass some of the hereditary forms, such as familial hyperparathyroidism, and parathyroid carcinoma. The latter condition is responsible for only 0.5% of cases of primary hyperparathyroidism, and is usually a slowly growing invasive neoplasm, which requires ipsilateral thyroidectomy, paratracheal tissue dissection and lymph node and thymus removal [48].

Multiple endocrine neoplasia (MEN) syndromes

Multiple endocrine neoplasia syndromes are a collection of autosomal dominant conditions in which the patient develops tumours in neuroendocrine tissues

(Chapter 6). The tumours can be non-functional or functional, in which case they secrete hormones. MEN 1 is a result of a mutation in the *MEN 1* gene, located on chromosome 11. MEN 2 is determined by mutations in the c-RET proto-oncogene, which encodes RET, a tyrosine kinase protein bound to cell membrane receptors.

Primary hyperparathyroidism is a feature of the MEN syndromes, especially MEN 1 in which almost 100% of patients develop parathyroid hyperplasia by the age of 50 years, compared with only 15–30% in MEN 2A [49]. Hyperparathyroidism is not a feature in MEN 2B. Primary hyperparathyroidism in MEN 1 is most often due to multinodular hyperplasia, though an adenoma can be found in some cases. Other tumours commonly described in MEN 1 include a gastrinoma or other enteropancreatic tumour, in up to 75% of patients (Chapter 6), and anterior pituitary tumours (Chapter 1). Also common are carcinoids (usually thymic or bronchial) and adrenocortical tumours which are usually non-functional. Phaeochromocytoma, a catecholamine-secreting tumour of the adrenal medulla, affects less than 1% of patients with MEN 1.

MEN 2 is characterised by medullary carcinoma of the thyroid (MTC) and phaeochromocytoma, and can be subdivided into MEN 2A and MEN 2B. MEN 2A differs from 2B in that primary hyperparathyroidism occurs in MEN 2A but not MEN 2B, and MTC occurs later and with less aggression in the former. A third subdivision of MEN 2 is familial medullary thyroid carcinoma, in which the thyroid carcinoma is the only feature, but it occurs in at least four family members [49].

Clinical features

The clinical presentation of primary hyperparathyroidism has altered over the past century. It is now a commonly recognised endocrine disorder, with the number of parathyroidectomies increasing each year. Originally, it was diagnosed only when the development of secondary complications became dramatic. There may have been recurrent renal calculi and osteopenia with bone resorption and the classical 'salt and pepper' appearance on the skull X-ray. The description of 'stones, bones, moans and groans' is less common today in patients with primary hyperparathyroidism. Features can involve many organ systems (Table 3.1).

With the more frequent use of readily accessible laboratory assays, the detection of primary hyperparathyroidism through initial detection of raised serum calcium has increased to the extent that patients are

Table 3.1 The organ systems that can be affected by primary hyperparathyroidism.

Organ system	Symptom/sign
Skeletal/articular	Osteopenia, gout, pseudogout
Neuropsychiatric	Depression, lethargy, fatigueability
Cardiovascular	Hypertension, vascular calcification
Gastrointestinal	Peptic ulcer disease, pancreatitis
Renal	Nephrolithiasis, nephrocalcinosis
Haematological	Anaemia

now often relatively asymptomatic at the time of diagnosis – apart from the non-specific findings of lethargy, weakness and depression. With the increased availability of bone densitometry, reduced mineral density of cortical (not cancellous) bone can be seen in most patients even with mild primary hyperparathyroidism [48]. Hyperparathyroidism is becoming recognised as a risk factor for increased mortality from cardiovascular disease, and in the development of impaired glucose tolerance. This supports surgical intervention by an experienced endocrine surgeon even in relatively asymptomatic patients [50].

Diagnosis

A raised serum calcium level is one of the primary diagnostic criteria of primary hyperparathyroidism. Whereas measurement of total serum calcium is widespread, there are potential advantages to be gained by measurement of the free ionised fraction. First, calcium in its ionised form gives rise to most of the clinical and physiological features of hyperparathyroidism. Second, it is not affected by posture or hypoalbuminaemia. Third, in mild primary hyperparathyroidism total serum calcium may be within the normal range, despite the ionised fraction being raised. Metabolic acidosis, as found in the critically ill, decreases the affinity of calcium for albumin and therefore increases the free ionised fraction [51].

In the past, the common immunoassays detected small fragments and metabolites of PTH. The increased availability of an immunoassay for intact PTH (amino acids 1–84) in the last decade has enhanced the diagnosis and management of primary hyperparathyroidism. A raised serum PTH with normal or raised serum calcium suggests primary hyperparathyroidism. Hypercalcaemia from another cause would lower the serum PTH by negative feedback. Plasma concentrations of intact PTH at the upper end of the normal

reference range in a patient with a mild elevation in serum calcium should raise suspicions of primary hyperparathyroidism. Hypomagnesaemia and vitamin D deficiency can also affect PTH levels. These should be corrected if abnormal before a diagnosis of primary hyperparathyroidism is made.

One of the main diagnostic differentials to be excluded when suspecting primary hyperparathyroidism is *familial hypocalciuric hypercalcaemia* (FHH). This is caused by any of a wide range of inactivating mutations in the gene encoding the calcium-sensing receptor and is inherited in an autosomal dominant fashion. The mutation reduces the sensitivity of tissues expressing the CaS receptor, specifically the parathyroid (leading to hypercalcaemia) and the kidney (leading to increased renal absorption of calcium). Urinary calcium excretion can be measured and expressed as a ratio of calcium clearance to creatinine clearance to improve the clarity of the diagnosis. Differentiating FHH from primary hyperparathyroidism requires knowledge of the family history, laboratory values and genetic testing [52]. The difference is an important one, as primary hyperparathyroidism responds to surgery, but FHH does not.

Management of primary hyperparathyroidism

The gold standard of treatment and the only hope of cure is surgical parathyroidectomy. Techniques vary, based on the experience of the surgeon and the nature of the disease process. Preoperative imaging has altered the surgical management. Following detection of a solitary parathyroid adenoma, patients can be offered minimally invasive resection under local or general anaesthesia in a day case setting. However, in biochemical terms, there are several pharmacological treatments which can first be of benefit to patients, either to optimise their surgical management or in lieu of surgery if it is declined or the patient is unfit.

Calcimimetics

Cinacalcet is a phenylalkylamine compound, and as a calcimimetic agent is a relative newcomer among drug treatments for hyperparathyroidism. By allosteric modulation of the transmembrane domains of the calcium-sensing receptor (Figure 3.3), it is able to enhance the sensitivity of the receptor to calcium. This reduces the output of PTH from the parathyroid chief cell. Most of the data supporting its use is in secondary hyperparathyroidism, but evidence is emerging of its usefulness in primary hyperparathyroidism [53, 54].

Bisphosphonates

These are pyrophosphate analogues which reduce bone resorption by inhibition of osteoclastic activity. They have been shown to improve bone mineral density with very few side effects. *Pamidronate* has been part of the standard treatment of severe hypercalcaemia for many years. *Alendronate* and the more potent *risedronate* are currently in use for the treatment of osteoporosis from any cause, but studies have highlighted their potential importance in the medical treatment of hyperparathyroidism [54].

The practice of withholding bisphosphonates prior to parathyroidectomy is controversial. Some point out the risk of bisphosphonates contributing to postoperative hypocalcaemia [54, 55]. However, severe post-parathyroidectomy hypocalcaemia is not only due to limiting the contribution from bone to the level of circulating calcium. It can be due to postoperative 'hungry bone syndrome', an important complication in which there is augmented uptake of calcium into bone for rapid mineralisation of the excessive amounts of osteoid tissue and to support osteoblast activity to repair resorption cavities. Several case reports and small studies show a protective effect of bisphosphonates against this enhanced osteoclastic activity [56, 57].

Other medical treatments and lifestyle modifications

Correction of any concurrent vitamin D deficiency is important in hyperparathyroidism. Vitamin D amplifies the expression of the gene encoding the calcium-sensing receptor and therefore suppresses the release of PTH. Oestrogen replacement and the oestrogen receptor modulator *raloxifene* also may be of benefit in postmenopausal women with primary hyperparathyroidism, by lowering serum calcium levels and markers of bone turnover [58].

Additional measures include regular exercise to minimise bone resorption and avoidance of hypovolaemia which would exacerbate any hypercalcaemia and nephrolithiasis. Certain drug therapies can exacerbate the effects of hyperparathyroidism. Thiazide diuretics enhance renal calcium reabsorption and should be avoided. Although the dihydropyridine class of calcium channel antagonists has been shown to block the calcium channels inserted by PTH in the kidney [29], a single dose of nifedipine was demonstrated to increase the level of circulating PTH in healthy volunteers [59]. The effects of calcium channel blockade in hyperparathyroidism have not yet been fully elucidated.

Secondary hyperparathyroidism

Hypocalcaemia from causes other than hypoparathyroidism, such as malabsorption or calcium or vitamin D deficiency, will trigger an increase in PTH levels. This is true secondary hyperparathyroidism, and treating the underlying cause will correct the hyperparathyroidism. Chronic renal failure can give rise to hyperparathyroidism from a more complex disease mechanism, which is more severe and more difficult to treat than other forms of secondary hyperparathyroidism.

Renal hyperparathyroidism

In this condition, hypocalcaemia occurs due to reduced calcium reabsorption in the diseased nephron as well as an inability to activate vitamin D in the diseased kidney, leading to a decreased absorption of dietary calcium. The parathyroid glands are stimulated to produce more PTH in an attempt to redress the imbalance. Hyperphosphataemia, due to declining glomerular filtration rate and renal phosphate retention, also stimulates parathyroid gland activity both indirectly, via further reductions in plasma calcium, and directly. The parathyroid glands hypertrophy. Left untreated, the production and release of PTH becomes uncoupled from the level of circulating calcium and proceeds autonomously. This was previously considered as a separate entity known as *tertiary hyperparathyroidism*. Standard medical treatments such as phosphate binders and vitamin D have often been tried before patients with renal hyperparathyroidism present for parathyroidectomy. Calcimimetic agents may also be used [60].

Fibroblast growth factor 23 (FGF23) and Klotho

Recently, there has been considerable development in the understanding of the mechanism of the disease process in secondary hyperparathyroidism. *FGF23* is a protein produced mainly in bone that has phosphaturic actions analogous to PTH in that both inhibit phosphate reabsorption in the proximal convoluted tubule. But they have opposing actions on renal activation of vitamin D: PTH promotes activation of vitamin D and thereby increases calcium absorption, whereas FGF23 inhibits the 1 hydroxylase enzyme [61].

Klotho is a membrane protein found in several tissues, including the parathyroids, pituitary and brain, but mainly in the kidney. It appears to enhance the binding of FGF23 to its receptor, and Klotho deficiency is associated with a significant increase in the plasma level of FGF23.

The primary process leading from renal failure to hyperparathyroidism seems to include these two factors. Chronic kidney disease leads to reduction in renal expression of Klotho and increased circulating levels of FGF23. The FGF23 levels are also raised in response to the hyperphosphataemia. The FGF23 then exerts its phosphaturic effect and inhibits the hydroxylation of vitamin D.

Medical management

In many patients, secondary hyperparathyroidism can be managed pharmacologically. Traditional medical treatment focused on the deficiency of vitamin D due to the renal disease and the resultant increase in circulating PTH concentrations. Vitamin D and its analogues were the first line treatment. The goal is to suppress further release of PTH. This is problematic as vitamin D also raises serum phosphate levels in the present of pre-existing hyperphosphataemia [62]. Additional therapies have included regulation of phosphate levels, either through limitation of dietary intake or through the use of phosphate binding agents. Several of these drugs have limitations: the aluminium-containing phosphate binders are avoided because of aluminium toxicity, and those containing calcium have been associated with hypercalcaemia, especially when taken with vitamin D [63]. Several recent studies adding the calcimimetic cinacalcet to the standard therapies have shown beneficial results in terms of PTH levels and calcium and phosphate regulation. No studies have been reported as yet with cinacalcet as the sole therapy [62].

Parathyroidectomy

There are several options available to the surgeon and the patient, depending upon their personal preference and the underlying pathology. In the past, a solitary adenoma could only be diagnosed histologically, rather than preoperatively. Surgical cure required bilateral neck exploration unless a large adenoma was discovered early in the procedure. Similarly, in multiglandular hyperplasia, resection of a large, predominantparathyroid gland may allow the remaining glands to shrink to normal size. But if the underlying reason for the hyperplasia is untreated, as in uraemic hyperparathyroidism, the remaining glands may become hyperplastic again over time, requiring re-operation. Controversy regarding the surgical management of renal hyperparathyroidism also exists: should a subtotal parathyroidectomy be undertaken leaving a small glandular remnant in the neck; or a total parathyroidectomy with autotransplantation

of glandular tissue into the forearm muscles? Total parathyroidectomy without autotransplantation can lead to adynamic bone disease and the need for long term calcium and vitamin D supplementation. However, reimplantation is rarely successful as revascularisation of the transplanted gland is not always established.

Surgical approaches

The classical incision for parathyroidectomy involving bilateral neck exploration is the transverse, midline cervicotomy used for thyroidectomy, and is optimal for patients with multigland disease (hyperplasia) or multiple adenomata. An alternative is a bilateral oblique approach. In this method, two symmetrical incisions are made above and lateral to the head of the clavicle [64]. This approach is also suitable for unilateral parathyroidectomy, which can easily be carried out under local anaesthesia, and results in reduced postoperative pain as incision through muscle is unnecessary.

Minimally invasive parathyroidectomy involves the use of small (10–12 mm) incisions through a lateral oblique approach or isolated incisions directly over the site of the parathyroid glands. It is only feasible for resection of small, pre-localised adenomas, but it is an attractive, safe option in the hands of an experienced endocrine surgeon. Other approaches for small adenomas include endoscopic parathyroidectomy. The endoscope can be inserted above the sternal notch or laterally; gas insufflation and multiple trochars are used through several small incisions. Severe and prolonged subcutaneous emphysema has been reported using this technique [65], but limiting insufflation under the strap muscles to 3–4 minutes at a time with pressures of no more than 12 mm Hg should reduce the likelihood of this adverse event. The use of xenon rather than carbon dioxide for insufflation may also be helpful in this regard. Repeat surgery is often complicated by marked fibrosis from the initial endoscopic surgery. Exploration of the neck in video-assisted parathyroidectomy involves insertion of a 5 mm scope via a small central or lateral incision. No gas is insufflated and surgical access is maintained by the use of small retractors. This can be particularly useful for glands lying in the upper chest [66]. Only rarely is thoracotomy or thoracoscopy required for excision of parathyroid tumours.

Preoperative localisation

The advent of new imaging modalities has allowed surgeons to offer localised surgery with limited dissection for some patients. There are several options, and

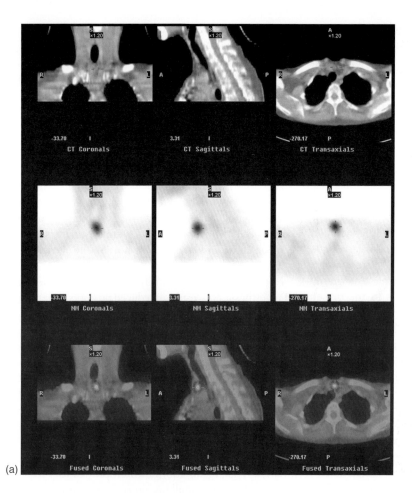

Fig. 3.4 (a) SPECT-MIBI localisation study of parathyroid adenoma showing the CT images, the scintigraphic images and the digitally fused result.

(a)

often multiple imaging modalities are used in the same patient [67]. This brings the advantages of reduced postoperative pain, a better cosmetic result, a shortened duration of surgery and a reduced hospital stay; for some patients the operation can then be undertaken as a day case procedure.

Ultrasonography of the neck is the most convenient method and can identify up to 90% of large parathyroid adenomas [68], though glands within the mediastinum will not be identified, and the smaller adenomas can prove elusive with this technique. Normal glands cannot be seen.

Both CT and MRI are more labour-intensive and costly than cervical ultrasound and may only have a similar accuracy [69], with normal glands again not easily detectable. They are particularly useful in the case of a mediastinal parathyroid adenoma, or detecting those glands lying in the tracheo-oesophageal groove.

Venous sampling combined with rapid PTH assay or arteriography can be used preoperatively to map the blood supply to the neck. This is usually reserved for patients requiring re-operation, and embolisation of vessels may be an alternative to surgery.

Radionuclide isotope scanning of the parathyroid glands has become the mainstay of preoperative localisation of parathyroid adenomas. The isotope used is Sestamibi radio-labelled with technetium 99m, which is taken up by parathyroid tissue. This isotope also has a role in myocardial perfusion studies (Figure 3.4) [70, 71]. This technique has become more advanced with the advent of *single photon emission computed tomography (SPECT)* in which the gamma camera rotates around the patient in a manner similar to a conventional CT. Additionally, the SPECT images can be overlayed on traditional CT images to display an accurate anatomical and functional, three-dimensional representation of the neck or mediastinum.

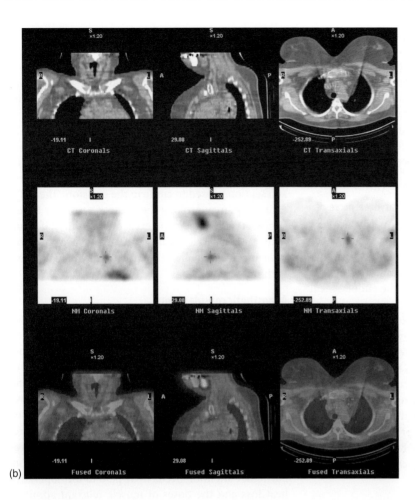

(b)

Fig. 3.4 (b) In this study, the parathyroid adenoma is highlighted in the mediastinum. Images courtesy of Dr L. Smith, Royal Liverpool University Hospital, Department of Nuclear Medicine.

Localisation studies are especially important in the case of re-operation for incomplete resection. Imaging studies may highlight a hitherto undiscovered ectopic gland, for example buried within the thyroid gland or deep in the mediastinum. The latter case may warrant referral to a thoracic surgical unit. Four-dimensional computed tomography (4D-CT) is an emerging imaging modality in which dynamic scanning is carried out in conjunction with contrast enhancement. This technique may prove valuable prior to re-operation [72].

The surgical management of renal hyperparathyroidism benefits very little from initial preoperative localisation. In these cases, all the glands are likely to be hyperplastic and scintigraphy may not differentiate between them. All the parathyroid tissue will need to be resected and there is thus less scope for minimising the operation. Reimplantation of parathyroid gland is rarely practised in these patients.

Intraoperative monitoring and localisation of the parathyroid glands

Methylene blue

Preoperative intravenous infusion of methylene blue was used to identify the parathyroid glands, and in open or minimally invasive surgery the operative times can be reduced. However, there have been several reports of neurological symptoms in patients receiving methylene blue up to 7.5 mg kg^{-1} [73], and delayed recovery when total intravenous anaesthesia (TIVA) has also been used [74]. Lower doses of methylene blue still allow glands to be identified, and this remains an aid to surgery in many centres.

Gamma probe

Radio-guided parathyroidectomy identifies the adenoma following injection of technetium 99m Sestamibi 1–4 hours prior to surgery. Surgeons use a hand-held gamma counter probe and counts are obtained in all four quadrants of the neck prior to skin incision, and then again after incision, below the strap muscles. Care is needed to avoid detection of radioactivity from the heart, and surgical exploration is undertaken where the counts are highest. This can reduce operative time. Radioactivity of the removed gland can be checked. This technique has not been widely embraced by experienced endocrine surgeons because of the risks involved [75].

Intraoperative identification of the recurrent laryngeal nerve

Recurrent and superior laryngeal nerve palsy rates vary depending on the skill of the surgeon, but should occur in less than 1% of cases following thyroid or parathyroid surgery. Intraoperative nerve monitoring is now widely available. A sensor placed on the endotracheal tube at the level of the vocal cords detects muscle contraction when the nerve is compressed or intentionally stimulated, giving an audible and visual signal confirming the nerve's integrity. This technique requires an unparalysed, intubated patient. A remifentanil infusion technique is useful if intraoperative nerve monitoring is to be undertaken, facilitating a good recovery and short hospital stay. Preoperative nasendoscopy should be considered as part of the preoperative assessment, especially in those patients who are having revision surgery, to document any pre-existing vocal cord palsy.

Intraoperative monitoring of parathyroid hormone

The availability of a rapid assay of intact parathyroid hormone (iPTH) has had a significant impact upon surgical treatment. Baseline venous samples are taken preoperatively and compared with intraoperative samples. Intraoperatively, samples are taken before excision of the glands and again after it. A reduction in iPTH values of more than 50% suggests that all hyperfunctioning parathyroid tissue has been excised [76]. There is no consensus as to the optimal site for venous sampling: some clinicians recommend peripheral sampling but others choose central venous sampling (with or without peripheral sampling) directly via the operative site and usually from the internal jugular veins.

The time interval between excision and sampling has also been disputed. While a decrease in iPTH levels of 50% within 5 minutes suggests an adequate parathyroidectomy, some clinicians aim for a return of the iPTH to within the normal range [77]. Central venous sampling gives higher values of iPTH, so those surgeons who prefer this measurement and a return to the normal range find that an interval of 15–30 minutes is required [78]. Certainly, in patients with chronic renal impairment, correct interpretation of post-resection iPTH necessitates an interval of 20–30 minutes to maintain accuracy [76]. Some surgeons consider that iPTH assay adds little to their ability to remove hyper-secreting tissue, particularly if frozen section is used to confirm the excision. The iPTH estimation may prolong the operative time, or falsely suggest that further gland excision is required if insufficient time has been allowed to lapse before sampling. Total intravenous anaesthesia techniques can interfere with this assay [79].

Anaesthetic considerations

Patients with primary hyperparathyroidism are often elderly with co-morbidities, and there continue to be a few deaths each year in the UK associated with parathyroid surgery. With preoperative localisation of adenomata and minimally invasive surgery, there is a trend to same day discharge of patients and more procedures being undertaken under local anaesthesia. However, the precise duration of surgery can be difficult to predict when intraoperative blood tests or pathology frozen section results are guiding the surgical dissection. Particular attention needs to be paid to intraoperative heat loss and the doses of muscle relaxant administered. Hypercalcaemia increases the requirement for non-depolarising muscle relaxants due to potentiation of presynaptic acetycholine release at the neuromuscular junction. Reduced duration of action of rocuronium has been reported in a normocalcaemic patient with hyperparathyroidism [80]. Routine monitoring of neuromuscular block during parathyroidectomy is advisable.

As for thyroid surgery, the anaesthetised patient should be placed in reverse Trendelenburg position (to minimise venous filling in the neck), with the neck carefully extended, especially in the elderly, and symmetry of the upper body maintained. The orbits should be protected and the head is supported on a ring with a 'sand bag' placed between the shoulder blades. Intravenous access is required throughout for fluid and drug administration, even during local anaesthesia, although major bleeding is only rarely encountered. As hyperparathyroidism is associated with an osmotic polyuria, adequate hydration with crystalloids is always necessary perioperatively, and intravenous fluids may be required preoperatively. If intraoperative PTH assay is to be undertaken, access may be required to a lower limb for venous sampling. Tracheal intubation may not always be necessary as minimally invasive surgery precludes marked retraction of the trachea and larynx, and a laryngeal mask airway may be appropriate for some patients.

Anaesthetists may be asked to simulate a Valsalva manoeuvre with the patient in a 'head down' position prior to wound closure to assess haemostasis. As patients only have mild to moderate pain postoperatively, nausea and vomiting are the major source of discomfort and should be avoided. Retching also increases the risk of postoperative bleeding, with a neck haematoma potentially causing airway obstruction and increasing the risk of recurrent laryngeal nerve palsy.

As adverse outcome events are rare, studies to date have not shown any differences between local and general (volatile or TIVA-based) anaesthetic techniques for parathyroidectomy. Local anaesthetic techniques can be employed unilaterally or bilaterally, with superficial rather than deep cervical plexus blocks, and many centres only use local infiltration by the surgical team. Surgical supplementation of regional anaesthesia is required for retraction of the upper pole of the thyroid when deep or superficial cervical block has been performed. Local anaesthetic techniques are usually accompanied by intravenous sedation [81].

Calcium supplementation is usually required postoperatively, and serum calcium is measured the evening after surgery and then the following day. Patients may become symptomatic with calcium concentrations within the normal range if levels drop rapidly. Short hospital stays are possible for solitary adenoma following minimally invasive surgery performed by a skilled surgeon who is confident not to insert drains or to remove them early, combined with a well-motivated patient. Those patients discharged early are instructed to take oral calcium supplements (up to 3 g per day) and to represent to hospital if they become symptomatic. This is safe practice where patients are discharged to adjacent hotel facilities, but in the UK one postoperative night as an inpatient is usual. Patients with renal parathyroid disease are more likely to require intravenous calcium supplementation and a longer duration of hospital stay [82].

References

1. Dubose J, Ragsdale T, Morvant J. 'Bodies so tiny': the history of parathyroid surgery. *Curr Sci* 2005; **62**: 91–5.
2. Carney JA. The glandulae parathyroideae of Ivar Sandstrom. Contributions from two continents. *Am J Surg Pathol* 1996; **20**: 1123–44.
3. Wang C. The anatomic basis of parathyroid surgery. *Ann Surg* 1976; **183**: 271–5.
4. Nanka O, Sedy J, Vitkova I, Libansky P, Adamek S. Surgical anatomy of parathyroid glands with emphasis on parathyroidectomy. *Prague Med Rep* 2006; **107**: 261–72.
5. Sadler TW, Langman J. *Langman's Medical Embryology*. Philadelphia, Lippincott Williams & Wilkins, 2006, pp. 261–4.
6. Xu P, Zheng W, Laclef C, et al. Eya1 is required for the morphogenesis of mammalian thymus, parathyroid and thyroid. *Development* 2002; **129**: 3033–44.
7. Mihai R, Farndon JR. Parathyroid disease and calcium metabolism. *Br J Anaesth* 2000; **85**: 29–43.
8. Gordon J, Wilson VA, Blair NF, et al. Functional evidence for a single endodermal origin for the thymic epithelium. *Nat Immunol* 2004; **5**: 546–53.
9. Graham A, Okabe M, Quinlan R. The role of the endoderm in the development and evolution of the pharyngeal arches. *J Anat* 2005; **207**: 479–87.
10. Cinti S, Sbarbati A. Ultrastructure of human parathyroid cells in health and disease. *Microsc Res Tech* 1995; **32**: 164–79.
11. Brewer HBJ, Fairwell T, Ronan R, Sizemore GW, Arnaud CD. Human parathyroid hormone: amino-acid sequence of the amino-terminal residues 1–34. *Proc Natl Acad Sci U S A* 1972; **69**: 3585–8.
12. Ganong W. *Review of Medical Physiology*. New York, McGraw-Hill Medical, 2005, pp. 390–1.
13. Gomperts B. *Signal Transduction*. Boston, Academic Press, 2003, pp. 56.
14. Kifor O, Kifor I, Brown EM. Signal transduction in the parathyroid. *Curr Opin Nephrol Hypertens* 2002; **11**: 397–402.
15. Chen RA, Goodman WG. Role of the calcium-sensing receptor in parathyroid gland physiology. *Am J Physiol Renal Physiol* 2004; **286**: 1005–11.
16. Brown EM, MacLeod RJ. Extracellular calcium sensing and extracellular calcium signaling. *Physiol Rev* 2001; **81**: 239–97.
17. Vetter T, Lohse MJ. Magnesium and the parathyroid. *Curr Opin Nephrol Hypertens* 2002; **11**: 403–10.
18. Shoback D. Clinical practice. Hypoparathyroidism. *N Engl J Med* 2008; **359**: 391–403.
19. Brown EM, Gamba G, Riccardi D, et al. Cloning and characterization of an extracellular Ca2+-sensing

receptor from bovine parathyroid. *Nature* 1993; **366**(6455): 575–80.

20. Brown EM. Calcium receptor and regulation of parathyroid hormone secretion. *Rev Endocr Metab Disord* 2000; **1**: 307–15.

21. Anderson P, May B, Morris H. Vitamin D metabolism: new concepts and clinical implications. *Clin Biochem Rev* 2003; **24**: 13–26.

22. Malluche HH, Koszewski N, Monier-Faugere MC, Williams JP, Mawad H. Influence of the parathyroid glands on bone metabolism. *Eur J Clin Invest* 2006; **36** Suppl 2: 23–33.

23. Talmage RV, Mobley HT. Calcium homeostasis: reassessment of the actions of parathyroid hormone. *Gen Comp Endocrinol* 2008; **156**: 1–8.

24. Poole KES, Reeve J. Parathyroid hormone – a bone anabolic and catabolic agent. *Curr Opin Pharmacol* 2005; **5**: 612–17.

25. Brunette MG, Hilal G, Mailloux J, Leclerc M. G proteins regulate calcium channels in the luminal membranes of the rabbit nephron. *Nephron* 2000; **85**: 238–47.

26. Suki W. Calcium transport in the nephron. *Am J Physiol* 1979; **237**: F1–6.

27. Friedman PA, Coutermarsh BA, Kennedy SM, Gesek FA. Parathyroid hormone stimulation of calcium transport is mediated by dual signaling mechanisms involving protein kinase A and protein kinase C. *Endocrinology* 1996; **137**: 13–20.

28. Lau K, Bourdeau JE. Parathyroid hormone action in calcium transport in the distal nephron. *Curr Opin Nephrol Hypertens* 1995; **4**: 55–63.

29. Bacskai BJ, Friedman PA. Activation of latent Ca2+ channels in renal epithelial cells by parathyroid hormone. *Nature* 1990; **347**(6291): 388–91.

30. Akhter S, Kutuzova GD, Christakos S, DeLuca HF. Calbindin D9k is not required for 1,25-dihydroxyvitamin D3-mediated Ca2+ absorption in small intestine. *Arch Biochem Biophys* 2007; **460**: 227–32.

31. Lee G, Lee K, Choi K, et al. Phenotype of a calbindin-D9k gene knockout is compensated for by the induction of other calcium transporter genes in a mouse model. *J Bone Miner Res* 2007; **22**: 1968–78.

32. Nemere I, Larsson D. Does PTH have a direct effect on intestine. *J Cell Biochem* 2002; **86**: 29–34.

33. Tenenhouse HS. Phosphate transport: molecular basis, regulation and pathophysiology. *J Steroid Biochem Mol Biol* 2007; **103**(3–5): 572–7.

34. Nemere I. Parathyroid hormone rapidly stimulates phosphate transport in perfused duodenal loops of chicks: lack of modulation by vitamin D metabolites. *Endocrinology* 1996; **137**: 3750–5.

35. Gensure RC, Gardella TJ, Juppner H. Parathyroid hormone and parathyroid hormone-related peptide, and their receptors. *Biochem Biophys Res Commun* 2005; **328**: 666–78.

36. Shprintzen RJ. Velo-cardio-facial syndrome: 30 years of study. *Dev Disabil Res Rev* 2008; **14**: 3–10.

37. Hieronimus S, Bec-Roche M, Pedeutour F, et al. The spectrum of parathyroid gland dysfunction associated with the microdeletion 22q11. *Eur J Endocrinol* 2006; **155**: 47–52.

38. Marx SJ. Hyperparathyroid and hypoparathyroid disorders. *N Engl J Med* 2000; **343**: 1863–75.

39. Erbil Y, Barbaros U, Issever H, et al. Predictive factors for recurrent laryngeal nerve palsy and hypoparathyroidism after thyroid surgery. *Clin Otolaryngol* 2007; **32**: 32–7.

40. Asari R, Passler C, Kaczirek K, Scheuba C, Niederle B. Hypoparathyroidism after total thyroidectomy: a prospective study. *Arch Surg* 2008; **143**: 132–7.

41. Heath D, Marx SJ. *Calcium Disorders.* London/Boston, Butterworth Scientific, 1982, p. 104.

42. Griffin J. *Textbook of Endocrine Physiology.* Oxford, Oxford University Press, 2004, p. 370.

43. Fuleihan GE, Rubeiz N. Dermatologic manifestations of parathyroid-related disorders. *Clin Dermatol* 2006; **24**: 281–8.

44. Horwitz MJ, Stewart AF. Hypoparathyroidism: is it time for replacement therapy. *J Clin Endocrinol Metab* 2008; **93**: 3307–9.

45. Winer KK, Sinaii N, Peterson D, Sainz BJ, Cutler GBJ. Effects of once versus twice-daily parathyroid hormone 1–34 therapy in children with hypoparathyroidism. *J Clin Endocrinol Metab* 2008; **93**: 3389–95.

46. Winer KK, Ko CW, Reynolds JC, et al. Long-term treatment of hypoparathyroidism: a randomized controlled study comparing parathyroid hormone-(1–34) versus calcitriol and calcium. *J Clin Endocrinol Metab* 2003; **88**: 4214–20.

47. Winer KK, Yanovski JA, Sarani B, Cutler GBJ. A randomized, cross-over trial of once-daily versus twice-daily parathyroid hormone 1–34 in treatment of hypoparathyroidism. *J Clin Endocrinol Metab* 1998; **83**: 3480–6.

48. Bilezikian JP, Silverberg SJ. Clinical spectrum of primary hyperparathyroidism. *Rev Endocr Metab Disord* 2000; **1**: 237–45.

49. Falchetti A, Marini F, Luzi E, Tonelli F, Brandt ML. Multiple endocrine neoplasms. *Best Pract Res Clin Rheumatol* 2008; **22**: 149–63.

50. Andersson P, Rydberg E, Willenheimer R. Primary hyperparathyroidism and heart disease – a review. *Eur Heart J* 2004; **25**: 1776–87.

51. Glendenning P. Diagnosis of primary hyperparathyroidism: controversies, practical issues and the need for Australian guidelines. *Intern Med J* 2003; **33**: 598–603.

52. Raue F, Frank-Raue K. Primary hyperparathyroidism – what the nephrologist should know – an update. *Nephrol Dial Transplant* 2007; **22**: 696–9.

53. Dong BJ. Cinacalcet: An oral calcimimetic agent for the management of hyperparathyroidism. *Clin Ther* 2005; **27**: 1725–51.

54. Mosekilde L. Primary hyperparathyroidism and the skeleton. *Clin Endocrinol (Oxf)* 2008; **69**: 1–19.

55. Phitayakorn R, McHenry CR. Hyperparathyroid crisis: use of bisphosphonates as a bridge to parathyroidectomy. *J Am Coll Surg* 2008; **206**: 1106–15.

56. Gurevich Y, Poretsky L. Possible prevention of hungry bone syndrome following parathyroidectomy by preoperative use of pamidronate. *Otolaryngol Head Neck Surg* 2008; **138**: 403–4.

57. Lee I, Sheu WH, Tu S, Kuo S, Pei D. Bisphosphonate pretreatment attenuates hungry bone syndrome postoperatively in subjects with primary hyperparathyroidism. *J Bone Miner Metab* 2006; **24**: 255–8.

58. Farford B, Presutti RJ, Moraghan TJ. Nonsurgical management of primary hyperparathyroidism. *Mayo Clin Proc* 2007; **82**: 351–5.

59. Wynne AG, Romanski SA, Klee GG, Ory SJ, O' Fallon WM, Fitzpatrick LA. Nifedipine, but not verapamil, acutely elevates parathyroid hormone levels in premenopausal women. *Clin Endocrinol (Oxf)* 1995; **42**: 9–15.

60. Elder GJ. Parathyroidectomy in the calcimimetic era. *Nephrology (Carlton)* 2005; **10**: 511–15.

61. Stubbs J, Liu S, Quarles LD. Role of fibroblast growth factor 23 in phosphate homeostasis and pathogenesis of disordered mineral metabolism in chronic kidney disease. *Semin Dial* 2007; **20**: 302–8.

62. Wetmore J, Quarles L. Calcimimetics or vitamin D analogs for suppressing parathyroid hormone in end-stage renal disease: time for a paradigm shift. *Nat Clin Pract Nephrol* 2009; **5**: 24–33.

63. de Francisco ALM. New strategies for the treatment of hyperparathyroidism incorporating calcimimetics. *Expert Opin Pharmacother* 2008; **9**: 795–811.

64. Chaffanjon PC, Brichon PY, Sarrazin R. Bilateral oblique approach to parathyroid glands. *Ann Surg* 2000; **231**: 25–30.

65. Reeve TS, Babidge WJ, Parkyn RF, et al. Minimally invasive surgery for primary hyperparathyroidism: systematic review. *Arch Surg* 2000; **135**: 481–7.

66. Miccoli P. Minimally invasive surgery for thyroid and parathyroid diseases. *Surg Endosc* 2002; **16**: 3–6.

67. Shah S, Win Z, Al-Nahhas A. Multimodality imaging of the parathyroid glands in primary hyperparathyroidism. *Minerva Endocrinol* 2008; **33**: 193–202.

68. Shaheen F, Chowdry N, Gojwari T, Wani A, Khan S. Role of cervical ultrasonography in primary hyperparathyroidism. *Indian J Radiol Imaging* 2008; **18**: 302–5.

69. Kabala JE. Computed tomography and magnetic resonance imaging in diseases of the thyroid and parathyroid. *Eur J Radiol* 2008; **66**: 480–92.

70. Maddahi J, Kiat H, Van Train KF, et al. Myocardial perfusion imaging with technetium-99m Sestamibi SPECT in the evaluation of coronary artery disease. *Am J Cardiol* 1990; **66**: 55E–62E.

71. Borley NR, Collins RE, O' Doherty M, Coakley A. Technetium-99m Sestamibi parathyroid localization is accurate enough for scan-directed unilateral neck exploration. *Br J Surg* 1996; **83**: 989–91.

72. Mortenson MM, Evans DB, Lee JE, et al. Parathyroid exploration in the reoperative neck: improved preoperative localization with 4D-computed tomography. *J Am Coll Surg* 2008; **206**: 888–95.

73. Majithia A, Stearns MP. Methylene blue toxicity following infusion to localize parathyroid adenoma. *J Laryngol Otol* 2006; **120**: 138–40.

74. Licker M, Diaper J, Robert J, Ellenberger C. Effects of methylene blue on propofol requirement during anaesthesia induction and surgery. *Anaesthesia* 2008; **63**: 352–7.

75. Sitges-Serra A, Rosa P, Valero M, Membrilla E, Sancho JJ. Surgery for sporadic primary hyperparathyroidism: controversies and evidence-based approach. *Langenbecks Arch Surg* 2008; **393**: 239–44.

76. Pellitteri PK. The role of intraoperative measurement of parathyroid hormone in parathyroid surgery. *ORL J Otorhinolaryngol Relat Spec* 2008; **70**: 319–30.

77. Inabnet WB. Intraoperative parathyroid hormone monitoring. *World J Surg* 2004; **28**: 1212–15.

78. Beyer TD, Chen E, Ata A, DeCresce R, Prinz RA, Solorzano CC. A prospective evaluation of the effect of sample collection site on intraoperative parathormone monitoring during parathyroidectomy. *Surgery* 2008; **144**: 504–9.

79. Sokoll LJ, Drew H, Udelsman R. Intraoperative parathyroid hormone analysis: A study of 200 consecutive cases. *Clin Chem* 2000; **46**: 1662–8.

80. Munir MA, Jaffar M, Arshad M, Akhter MS, Zhang J. Reduced duration of muscle relaxation with

rocuronium in a normocalcaemic hyperparathyroid patient. *Can J Anaesth* 2003; **50**: 558–61.

81. Pintaric TS, Hocevar M, Jereb S, Casati A, Jankovic VN. A prospective, randomized comparison between combined (deep and superficial) and superficial cervical plexus block with levobupivacaine for minimally invasive parathyroidectomy. *Anesth Analg* 2007; **105**: 1160–3.

82. Mittendorf EA, Merlino JI, McHenry CR. Post-parathyroidectomy hypocalcemia: incidence, risk factors, and management. *Am Surg* 2004; **70**: 114–19.

83. Suliburk JW, Perrier ND. Primary hyperparathyroidism. *Oncologist* 2007; **12**: 644–53.

Adrenal disease: cortex and medulla

Charles S. Reilly

The adrenal glands are located at the upper margin (antero-superior) of the kidneys about the level of the 12th thoracic vertebra. They are composed of two functional parts, the medulla and the cortex.

The medulla is essentially an integral part of the sympathetic nervous system containing chromaffin cells which produce catecholamines. The cells receive pre-ganglionic sympathetic nerve fibres and are, functionally, modified sympathetic ganglia. The cells synthesise catecholamines (epinephrine [adrenaline], norepinephrine [noradrenaline] and dopamine) which are released systemically into their rich blood supply in response to sympathetic stimulation (fight or flight).

The cortex surrounds the medulla and can be divided functionally into three zones. Progressing in from the outer capsule is the *zona glomerulosa* which produces mineralocorticoids (aldosterone), then the *zona fascicularis* which produces glucocorticoids (cortisol) and finally the *zona reticularis* which produces androgens.

All the adrenocortical hormones share a common stem for synthesis from cholesterol which is converted in the mitochondria to pregnenolone (Figure 4.1). Subsequently, dehydrogenation produces progesterone which is the precursor for the gluco- and mineralocorticoids. Hydroxylation of pregnenolone produces the precursors of the androgens.

The mineralocorticoids, principally aldosterone, are produced in the zona glomerulosa. They have a homeostatic role in the control of blood volume and the body's sodium and potassium content. Aldosterone promotes renal sodium and water retention and potassium loss. Secretion of aldosterone is controlled by the renin-angiotensin system. Renin is released by the juxta-glomerular apparatus in the kidney in response to a variety of stimuli including hypotension, hyponatraemia and hyperkalaemia. Renin converts angiotensinogen to angiotensin I that is converted in the lung capillaries to the active component angiotensin II. Angiotensin II stimulates aldosterone secretion. Adrenocorticotrophic hormone (ACTH) also produces some increase in aldosterone secretion.

The primary glucocorticoid is cortisol. It has a wide range of essential metabolic and homeostatic effects which are essential for life – bilateral adrenalectomy without replacement of cortisol would result in death within a few days. It has key roles in protein, lipid and carbohydrate metabolism including gluconeogenesis and lipolysis. It also has important roles in response to inflammation and allergy. Secretion is controlled by ACTH which is released from the anterior pituitary. In turn ACTH is controlled by corticotrophin releasing hormone which is released from the hypothalamus as part of the circadian rhythm (high in the morning, low in the evening) and in response to physical or emotional stress. Circulating cortisol produces a negative feedback mechanism for this system.

Androgens are produced in the zona reticularis in males and females. The hormones produced include androstenedione and dehydroepiandrosterone (Figure 4.1). Adrenal hyperplasia and androgen-secreting adenomas can result in excess circulating androgens.

Disease processes of the adrenal glands that may require surgical intervention result from excessive secretion of one or more of these hormones. A secretory tumour of the medulla is known as a phaeochromocytoma, which produces high circulating concentrations of catecholamines. In the cortex, benign secretory adenomas can produce cortisol resulting in high circulating levels (Cushing's disease) or secrete aldosterone (Conn's syndrome).

These three conditions (phaeochromocytoma, Conn's and Cushing's) may present for surgery to remove the tumour and each present specific anaesthetic problems which will be dealt with in this chapter.

Core Topics in Endocrinology in Anaesthesia and Critical Care, eds. George M. Hall, Jennifer M. Hunter and Mark S. Cooper. Published by Cambridge University Press. © Cambridge University Press 2010.

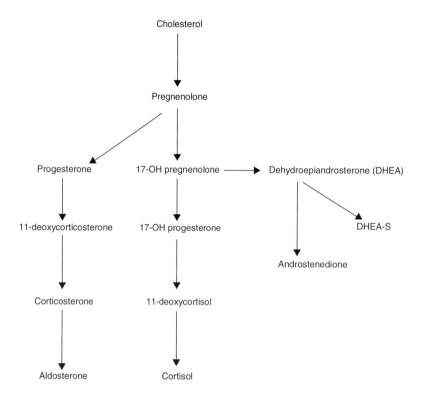

Fig. 4.1 Adrenal steroid synthesis.

The number of adrenal masses presenting for surgery may be increasing as they are detected during imaging studies done for other, non-adrenal, problems. These fortuitously found masses have been given the rather clumsy label of 'incidentalomas'. Adrenal masses are found as incidental findings at autopsy in up to 8% in some studies and the incidence appears to increase with age. Some recent imaging studies have had incidences as high as 4% if small (< 1 cm) masses are included [1]. A strategy for subsequent investigation of these patients to determine whether these are secretory or malignant masses which may require surgical intervention has been described [1]. Primary adrenal carcinoma is rare, but the rate in incidentalomas increases with increasing size of the detected mass, with some series quoting 25% of masses > 6 cm being malignant.

Surgery for adrenal disease

A laparoscopic approach was first used in the early 1990s and it has now become the standard surgical technique for adrenalectomy. Initially, an upper-size limit of 6 cm diameter masses was used [2], but with wider experience masses up to 15 cm have been resected by this route. A review of the laparoscopic approach for adrenalectomy analysed techniques and outcome of the larger published studies [3]. The authors found that the transperitoneal approach was still the most widely used with the retroperitoneal route second. In over 2500 patients from a total of 19 published studies, average operative time was about 140 minutes with a blood loss averaging 80 ml. Complication rates varied from 3 to 15%, with bleeding accounting for 40% of these. Conversion to an open approach ranged from 0–13% (mean 2%).

Phaeochromocytoma

Phaeochromocytoma is a rare tumour which is estimated to have an incidence in a general population of 1 in 1.5–2.0 million per year. It accounts for a very small number (< 0.6%) of patients presenting at clinic with hypertension [4]. It can present at any age (a range from neonates [5] through to 75+ years has been described) but is commonest in the range of 20–50 years and is slightly more common in females than in males. Presentation during pregnancy has been described [6]. Some phaeochromocytoma clearly have a hereditary basis and are linked with disease states including multiple endocrine neoplasia (MEN) type 2 (Chapter 6) and neuroectodermal dysplasias, such as neurofibromatosis, Sturge–Weber syndrome and von Hippel–Lindau syndrome (Table 4.1).

Table 4.1 Syndromes associated with phaeochromocytoma.

Multiple endocrine neoplasia (MEN)
Type 2A (Sipple's syndrome):
Medullary carcinoma of the thyroid
Parathyroid hyperplasia or adenoma
Phaeochromocytoma
Type 2B – MEN type 2A plus:
Mucosal neuromata
Marfanoid habitus
Phaeochromocytoma
Neuroectodermal dysplasias
Neurofibromatosis type 1
Paraganglioma syndromes
Sturge–Weber syndrome
Von Hippel–Lindau syndrome

Table 4.2 Frequency of signs and symptoms (%) of phaeochromocytoma.

Signs	Symptoms (%)
Headache	60–90
Palpitations	50–70
Sweating	55–75
Pallor	40–45
Nausea	20–40
Flushing	10–20
Weight loss	20–40
Tiredness	25–40
Anxiety, panic	20–40
Sustained hypertension	50–60
Paroxysmal hypertension	30
Orthostatic hypotension	10–50
Hyperglycaemia	40

From Lenders et al. [4] with permission.

The majority of phaeochromocytoma arise in the adrenal gland but they can occur in other sites where they may be classified as *paragangliomas*. The majority of other primary sites are within the abdominal cavity and include the para-aortic, mesenteric and pelvic ganglia. However, intrathoracic tumours are well described, as are those arising in the bladder and urogenital tract [7, 8]. The traditional teaching of the '10' rule for phaeochromocytoma suggested that 10% were extra-adrenal, 10% were malignant and 10% bilateral. This, however, with the development of genetic testing, appears to be an underestimate. It has been generally held that around 10% of phaeochromocytoma patients had genetically linked (familial) disease, but recent work suggests that up to 30% of phaeochromocytoma may have a hereditary basis [9], and 5 mutations linked to familial phaeochromocytoma have been identified so far, (Chapter 6). For example, in paraganglioma syndrome, a specific germline mutation in the *SDHB* gene (succinate dehydrogenase complex subunit B) appears to be associated with a higher risk of malignancy and with a poorer prognosis. The hereditary forms have a higher incidence of bilateral tumours and of extra-adrenal primaries, which may occur in up to 20% of these patients, and, in addition, the risk of malignancy may be as high as 40%.

The pattern of incidence is well illustrated by a recent retrospective analysis of a group of 115 American patients with phaeochromocytoma which found that 90 had adrenal tumours, 18 had extra-adrenal sites only, and 7 had both [10]. Of the 115 tumours, 10 were malignant. A total of 29 had familial associated phaeochromocytoma, comprising of 8 with von Hippel–Lindau disease, 17 with MEN2, and 4 with von Recklinghausen's disease.

Presentation and diagnosis

The patient experiences symptoms as a result of the episodic release of catecholamines which is often provoked by minor stimuli. The classic symptoms of headache, sweating, pallor, anxiety and palpitation provoked by stress (exercise, pain, posture) (Table 4.2) occur in only 50% of patients [4]. As the other symptoms are non-specific there may be a considerable delay in diagnosis. There may therefore have to be an index of suspicion in triggering investigations. As mentioned above, there is quite a strong association between MEN type 2, neuroectodermal dysplasias and phaeochromocytoma (Table 4.1). In patients with these conditions, development of any of these symptoms requires immediate investigation. There is an argument for regular screening in these individuals. In the general population, the increased use of imaging techniques has led to an increasing number of adrenal masses being detected during screening. Around 5% of incidentalomas are asymptomatic or undiagnosed phaeochromocytoma, and this unrelated screening accounts for up to 25% of all phaeochromocytoma diagnoses.

A specific diagnosis of phaeochromocytoma is made biochemically based on the presence of elevated catecholamines or their metabolites in plasma or

Table 4.3 Biochemical tests used in the diagnosis of phaeochromocytoma, and their efficacy according to the concentrations determined in aiding the diagnosis.

Diagnosis of phaeochromocytoma	Unlikely	Likely
Urine tests (nmol/24 h)		
Norepinephrine (noradrenaline)	< 500	> 1180
Epinephrine (adrenaline)	< 100	> 170
Normetanephrine	< 3000	> 6550
Metanephrine	< 1000	> 2880
VMA (μmol/24 h)	< 40	> 55
Blood tests (nmol l^{-1})		
Norepinephrine (noradrenaline)	< 3.0	> 7.7
Epinephrine (adrenaline)	< 0.45	> 1.7
Normetanephrine	< 0.6	> 1.4
Metanephrine	< 0.3	> 0.42

Based on Lenders et al. [4].

urine. (Table 4.3) The nature of the disease process and the normal fluctuation in catecholamine concentrations can make diagnosis difficult. There is a considerable risk of false positive results. This means that the tests must have high sensitivity and specificity to be of use. For example, measurement of the catecholamine metabolite, vanillyl mandelic acid (VMA), has high specificity but relatively low sensitivity. The current recommendations are that initial screening for phaeochromocytoma should include the measurement of fractionated metanephrines in urine and/or plasma [11]. Plasma catecholamines may be raised but this is not a consistent finding. A recent review [4] banded the utility of the results of urine and plasma measurements in making a diagnosis of phaeochromocytoma into likely and unlikely (Table 4.3). There is, however, a range between where a 'possible' diagnosis is the only conclusion.

After a biochemical diagnosis has been made, the site of the phaeochromocytoma must be established. The majority can be identified by MRI or CT, with MRI being more accurate for detection of the extra-adrenal tumours [12]. If there is a suspicion of multiple sites or metastases, scintigraphy with radiolabelled I- MIBG (meta-iodobenzylguanidine) has high specificity and sensitivity for their detection.

Preoperative preparation

The chronic elevation of catecholamines and rapid fluctuations in circulating catecholamine levels produce a number of significant cardiovascular changes which require attention preoperatively. Most obviously

there are abrupt marked changes in arterial pressure often accompanied by a tachycardia.

These changes can be extreme with systolic pressures in excess of 200 mm Hg and diastolic pressures over 100 mm Hg. In patients with co-existing heart disease these pressures, particularly in association with a heart rate in excess of 100 beats per minute, impose a considerable workload on the heart and can lead to myocardial ischaemia (as a result of the high intraventricular pressures and shortening of diastole, during which the myocardium is perfused). In contrast, postural hypotension can also occur during periods when there is no catecholamine release. This is in part due to the relative hypovolaemia which results from prolonged alpha-adrenergic stimulation. That is, chronic peripheral vascular vasoconstriction adjusts the 'normal' intravascular volume to a lower value. In addition, chronic stimulation of the alpha-adrenergic receptors will lead to a change in receptor density and responsiveness which blunts the normal homeostatic response to postural change. Preoperative preparation is therefore aimed at controlling the surges and drops in arterial pressure and restoring blood volume to normal. It is useful for the anaesthetist to be involved at an early stage in the preoperative preparation.

Preoperative drug therapy

The initial therapy is the use of alpha-adrenergic blockade, usually phenoxybenzamine but other alpha-blockers such as doxazosin or prazosin have also been used. This controls surges in arterial pressure and restores the blood volume by blocking the chronic vasoconstriction. Following alpha-adrenergic blockade it may be necessary to introduce beta-adrenergic blockade (e.g., atenolol) to control reflex tachycardia. Labetolol has a theoretical advantage in producing some alpha blockade as well but this is insufficient on its own. Virtually every class of antihypertensive drugs has been used in the control of hypertension in patients with phaeochromocytoma but, other than alpha blockade, there are no particular indications based on mechanism of action. Due to the relative rarity of this disease, there is an overall lack of randomised studies comparing the different pharmacological approaches.

Alpha-adrenergic block

Phenoxybenzamine is the 'traditional' agent used preoperatively in phaeochromocytoma patients and it is still the most widely used. It is a long-acting agent which produces blockade of both α_1- and α_2-adrenergic receptors and thus acts both pre- and post-synaptically. It is usually started at a dose of 10 mg twice daily, but it may require a total daily dose of up to 100 mg. It has a relatively slow onset and the dose should be adjusted only every 2–3 days to allow for this. Various guidelines have been proposed as the target for preoperative alpha blockade. These include: maintenance of normotension at rest; pressures less than 160/90 mm Hg for 24 hours; the presence of orthostatic hypotension; and a systolic arterial pressure > 90 mm Hg on standing. These effects usually take at least seven days to be established and thus treatment for two weeks before the operation is generally recommended. Phenoxybenzamine is associated with several side effects, including tachycardia, miosis, gastrointestinal upsets and postural hypotension.

Doxazosin and prazosin are quinazoline derivatives which have selective post-junctional α_1 inhibitory activity. They therefore produce a fall in arterial pressure with less of an increase in heart rate than is seen with phenoxybenzamine. Doxazosin is given in a dose of 2–16 mg per day in a once daily dose, and prazosin over a similar range up to a maximum of 20 mg per day in divided doses. Both drugs will produce postural hypotension at higher doses. Both have been used successfully in the preoperative preparation of patients with phaeochromocytoma.

Several studies have compared the use of phenoxybenzamine, doxazosin and prazosin in the preparation of patients with phaeochromocytoma [13, 14]. The rarity of the disease means that these studies are of relatively small numbers. However, the preoperative haemodynamic stability achieved is comparable with all the agents. The argument is put forward that the longer duration of action of phenoxybenzamine may lead to greater postoperative haemodynamic instability, but this is not a consistent finding.

Urapidil is a short-acting, post-junctional, competitive α_1-antagonist which also has a central 5-HT (serotonin) agonist action. It can be given orally or by intravenous infusion. This drug has been available in some European and Asian countries for several years but not in the UK or the USA [15]. However, it is a potentially interesting drug for wider use in the management of phaeochromocytoma. Several studies from France have described its use in the acute management of phaeochromocytoma, with an infusion of 10–15 mg h^{-1} for 3 days preoperatively providing reasonable haemodynamic stability [16]. A recent study has evaluated the use of an even higher dosage regimen [17].

Beta-adrenergic blockade may be required following establishment of alpha blockade. Alpha blockade, particularly with phenoxybenzamine (α_1 and α_2), can produce significant tachycardia and even tachyarrhythmias. However, it is important that beta blockade is not started before alpha blockade as this will result in severe hypertension – alpha-mediated peripheral vasoconstriction without the modulation of the beta-mediated vasodilation in other vessel beds. Atenolol 25–50 mg daily is appropriate and this has largely replaced the use of propranolol. There is potentially some attraction in the use of labetolol in these patients as it has both alpha- and beta-adrenergic blocking effects. However, the beta effect outweighs that of the alpha effect by a considerable margin and, while it may be a useful alternative for controlling tachycardia following alpha blockade, it should not be used as the first line treatment for the reasons stated above.

Calcium channel blockers have been used in the preoperative preparation. They exert their effect by inhibiting calcium transport in vascular smooth muscle. The most widely used agent is nicardipine, which has the advantage that it can be used orally preoperatively and by infusion peroperatively. Orthostatic hypotension is much less of a problem than with the use of alpha-adrenergic blockade. Preoperative control similar to that achieved with adrenergic blockade has been claimed [18]. Calcium channel blockers have also been used as an additional agent when adrenergic blockade (alpha and beta) has not produced adequate control of arterial pressure.

Metyrosine: an alternative, or additional, method of reducing the effect of circulating catecholamines is to interfere with their synthesis. Metyrosine is a competitive inhibitor of tyrosine hydroxylase, a key enzyme in catecholamine synthesis. It acts to deplete the catecholamine stores in the body and thus to minimise surges in arterial pressure. The dose is 1–2 g per day in divided doses. It is not widely used as a sole agent but is given in some centres as additional therapy in patients who still have poor control despite adrenergic blocking drugs. Unfortunately, it has quite marked systemic side effects as it can cross the blood brain barrier, particularly at higher doses, and these include sedation, depression, anxiety and diarrhoea [19].

In summary, alpha-adrenergic blockade is the mainstay of preoperative control in patients with phaeochromocytoma. Phenoxybenzamine is still the most widely used agent for this in the UK. Beta-adrenergic blockade is often added to control the heart rate after alpha blockade is established. Alternatively, calcium channel blockade can be used successfully. As noted earlier, there is a need for randomised controlled studies comparing these treatment options.

Perioperative management

It is important that the team involved in the management of a patient (physician, surgeon and anaesthetist) communicate well and are all involved in preparing the patient for surgery. In most countries, phaeochromocytoma are referred to specialist centres for management and this is to be commended. It is obviously more appropriate that these relatively rare cases are dealt with by a team that manage 10–20 per year rather than a team that see only 1 case every 5–10 years. For an anaesthetist managing a phaeochromocytoma patient for the first time it is sensible to use techniques and drugs that they are familiar with as this reduces the variables involved.

Surgical management

The advent of laparoscopic surgery has changed the surgical approach to resection of phaeochromocytoma [20]. The majority of tumours are now resected laparoscopically but large, bilateral or malignant tumours may require laparotomy. The majority of phaeochromocytoma can be removed laparoscopically using a retroperitoneal approach with the patient in a lateral position with some break on the operating table. Larger or bilateral tumours may require a supine transperitoneal approach. The same positioning options are required for open surgery. When laparoscopic resection was first introduced 15 years ago the upper-size limit of resectable tumour was set at 6 cm. However, with increasing experience tumours up to 15 cm in diameter have been removed laparoscopically. The surgical options and techniques have been reviewed [2, 3].

Anaesthetic management

Premedication

The patient's medication, including antihypertensive therapy, should be continued through to the operation. However, if phenoxybenzamine is being used, the last dose should be given the day before surgery. As stressful situations can be a trigger to catecholamine release, it is appropriate to prescribe an anxiolytic (benzodiazepine) preoperatively.

Monitoring

The physiological changes and stress involved in induction of anaesthesia can trigger catecholamine release. It is therefore essential that good cardiovascular monitoring (ECG, oximetry and invasive arterial pressure) is in place before induction. Central venous access for monitoring and for administration of vasoactive drugs is required. In patients with compromised cardiovascular function, either secondary to the phaeochromocytoma or from any other cause, it may be of value to include a method of measuring cardiac output as the operation can entail marked changes in intravascular volume, sympathetic activity and venous return. It is essential to check arterial gases and blood glucose at regular intervals throughout surgery.

Induction of anaesthesia and tracheal intubation can trigger severe hypertension in patients with phaeochromocytoma. It is essential that induction is carried out in a smooth unhurried manner to minimise the risk of stimuli such as hypotension or the pressor response to intubation. A technique using propofol and a short-acting opioid such as remifentanil is appropriate. Drugs which have the potential to produce histamine release should be avoided. Following muscle relaxation with a non-depolarising agent, adequate time should be allowed for the block to develop before attempting tracheal intubation to prevent a pressor response. The use of suxamethonium is best avoided as both the potential for histamine release and the effect of muscle fasciculation can trigger massive catecholamine release from the phaeochromocytoma. If a rapid sequence induction is essential, e.g., severe reflux, high dose rocuronium is the best option. Due to its sympathomimetic effects, ketamine is not appropriate in these patients.

Maintenance

It is usual to use a balanced technique to maintain anaesthesia with an inhalational agent and short-acting opioids. The vasodilatory effects of isoflurane and sevoflurane may be of some benefit and both have been used successfully in these patients. Similarly, all of the short-acting opioids have been used, including remifentanil.

The role of epidural anaesthesia in patients with phaeochromocytoma is less clear. With the majority of surgical procedures now being laparoscopic there is less need for extensive intra and postoperative analgesia. The arguments for the use of an epidural perioperatively are: provision of good intra and postoperative analgesia (especially in open procedures);

the vasodilatory effect requires correction with a fluid load which can minimise the likelihood of hypotension after the tumour is resected (see below); and that the lower arterial pressure from vasodilatation helps to minimise surges in pressure during tumour handling. The arguments against are: placement of the epidural catheter (positioning of the patient, direct pressure and accompanying stress) may trigger a catecholamine surge; hypotension from vasodilatation may also do this; it introduces another (?unnecessary) variable to the patient's haemodynamic status; and that after laparoscopic surgery extensive analgesia is not required. A reasonable synthesis of these arguments may be that the use of an epidural should be considered for open surgical procedures with limited use before resection of the tumour but then used to provide good postoperative analgesia.

Intraoperative problems

There are two major problems that will be encountered intraoperatively: hypertension during resection, and hypotension following devascularisation of the tumour. While preoperative preparation may minimise the incidence of the latter, the former is a consistent problem in phaeochromocytoma surgery [21].

Hypertension

Severe hypertension can abruptly occur at several stages of the procedure including induction, retroperitoneal insufflation and tumour handling. The rise in arterial is abrupt and severe with systolic pressures in excess of 200 mm Hg and diastolic pressures over 100 mm Hg being not uncommon[22]. This may be accompanied by a tachycardia, particularly if the patient has not been given beta-adrenergic blockers preoperatively (Figure 4.2). Tumour handling or manipulation is the most consistent stimulus and can produce life-threatening rises in arterial pressure, which can precipitate myocardial infarction, cardiac failure, pulmonary oedema and cerebrovascular effects. However, this can occur in some patients before surgery during placement of lines, tracheal intubation, movement and positioning of the patient (e.g., into the lateral position for surgery), or insufflation with carbon dioxide (Figure 4.2). It is essential, therefore, that the anaesthetist has a strategy to deal with these complications well before inducing anaesthesia and has an antihypertensive agent available immediately for infusion (preferably using a central line).

Many drugs have been used successfully including: sodium nitroprusside, phentolamine, esmolol,

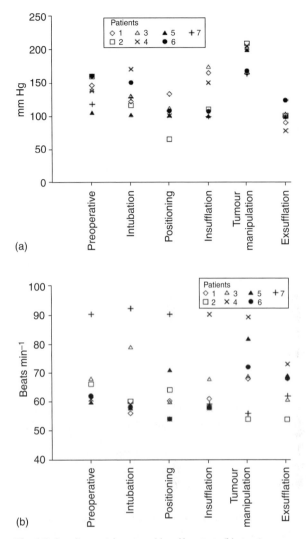

Fig. 4.2 Systolic arterial pressure (a) and heart rate (b) at various stages of laparoscopic resection of phaeochromocytoma in seven patients. From Atallah et al. [22] with permission.

nicardipine, magnesium sulphate and urapidil (Table 4.4). Again, using an agent that the anaesthetist is familiar with is probably more important than the mechanism of action. It is important to remember that the action of these agents may be altered by the antihypertensive drugs given preoperatively.

Sodium nitroprusside (SNP) is an inorganic ferrous salt which is a potent vaso- and venodilator, producing its action through release of nitric oxide (NO). In contact with blood it rapidly decomposes to produce NO. As NO is a potent but short-acting dilator, SNP must be given by continuous infusion. Its potential advantages are a rapid onset and offset, and its potency. Disadvantages include severe hypotension with a compensatory

Table 4.4 Antihypertensive drugs used during phaeochromocytoma surgery.

Sodium nitroprusside	0.5–1.5 µg kg^{-1} min^{-1}, max. 8 µg kg^{-1} min^{-1}
Phentolamine	1–5 mg bolus, 0.5–1.0 mg min^{-1}
Esmolol	250–500 µg kg^{-1} min^{-1}, then 25–250 µg kg^{-1} min^{-1}
Nicardipine	1–2 µg kg^{-1} min^{-1}, up to 7.5 µg kg^{-1} min^{-1}
Magnesium sulphate	2–4 g bolus, then 1–2 g h^{-1}
Urapidil	10–15 mg h^{-1}

tachycardia (which may be exaggerated by other drugs e.g., adrenergic blockers attenuating the compensatory mechanisms), toxicity from the iron metabolites which produce thiocyanate and tachyphylaxis.

Phentolamine is a competitive α_1 and α_2 antagonist which has been widely used to control hypertensive episodes in phaeochromocytoma patients. It has a relatively rapid onset and a duration of action of around one hour. It is given by infusion. It is potentially of use in the alarming situation of dealing with a previously undiagnosed phaeochromocytoma in an anaesthetised patient undergoing surgery. The infusion should be started cautiously as severe hypotension can occur.

Esmolol is a short-acting (nine minute half-life) cardioselective beta-adrenergic blocker which has been used, often in combination with one of the other drugs described here, to control intraoperative hypertension and tachycardia. Its short action is of benefit following removal of the tumour as prolonged beta-adrenergic blockade is a disadvantage at that stage (see below).

Nicardipine: the mechanism of action of this drug has been discussed earlier.

Magnesium sulphate has a number of antiadrenergic effects which are mediated mainly through its actions on calcium channels [23]. Calcium is required for the release of catecholamines from the adrenal medulla and magnesium appears to block its action. Magnesium has effects on L-type calcium channels in membranes and the sarcoplasmic reticulum. It also has vasodilatory and antiarrhythmic effects and a small, dose-dependent myocardial depressant effect. Magnesium sulphate has been used successfully to control arterial pressure intraoperatively in phaeochromocytoma patients [24]. In patients pretreated with phenoxybenzamine or prazosin, a bolus loading dose of magnesium (40–80 mg kg^{-1}) was followed by an infusion of 1–2 g h^{-1}.

Urapidil: see above.

The onset of hypertensive episodes is abrupt and is triggered by events such as induction of anaesthesia, movement of the patient, insufflation and, in particular, handling of the tumour. These episodes are accompanied by surges of catecholamines which may achieve very high concentrations. For example, during one study peak norepinephrine (noradrenaline) concentrations of 200–300 ng ml^{-1} (normal < 510 pg ml^{-1}) and epinephrine (adrenaline) concentrations of 150–200 ng ml^{-1} (normal < 170 pg ml^{-1}) were measured during insufflation and tumour handling [16]. As catecholamines have a short duration of action the episodes are self-limiting, if the stimulus is removed. Thus all procedures must be done in a controlled manner; for example, insufflation should be done gradually and unnecessary manipulation of the tumour avoided. The surgeon must be prepared to stop operating for several minutes to allow severe arterial pressure/heart rate increases to be brought back under control.

Hypotension

Following ligation of the tumour's venous drainage, there is an abrupt removal of sympathetic activity. This can result in severe and refractory hypotension, particularly if the patient has had incomplete alpha blockade preoperatively. Some patients may require a vasoconstrictor/inotropic infusion (e.g., norepinephrine) for some hours postoperatively. One of the arguments for the use of alpha-adrenergic blockade for a sufficiently long period preoperatively is to allow restoration of intravascular volume, which can help to minimise the immediate hypotensive effect of withdrawal of catecholamines. Treatment of the hypotension should include intraoperative volume loading and minimising the infusion of antihypertensive drugs. As mentioned briefly above, there are good reasons not to use long-acting hypotensive drugs to control arterial pressure during the earlier part of surgery. Similarly, it is advisable to avoid the use of long acting alpha- and beta-adrenergic blockade immediately pre and perioperatively; for example, the last dose of phenoxybenzamine is given the day before surgery. It is the author's experience that with good preoperative alpha blockade using phenoxybenzamine (with beta blockade if required) and intraoperative fluid replacement, the need for postoperative inotropes is rare.

Postoperative care

In addition to routine postoperative care, it is appropriate to have the patient in a high dependency unit (HDU) (level 2) setting. Intra-arterial pressure monitoring should be continued to detect any episodes of hyper- or hypotension. Likewise, central venous pressure monitoring should be used to direct fluid and (if required) inotrope therapy. Blood glucose should be monitored as insulin levels may rise following removal of the suppression caused by the catecholamines. Postoperative analgesia can be provided with opioids or, if the procedure was an open one, with epidural analgesia.

Primary hyperaldosteronism (Conn's syndome)

The classic presentation of hyperaldosteronism is of a relatively young patient with severe hypertension and marked hypokalaemia. However, it is recognised that hyperaldosteronism can be present without accompanying hypokalaemia [25]. A recent review [26] recommended that investigation to exclude hyperaldosteronism should be considered in several groups of patients (in addition to those with hypertension and hypokalaemia) including hypertension in young patients (< 20 years), severe or refractory hypertension and an incidentaloma and hypertension.

The hypokalaemia is a result of increased urinary loss of potassium. This is a direct effect of the raised aldosterone. Aldosterone acts on the mineralocorticoid receptors in the distal convoluted tubule of the nephron and collecting ducts to promote sodium and water retention and loss of potassium.

The most common forms of primary hyperaldosteronism are idiopathic hyperaldosteronism due to hyperplasia which is usually bilateral, and an aldosterone producing adenoma which is more usually unilateral. The latter is responsive to adrenalectomy with correction of the hypokalaemia in all and arterial pressure in the majority of patients. However, in the idiopathic form, adrenalectomy does not usually completely cure the hypertension.

Diagnosis can usually be made by measuring the plasma aldosterone:renin activity ratio in a morning blood sample. However, to distinguish between the idiopathic and aldosterone-secreting types, and hence the suitability for surgical intervention, further investigation is necessary. A CT scan may be of value but is not very accurate at differentiating between the two types; for example, between a small unilateral aldosterone secreting adenoma and bilateral more diffuse changes. In some cases, adrenal vein sampling for aldosterone concentrations with angiographic guidance may be required [27].

Treatment for both forms is with an aldosterone antagonist. *Spironolactone* (initial dose 12.5–25.0 mg day^{-1}) is still used commonly but a newer antagonist, *eplerenone* (up to 100 mg day^{-1}) has been introduced in the past few years. Eplerenone is a steroid nucleus-based aldosterone antagonist which is more specific for aldosterone and has less effect on glucocorticoid and androgen synthesis and therefore fewer side effects, such as gynaecomastia in males, than spironolactone. This fairly rapidly corrects the hypokalaemia but the hypertension may take 1–2 months to control. In the idiopathic form, spironolactone may be the only treatment required but some may need an additional antihypertensive drug. In the patient with an isolated adrenal adenoma secreting aldosterone, unilateral adrenalectomy after initial treatment with spironolactone or epleronone is usually appropriate.

Anaesthetic management

Preoperative correction of the hypokalaemia and control of the arterial pressure is essential. The anaesthetist should be aware that the diuretic action of spironolactone can produce a degree of hypovolaemia. Appropriate monitoring should include direct arterial and central venous pressure measurement. Plasma potassium should be measured regularly and supplemented as required. The majority of cases will be for unilateral removal of an adenoma and thus suitable for laparoscopic surgery.

Excess glucocorticoid secretion (Cushing's syndrome)

Cushing's syndrome is a rare condition (1/100 000 per year) in which there is increased secretion of glucocorticoids from the adrenal cortex. This mainly involves cortisol but androgens may also be increased. The majority of cases result from increased ACTH arising from a pituitary tumour and a smaller number from 'ectopic ACTH' secretion from a source such as a lung oat-cell tumour. Around 10% of cases are not ACTH dependent and arise from a secretory adenoma or carcinoma of the adrenal [28].

The clinical effects of excess glucocorticoids are widespread and include weight gain (classically truncal obesity), hypertension, muscle weakness, facial changes and easy bruising. Glucose intolerance and diabetes are often present and increased mineralocorticoid activity may cause hypokalaemia. Hypokalaemia is most commonly associated with ectopic ACTH secretion syndrome.

An initial diagnosis can be made by biochemical tests including a dexamethasone suppression test, which measures the effect of an overnight dose of dexamethasone on the morning cortisol level, and 24-hour urinary cortisol. In patients with a high cortisol and failure of suppression by dexamethasone, the next stage of tests will be directed at establishing the cause of the cortisol excess (pituitary, adrenal or ectopic) and will involve further biochemical and radiological investigations [29].

Anaesthetic considerations

Anaesthetic management will be tailored to the problems presenting in an individual patient. That is, to address the specific mixture of hypertension, diabetes and electrolyte imbalance present in the patient. Monitoring of neuromuscular function is recommended because of the associated muscle wasting effects.

Movement and handling of the anaesthetised patient should be particularly carefully done because of the risk of bruising, skin fragility and also the frequent presence of osteoporosis in this group.

Steroid replacement therapy and surgery

Prolonged treatment with steroids such a prednisolone can produce secondary adrenocortical insufficiency due to suppression of the normal control mechanisms (ACTH secretion). This can result in profound cardiovascular collapse in the perioperative period. This severe complication can be avoided by supplementation with cortisol. In patients taking steroids as immunosuppressive therapy, failure to supplement in the perioperative period can result in an exacerbation of auto-immune disease. However, there has been considerable discussion over the years as which patients require replacement therapy and at what dose. In the past large doses (e.g., hydrocortisone 100 mg 3–4 times per day) were given. These are now thought to be excessive and current recommendations are: for minor surgery, hydrocortisone 25 mg at induction; moderate surgery, hydrocortisone 25 mg at induction and 100 mg in divided doses over the next 24 hours; and, for major surgery, hydrocortisone 25–50 mg at induction with 100 mg per 24 hours in divided doses for 3 days. This should apply to patients who have been taking at least prednisolone 10 mg per day (or the equivalent in other therapeutic steroid drugs, such as dexamethasone 6 mg, beclomethasone 1.5 mg or cortisone 40 mg daily)

within the last 3 months. It also will apply to patients with Addison's disease [30].

References

1. Singh PK , Buch HN. Adrenal incidentaloma; evaluation and management. *J Clin Pathol* 2008; **61**: 1168–73.

2. Lal G , Duh QY. Laparoscopic adrenalectomy – indications and technique. *Surg Oncol* 2003; **12**: 105–23.

3. Gumbs AA , Gagner M. Laparoscopic adrenalectomy. *Best Pract Res Clin Endocrinol Metab* 2006; **20**: 483–99.

4. Lenders JWM , Eisenhofer G , Mannelli M , Pacak K. Phaeochromocytoma. *Lancet* 2005; **366**: 665–75.

5. Armstrong R , Stidhar M , Greenhalgh KL, et al. Phaeochromocytoma in children. *Arch Dis Child* 2008; **93**: 899–945.

6. Brunt LM. Phaeochromocytoma in pregnancy. *Br J Surg* 2001; **88**: 481–3.

7. Disick GI , Palese MA. Extra-adrenal pheochromocytoma: diagnosis and management. *Curr Urol Rep* 2007; **8**: 83–8.

8. Ilias I , Pacak K. A clinical overview of pheochromocytomas/paragangliomas and carcinoid tumors. *Nucl Med Biol* 2008; **35**: 27–34.

9. Gimenez-Roqueplo AP, Burnichon N, Amar L, et al. Recent advances in the genetics of phaeochromocytoma and functional paraganglioma. *Clin Exp Pharmacol Physiol* 2008; **35**: 376–9.

10. Safwat AS, Bissada NK, Seyam RM, Al Sobhi S, Hanash KA. The clinical spectrum of phaeochromocytoma: analysis of 115 patients. *BJU Int* 2008; **101**: 1561–4.

11. Peaston RT , Ball S. Biochemical detection of phaeochromocytoma: why are we continuing to ignore the evidence? *Ann Clin Biochem* 2008; **45**: 6–10.

12. Adler JT, Meyer-Rochow GY, Chen H, et al. Phaeochromocytoma: current approaches and future decisions. *Oncologist* 2008; **13**: 779–93.

13. Kocak S, Aydintug S, Canakci N. Alpha blockade in preoperative preparation of patients with pheochromocytomas. *Int Surg* 2002; **87**: 191–4.

14. Prys-Roberts C, Farndon JR. Efficacy and safety of doxazosin for perioperative management of patients with pheochromocytoma. *World J Surg* 2002; **26**:1037–42.

15. Dooley M, Goa KI. Urapidil. A reappraisal of its use in the management of hypertension. *Drugs* 1998; **56**: 929–55.

16. Tauzin-Fin P, Sesay M, Gosse P, Ballanger P. Effects of perioperative a1 block on haemodynamic control during laparoscopic surgery for phaeochromocytoma. *Br J Anaesth* 2004; **92**: 512–17.

17. Gosse P, Tauzin-Fin P, Sesay MB, Sautereau A, Ballanger P. Preparation for surgery of phaeochromocytoma by blockade of alpha-adrenergic receptors with urapidil: what dose? *J Hum Hypertens* 2009; **23**(9): 605–9.

18. Combemale F, Carnaille B, Tavernier B, et al. Exclusive use of calcium channel blockers and cardioselective beta-blockers in the pre- and peri-operative management of pheochromocytomas: 70 cases. *Ann Chir* 1998; **52**: 341–5.

19. Pacak K. Preoperative management of the pheochromocytoma patient. *J Clin Endocrinol Metab* 2007; **92**: 4069–79.

20. Tiberio GAM, Baiocchi GL, Arru Luca, et al. Prospective randomized comparison of laparoscopic versus open adrenalectomy for sporadic pheochromocytoma. *Surg Endosc* 2008; **22**: 1435–9.

21. Weismann D , Fassnacht M , Weinberger F, et al. Intraoperative haemodynamic stability in patients with phaeochromocytoma – minimally invasive versus conventional open surgery. *Clin Endocrinol (Oxf)* 2006; **65**: 1365–2265.

22. Atallah F, Bastide-Heulin T , Soulié M, et al. Haemodynamic changes during retroperitoneoscopic adrenalectomy for phaeochromocytoma. *Br J Anaesth* 2001; **86**: 731–3.

23. Fawcett WJ, Haxby EJ, Male DA. Magnesium: physiology and pharmacology. *Br J Anaesth* 1999; **83**: 302–20.

24. James MFM. Use of magnesium sulphate in the anaesthetic management of phaeochromocytoma: a review of 17 anaesthetics. *Br J Anaesth* 1989; **62**: 616–23.

25. Mulatero P, Stowasser M, Loh KC, et al. Increased diagnosis of primary aldosteronism, including surgically correctable forms, in centers from five continents. *J Clin Endocrinol Metab* 2004; **89**: 1045–50.

26. Young WF. Adrenal causes of hypertension: pheochromocytoma and primary aldosteronism. *Rev Endocr Metab Disord* 2007; **8**: 309–20.

27. Young WF, Stanson AW, Thompson GB, Grant CS, Farley DR, van Heerden JA. Role for adrenal venous sampling in primary aldosteronism. *Surgery* 2004; **136**: 1227–35.

28. Biller BM, Grossman AB, Stewart PM, et al. Treatment of adrenocortical-dependent Cushing's syndrome: a consensus statement. *J Clin Endocrinol Metab* 2008; **93**: 2454–62.

29. Elamain MB, Murad MH, Mullan R, et al. Accuracy of diagnostic tests for Cushing's syndrome: a systematic review and metanalysis. *J Clin Endocrinol Metab* 2008; **93**: 1553–62.

30. Hahner S, Allolio B. Management of adrenal insufficiency in different clinical settings. *Expert Opin Pharmacother* 2005; **6**: 2407–17.

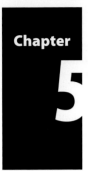

Pancreatic neuroendocrine tumours including carcinoid

Christopher J. R. Parker

Introduction and overview

Pancreatic islet cell tumours and carcinoids are rare, and patients with these tumours form a small part of the caseload of the anaesthetist who regularly undertakes anaesthesia for major abdominal surgery. The importance of these tumours depends on the following:

(a) They have a better prognosis than the pancreatic exocrine tumours that form the majority of the work of the pancreatic surgical service; more aggressive surgical resection is warranted than for pancreatic adenocarcinoma.

(b) They may secrete a number of hormones giving rise to distant metabolic effects.

The rarity of the tumours means that recommendations are based on relatively small series. This fact, together with their complex associations, variable biology, and the importance of imaging and follow up, calls for a multidisciplinary approach. Surgery is but one brief, though crucial, interlude on the patient's journey, and the involvement of gastroenterologists, surgeons, radiologists, oncologists and chemical pathologists needs to be co-ordinated, together with the availability of intensive care backup (Figure 5.1).

No anaesthetist can have an extensive personal experience. Anaesthetic aspects were reviewed in 2000 [1], and recent general guidelines are available [2]. This chapter highlights some points relevant to the anaesthetist. A broad distinction can be drawn between islet cell tumours and carcinoids.

Islet cell tumours

This group of tumours, which has been reviewed recently [3], includes:

(a) Insulinoma – which produces hypoglycaemia.

(b) Gastrinoma – leading to duodenal ulcers – the Zollinger–Ellison syndrome.

(c) Non-functioning endocrine tumours; this is the least dramatic but most common group of islet cell tumours.

There are three others, which are even more rare:

(d) Somatostatinoma – which can produce gallstones, diarrhoea and diabetes mellitus.

(e) Glucagonoma – leading to diabetes mellitus and a necrolytic rash.

(f) VIPoma – leading to diarrhoea – the Werner–Morrison syndrome.

Carcinoid tumours

These tumours arise from enterochromaffin cells and occur in the gastrointestinal tract and lung, and are characterised by the secretion of serotonin and production of kinins.

General characteristics of the tumours

The individual characteristics of some of these tumours will be surveyed below, but they share the following features:

(a) They have a variable level of malignancy.

(b) They can present as a sporadic case or with a familial history.

(c) They are associated with a variety of familial syndromes – such as multiple endocrine neoplasia type 1 (MEN 1), multiple endocrine neoplasia type 2 (MEN 2), neurofibromatosis and von Hippel–Lindau syndrome.

(d) They can be small and multiple, and localisation can be difficult.

Insulinoma

Insulinoma is the commonest functioning pancreatic neuroendocrine tumour.

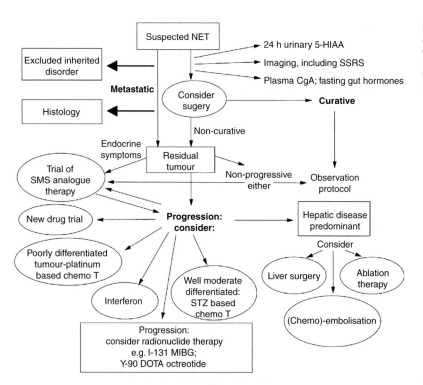

Fig. 5.1 Algorithm of the investigation and treatment of gut endocrine tumours. CgA, chromogranin A; 5-HIAA, 5-hydroxy-indoleacetic acid; NET, neuroendocrine tumour. From Ramage et al. [2] with permission.

Case vignette

A patient aged 64 years was admitted for total hip replacement. Her preoperative condition included advanced chronic obstructive pulmonary disease, and her postoperative course was complicated by acute myocardial infarction and an episode of acute renal failure; she also had several episodes of impaired consciousness associated with low blood glucose. Insulinoma was diagnosed, and localised to a 2.4 cm lesion in the pancreatic head, but the patient was thought unfit for surgery. Symptoms were controlled with diazoxide.

The diagnosis of insulinoma is based upon Whipple's triad:

(a) Symptoms of neuroglycopaenia.
(b) Blood glucose < 2.8 mmol l⁻¹.
(c) Relief of symptoms with glucose administration.

The symptoms of hypoglycaemia include those of neuroglycopaenia (e.g., dizziness, drowsiness, loss of consciousness) and also those of consequent sympathetic over-activity (e.g., tachycardia, sweating). There are many causes of hypoglycaemia [4], which can be classified according to the general health of the patient.

The patient with insulinoma generally appears well, and although this patient had life-threatening system disorders, the diagnosis was confirmed by laboratory testing.

The differential diagnosis of insulinoma includes factitious administration of sulphonylurea or exogenous insulin. In a case of doubt, symptoms can be evoked by a monitored prolonged fast – up to 72 hours, with regular monitoring of blood glucose, plasma insulin and C-peptide (which is cosecreted with insulin by pancreatic beta cells, but absent from exogenous insulin) levels. The combination of the following features is diagnostic [5]:

(a) Blood glucose < 2.2 mmol l⁻¹.
(b) Simultaneous insulin levels of 43 pmol l⁻¹ or greater.
(c) C-peptide levels of 200 pmol l⁻¹ or greater.
(d) An absence of sulphonylurea.

There was no family history of endocrine disorder in this case vignette, and though insulinoma can be associated with MEN 1 (in 1–16% of cases), the majority are sporadic. Usually insulinoma is solitary, but in familial syndromes the majority are multiple [6].

Like this patient, about 60% are female, and while the mean age is in the fifth decade, insulinoma can present at any age from 13 to over 80 years.

Localisation was possible here with a CT scan, but localisation of an insulinoma is often problematic because they are usually small – the majority are under 2 cm in diameter. Insulinoma is unusual in that only 50% express somatostatin receptors and thus somatostatin receptor scintigraphy is of less value than in other gastroenteropancreatic neuroendocrine tumours. A variety of other techniques have been recommended including preoperative portal venous blood sampling with calcium stimulation, and intraoperative ultrasound.

Unlike other pancreatic neuroendocrine tumours (especially gastrinoma), which can also occur in the duodenum, insulinoma is confined to the pancreas. Tumours can be located in the head (47%), body (32%) or tail (22%); vigorous efforts to accurately localise the tumour are highly recommended; blind pancreatic resection is not appropriate [7]. Medical management with diazoxide, which inhibits insulin release, is possible, and was done in this case. There are side effects, including hirsutism, and symptom control is not complete. Patients often gain weight as they learn to control symptoms with a carbohydrate snack.

Surgery is preferred as the definitive treatment – it obviates the need for diazoxide. Only 10% of insulinomas are malignant, and surgery potentially offers a complete cure. Moreover the risk of malignancy and metastasis in neuroendocrine tumours is related to size; the tumour size here (over 2 cm diameter) is such that malignant potential is a consideration. The operation performed will depend on location, and enucleation is often possible.

The chief concern of the anaesthetist caring for the patient undergoing surgery for insulinoma is controlling the blood glucose level. There have historically been two themes:

(a) The avoidance of profound hypoglycaemia, arising from excessive insulin secretion.

(b) The use of blood glucose monitoring to assist localisation, and provide evidence that resection has been completed.

Early case reports highlighted the fear of hypoglycaemia and advocated generous glucose administration [8]. The development of rapid near-patient blood glucose analysis obviated the risk of hypoglycaemia, and raised the possibility that careful monitoring of blood glucose might demonstrate a 'hyperglycaemic rebound', and confirm the completeness of resection. This approach was advocated by Schnelle et al. [9], and put on a more formal basis with the development of

an 'artificial pancreas' with continuous blood glucose monitoring and automatic control of insulin and glucose infusions [10]. It was subsequently realised that this approach is unreliable [11]. On average the blood glucose does rise after insulinoma resection, but there is great inter-individual variability, and in 23% of patients the glucose rebound was delayed – a false negative response that would, if it was relied upon, lead to excessive surgical exploration.

It is currently recommended that glucose should be measured every 20 minutes [11]. Of all glucose estimations, only 4 of 526 readings were more than 1.1 mmol l^{-1} below the previous value, and if the value of blood glucose was greater than 3.3 mmol l^{-1}, a value taken 20 minutes later was never less than 2.8 mmol l^{-1}. It was possible to avoid dangerous hypoglycaemia without more frequent measurement, and without excessive glucose loading.

Laparoscopic surgery might be considered in this case to lessen the impact of the extensive laparotomy (with bilateral subcostal incision) necessary for a conventional approach in such a high-risk patient. Enucleation of insulinoma has been undertaken laparoscopically [12]. A high rate of pancreatic fistula may be a limitation of the technique.

Gastrinoma

Gastrinoma is the second commonest functioning pancreatic neuroendocrine tumour, and contrasts with insulinoma in several respects.

Case vignette

A 50-year-old patient was admitted for surgical treatment of pancreatic gastrinoma. His father had died of gastrointestinal haemorrhage. He had a history of peptic ulcer disease, with previous admission for bleeding duodenal ulcer. A gastrinoma in the pancreatic head was diagnosed. A pylorus preserving pancreaticoduodenectomy was undertaken. The initial postoperative course was uneventful, but at day 10 there was severe gastric haemorrhage. A completion pancreatectomy, splenectomy and total gastrectomy was performed. Histology showed a further gastrinoma in the tail of the pancreas.

This patient is typical in that gastrinoma is slightly more common in men, and presents on average at 50 years. He had a family history of gastrointestinal haemorrhage. Gastrinoma accounts for 1 in 1000 cases of duodenal ulcer, so while this is not diagnostic of a familial episode, it highlights the link between gastrinoma and the MEN 1 syndrome. Between 25 and 40% of patients with gastrinoma will have MEN 1 [2], and up to 67% of MEN 1 patients develop Zollinger–Ellison syndrome due to a gastrinoma [6].

Guidelines recommend taking a detailed family history, clinical examination and appropriate biochemical and radiological investigations to search for a familial syndrome [2]. Diagnosis of MEN 1 requires two typical tumours, or a positive family history and one typical tumour [6]. There are detailed guidelines for investigation of MEN 1 [13].

Gastrin levels are raised in several conditions, including treatment with H_2 receptor antagonists and proton pump inhibitors (PPI), as well as atrophic gastritis. The diagnosis is made by high gastrin levels and basal acid output [14]. Treatment with PPI itself causes gastrin levels to be raised, and diagnosis requires PPI to be stopped for at least a week if possible (though risking clinical deterioration) [15]. The consequences of hypergastrinaemia include not only aggressive peptic ulcer disease and gastric mucosal hypertrophy, but also diarrhoea and malabsorption (due to acidification of pancreatic enzymes), and the risk of emergence of gastric carcinoids, especially in patients with MEN 1 [16]. Localisation techniques for gastrinomas include somatostatin receptor scintigraphy (which can miss 30% of gastrinomas, particularly in the pancreatic tail [3]) and endoscopic ultrasound, which however has a poor sensitivity for detecting duodenal gastrinomas [16].

The case history also highlights the potential for multiplicity of gastrinomas, and the failure to achieve surgical control with a standard Whipple's resection. Multiplicity of tumours is a more common feature in MEN 1-associated gastrinomas, where over 50% are multiple, than in sporadic cases where 80% are solitary [3]. Symptom control can be achieved with a PPI, and so gastrectomy is not indicated for symptom control. In contrast to insulinoma, most gastrinomas are malignant, and surgery is recommended for prognostic reasons in all patients with sporadic gastrinoma, as long-term cure is possible in some patients [17].

Surgery for gastrinoma in MEN 1 is less likely to offer a cure and the timing and indications are not agreed; tumour size > 2.5 cm is an indication, with the risk of metastasis being related to tumour size. Surgical strategies recognise the possibility that gastrinomas can be occult, small, multiple, and located in the duodenum or the pancreas including the tail. Occult tumours may be found in the 'gastrinoma triangle', which is defined by: the junction of the cystic duct and common bile duct superiorly; the junction of the second and third parts of the duodenum inferiorly; and the junction of the neck and body of the pancreas medially [18]. The surgery is complex, and may involve duodenotomy to search for duodenal tumours, enucleation of identified pancreatic tumours, left pancreatectomy and lymph node dissection [3]. Aggressive surgery including vascular reconstruction and liver resection has been advocated [19]. Gastrinomas are not suitable for laparoscopic surgery.

In preparation for anaesthesia and surgery, antacid therapy should be continued up to the time of induction, and the anaesthetist should be aware that the stomach may not be empty. Antacid therapy should be continued without interruption in the postoperative period. If splenectomy is required, then appropriate antibiotic prophylaxis is needed, and arrangements must be made for pneumococcal vaccination.

Non-functional neuroendocrine tumours

Case vignette

A patient aged 56 years had a routine 'life-check' CT scan. This revealed a 4 cm hypervascular mass in the pancreatic head. There were no symptoms. Plasma sampling was positive for chromogranin A, but investigation revealed no other endocrine abnormality. A non-functioning neuroendocrine tumour was diagnosed. Preoperative evaluation revealed a solitary hepatic metastasis. Surgical resection of the primary tumour (Whipple's operation) was undertaken.

The absence of symptoms is characteristic of non-functioning tumours. When symptoms are present, the most common is pain; nausea and fatigue are less common, and a minority present with a picture of obstructive jaundice.

The identification of this mass as a neuroendocrine tumour (NET) depended on the presence of the marker chromogranin A. This is an acidic polypeptide that is very widely distributed in all tissues derived from the neural crest [2]. It is secreted by otherwise non-secreting tumours, and thus is useful for diagnosis of a non-functioning tumour. Chromogranin A, like other peptide markers, is measured at reference centres in London and Belfast.

Another clue to the diagnosis was the vascularity of the lesion on contrast-enhanced CT scan, which is highly characteristic of a NET. The size of the primary tumour (4 cm in this case) correlates with the presence of metastasis. About 37–70% of sporadic non-functioning NETs have metastasis at presentation; in MEN 1 non-functioning NETs are common and the presence of metastasis correlates with the size of the primary tumour.

Overall survival in patients with non-functioning NET is much better than pancreatic ductal adenocarcinoma [3], for which such a radical approach of resection in the presence of metastasis would not be undertaken. Amongst a large ($n = 163$) series of non-functioning islet cell carcinomas, of 16 patients who presented with metastatic disease and underwent primary tumour resection, 9 died at a median of 2.2 years and 7 remained alive between 1 and 8 years after diagnosis [20]. Median survival in those without metastatic disease was 7.1 years. In another series of 37 patients with a non-functioning neuroendocrine carcinoma however, mean survival time was not affected by the presence of metastases – being 153 months in patients with metastatic disease [21]. Hepatic metastases are the main cause of death, and modalities of treatment include surgical resection; agents such as somatostatin analogues and interferon; chemotherapy; targeted radionuclides; and ablation therapy [2, 3].

Somatostatinoma

Case vignette

A 46-year-old man presented with a history of abdominal pain; gallstones were present on ultrasound scan, and at laparoscopic cholecystectomy the cholangiogram showed a dilated common bile duct with stones. A follow-up ERCP revealed a polyp in the second part of the duodenum. This was biopsied, and showed a NET that stained positive for somatostatin. Clinical examination showed café-au-lait spots and cutaneous neurofibromas. Blood pressure and blood glucose were normal. Whipple's resection of the primary tumour was undertaken.

Somatostatinomas are very rare – comprising 1% of all NETs of the gastrointestinal tract and pancreas.

Clinical features include gallstones, diarrhoea and weight loss. Diabetes mellitus is a common feature, arising from inhibition of insulin secretion. It was absent in this case, and this is consistent with the duodenal origin; a somatostatinoma of duodenal origin is less likely to secrete high levels of somatostatin than one of pancreatic origin [22, 23].

This unusual presentation highlights that NETs may occur as part of a familial syndrome: the MEN 1 or MEN 2 syndromes, neurofibromatosis type 1 or von Hippel–Lindau syndrome [2]. Neurofibromatosis is a common autosomal dominant condition – affecting 1 in 4000 births with the gastrointestinal tract involved in 20% [6]. A minority of somatostatinomas are familial [22], but the association with neurofibromatosis is much stronger for duodenal somatostatinomas (43%) than for those of pancreatic origin (1%) [22]. Over 50% metastasize, but complete resection has been associated with a 5-year survival of 95% [2]. The origin in the duodenum and the association with neurofibromatosis are both relatively good prognostic features. Duodenal somatostatinomas have less malignant potential than those arising in the pancreas, while those with an origin outside the pancreas or duodenum are the most malignant [23].

Other islet cell tumours: VIPoma and glucagonoma

VIPoma is a rare tumour. Secretion of Vasoactive Intestinal Polypeptide produces watery diarrhoea. There is loss of bicarbonate and potassium, which is severe – the potassium level being less than 2.5 mmol l^{-1} at some point in most patients [24].

Glucagonoma is a rare tumour of pancreatic alpha cells that secretes glucagon resulting in diabetes mellitus, and the propensity for cardiovascular complications. There is a necrolytic migratory rash and diarrhoea.

Both glucagonoma and VIPoma are likely to be malignant, with metastases in more than 60% and 70% of cases respectively [2]. Despite that, long-term survival is reported even in patients with metastatic disease. Surgery can provide complete relief of diarrhoea in patients with VIPoma and is recommended [3, 24]. Adequate fluid resuscitation and correction of electrolyte imbalance and metabolic acidosis is needed. Uneventful anaesthetic management of glucagonoma resection has been reported [25].

Carcinoid tumours

Carcinoid tumours have been reviewed by Caplin et al. [26]. Though rare, they are the commonest NETs. The annual incidence is 10–20 per million of population. They are an incidental finding in 1% of postmortems. Extensive epidemiological data from cancer registries [27] indicates a 50% 5-year survival overall, but with considerable variation depending on the site of the primary tumour. Carcinoids may be multiple, and associated with a second gastrointestinal malignancy. Foregut (bronchial, thymic and gastroduodenal) carcinoid is part of the spectrum of MEN 1, in which they occur in about 10% of cases [13].

Carcinoid tumours are noteworthy because they secrete a variety of substances including kinins and serotonin. Indeed, serotonin secretion is the hallmark of carcinoid tumours. The uptake and metabolism of these agents from the portal circulation by the liver means that the carcinoid syndrome does not become apparent until metastatic spread to the liver has occurred, unless the primary tumour is located outside the portal system (for example a bronchial carcinoid). There are two main features of the carcinoid syndrome:

(a) Carcinoid crises, comprising attacks of flushing, diarrhoea, bronchospasm and episodes of hypotension or hypertension.
(b) Cardiac valvular disease, usually of the tricuspid and pulmonary valves, that are exposed to hepatic venous blood. This leads to right ventricular failure. Mitral and aortic valves are affected when the lesion drains into the bronchial circulation or there is an atrial septal defect.

The anaesthetist will meet patients with carcinoid tumours undergoing abdominal surgery to relieve small or large bowel obstruction, reduce tumour burden, or treat hepatic metastases by resection, cryotherapy or hepatic artery ligation. Less commonly, cardiac surgery is undertaken, usually to replace or repair diseased right heart valves.

The risk of anaesthesia and surgery is related to the presence of carcinoid heart disease, and high preoperative urinary 5-hydroxyindoleacetic acid (5-HIAA) excretion [28]. Thus in the series of Kinney et al., the 15 patients who developed perioperative complications or death had a median urinary 5-HIAA excretion of 200 mg/24 h compared to 78 mg/24 h in the 104 patients who did not (normal value: < 6 mg/24 h) [28]. Two of the three deaths were in patients with advanced heart disease.

Carcinoid tumours express somatostatin receptors. These can be utilised for imaging by somatostatin scintigraphy [29], and provide responsiveness to octreotide. Administration of octreotide is the cornerstone of perioperative management of patients with carcinoid syndrome. Octreotide, a synthetic analogue of somatostatin, is given preoperatively either subcutaneously in repeated doses three times daily, or as a long-acting depot preparation every four weeks. Lanreotide is a long-acting analogue, also given by deep intramuscular injection every 14 days. At the time of surgery, octreotide can be given by continuous intravenous infusion, and additional intravenous bolus doses can be given if signs of a carcinoid crisis occur.

Following adoption of the use of octreotide in a large series spanning the years 1983 to 1996 [28], none of the 45 patients so treated developed a carcinoid crisis, compared with 8 of 73 patients who were not treated. The use of octreotide has effectively rendered the use of agents such as ketanserin and methysergide obsolete. Side effects are few, but somatostatin is found in the vagus nerve, and affects cardiac rhythm and conduction. Given by intravenous bolus, octreotide can produce a bradycardia and heart block [30].

Triggers to a carcinoid crisis include preoperative anxiety, intubation of the trachea, inadequate analgesia and manipulation of the tumour. Direct intra-arterial pressure monitoring is indicated, and the anaesthetist should prepare a range of drugs, such as phenylephrine and a nitrate so as to be able to respond promptly to intraoperative blood pressure fluctuations. Traditional advice has been to avoid the use of catecholamines because of the possibility that they would release mediators from the carcinoid tumour, and paradoxically cause hypotension. This advice predates the use of octreotide and is outdated [28, 31, 32]. If they are required, alpha agonists may be given safely.

A suitable anaesthetic technique [28, 30, 31, 33] includes sedation with a benzodiazepine to relieve anxiety. For induction of anaesthesia, thiopentone, etomidate and propofol have all been used, and etomidate recommended for patients undergoing cardiac surgery. Fentanyl can be used for intraoperative analgesia, and remifentanil has been reported to produce stable cardiovascular parameters [33]. Muscle relaxation with vecuronium, rocuronium or cisatracurium has been described. Thoracic epidural analgesia has been uneventful [33].

Table 5.1 Preoperative checklist for major pancreatic endocrine surgery.

	Management
Medical syndromes	
Insulinoma	Glucose, diazoxide
Gastrinoma	Proton-pump inhibitors and H$_2$ receptor blockers preoperatively
VIPoma	Somatostatin analogues
Glucagonoma	Somatostatin analogues
Somatostatinoma	Somatostatin analogues
Carcinoid	Somatostatin analogues, serotonin antagonists
Surgical diagnosis	Localisation, peptide secretion identified
Stomach	Nasogastric tube sited at induction
Emergency obstruction	Preoperative nasogastric suction and drainage, rapid sequence induction
Large surgical exposure	
Blood loss	Cross-match, coagulation screen, large-bore cannulae (e.g.13 G), central venous and arterial catheters with direct pressure monitoring, blood warmers and infusors (capacity 1 l min^{-1})
Potential hypothermia	Active and passive warming, temperature monitoring (core and periphery)
Pain	Epidural (thoracic) or patient-controlled analgesia, consent for
Cardiorespiratory	Facilities for positive end expiratory pressure, blood gases and acid–base measurements hourly perioperatively
System assessments	
Cardiovascular right (left) heart disease (carcinoid syndrome)	Prepare for hypo- and hypertension, consider intra-arterial catheter before induction, echocardiogram, ECG
Anaemia	Additional iron or transfusion
Respiratory	
Bronchospasm (carcinoid)	Somatostatin analogues, steroids, ventilator characteristics
Dyspnoea	Chest radiograph, echocardiography, blood gases
Liver/metabolism	
Coagulation	Prothrombin time, thrombin time, activated partial thromboplastin time
Biliary obstruction	Stent, fluids, maintain urine output with diuretics/dopamine
Albumin/proteins	Nutritional assessment
Glucose	Diabetic assessment and facilities for hourly blood glucose monitoring
Portal hypertension	Expect increased blood loss
Renal/fluids	Normalise electrolytes, catheterise
Risk assessment	Explain risks, record in patient's notes
Intensive care	Booked admission
Medications	Prophylaxis: antithrombosis (after epidural), antibiotics. Cautions in carcinoid: sedatives, drugs releasing histamine, (e.g., morphine, thiopental, atracurium)

From Holdcroft [1] with permission.

Aprotinin has been traditional in carcinoid syndrome for two reasons. First, to inhibit kallikrein released from the tumour, and second to decrease bleeding in cardiac surgery. The use of aprotinin does not reduce the intraoperative requirement for octreotide, and does not affect mortality [31]. Recent evidence on the renal complications of aprotinin, and its withdrawal make this unimportant.

General considerations

Major upper abdominal surgery involves a bilateral subcostal incision, may last for several hours, requires dissection of lymphatic tissue and causes fluid shifts; it will occasionally result in severe blood loss. A standard approach to such patients should be routine. Holdcroft has described a preoperative checklist for the additional problems of the patient with a NET (Table 5.1) [1]. Preoperative investigations include pulmonary function tests, ECG, full blood count, clotting screen, electrolytes and liver function tests.

Thoracic epidural analgesia should be discussed with the patient preoperatively. It does not improve overall mortality in high-risk patients [34], and carries the specific hazards of epidural abscess and haematoma, but it does offer the probability of high quality pain relief.

The general anaesthetic technique is based upon muscle relaxation with a non-depolarising neuromuscular blocking drug, and artificial ventilation; an air, oxygen and sevoflurane mixture is a reasonable choice. Good vascular access is essential, and will include two intravenous cannulae attached to warmed fluid infusions, central venous pressure monitoring and an arterial pressure line. Invasive monitoring facilitates a rapid response to haemodynamic change; arterial access allows intraoperative analysis of arterial blood gases and the lactate level, and in the case of insulinoma, frequent blood glucose estimation.

Use of oesophageal Doppler monitoring of cardiac output to adjust fluid therapy has been shown to improve outcome in colonic surgery, and it is reasonable to apply this approach in upper abdominal surgery as well. Unselective application of dopexamine [35] does not improve outcome, but fluid and inotrope therapy targeted to cardiovascular parameters in the postoperative period is beneficial [36]. It seems reasonable to apply these goals intraoperatively with selective use of dopexamine as indicated by the cardiac index. If liver resection is undertaken, then goals are different;

attention is given to minimising systemic venous pressure, thus decreasing blood loss and facilitating dissection of the liver.

Maintenance of the patient's temperature is vital to preserve haemostasis, minimise blood loss, reduce wound infection and postoperative shivering, and promote patient comfort. It is achieved by wrapping the lower limbs in insulating material, forced warm air convection, a heat moisture exchanger in the breathing system, and warming all intravenous fluids. To maximise surgical access, arms will be placed away from the side of the patient on arm boards; attention to detail while positioning the patient should protect against pressure palsy to the radial, ulnar and median nerves. If the patient is kept warm, blood loss less than one circulating volume and analgesia adequate, patients can be routinely extubated at the end of surgery.

References

1. Holdcroft A. Hormones and the gut. *Br J Anaesth* 2000; **85**: 58–68.
2. Ramage JK, Davies AHG, Ardill J, et al. Guidelines for the management of gastroenteropancreatic neuroendocrine (including carcinoid) tumours. *Gut* 2005; **54**: iv, 1–16.
3. Alexakis N, Neoptolemos JP. Pancreatic neuroendocrine tumours. *Best Practice & Research* 2008; **22**: 183–205.
4. Service FJ. Hypoglycemic disorders. *N Engl J Med* 1995; **332**: 1144–52.
5. Grant CS. Gastrointestinal endocrine tumours. Insulinoma. *Baillières Clin Gastroenterol* 1996; **10**: 645–71.
6. Alexakis N, Connor S, Ghaneh P, et al. Hereditary pancreatic endocrine tumours. *Pancreatology* 2004; **4**: 417–33; discussion 34–5.
7. Hirshberg B, Libutti SK, Alexander HR, et al. Blind distal pancreatectomy for occult insulinoma, an inadvisable procedure. *J Am Coll Surg* 2002; **194**: 761–4.
8. Bourke AM. Anaesthesia for the surgical treatment of hyperinsulinism. Case reports. *Anaesthesia* 1966; **21**: 239–43.
9. Schnelle N, Molnar GD, Ferris DO, Rosevear JW, Moffitt EA. Circulating glucose and insulin in surgery for insulinomas. *JAMA* 1971; **217**: 1072–8.
10. Schwartz SS, Horwitz DL, Zehfus B, Langer BG, Kaplan E. Continuous monitoring and control of plasma glucose during operation for removal of insulinomas. *Surgery* 1979; **85**: 702–7.
11. Muir JJ, Endres SM, Offord K, van Heerden JA, Tinker JH. Glucose management in patients undergoing

operation for insulinoma removal. *Anesthesiology* 1983; **59**: 371–5.

12. Fernandez-Cruz L, Blanco L, Cosa R, Rendon H. Is laparoscopic resection adequate in patients with neuroendocrine pancreatic tumors? *World J Surg* 2008; **32**: 904–17.

13. Brandi ML, Gagel RF, Angeli A, et al. Guidelines for diagnosis and therapy of MEN type 1 and type 2. *J Clin Endocrinol Metab* 2001; **86**: 5658–71.

14. Orlando LA, Lenard L, Orlando RC. Chronic hypergastrinemia: causes and consequences. *Dig Dis Sci* 2007; **52**: 2482–9.

15. Jensen RT, Niederle B, Mitry E, et al. Gastrinoma (duodenal and pancreatic). *Neuroendocrinology* 2006; **84**: 173–82.

16. Norton JA, Jensen RT. Resolved and unresolved controversies in the surgical management of patients with Zollinger–Ellison syndrome. *Ann Surg* 2004; **240**: 757–73.

17. Norton JA, Fraker DL, Alexander HR, et al. Surgery to cure the Zollinger–Ellison syndrome. N *Engl J Med* 1999; **341**: 635–44.

18. Stabile BE, Morrow DJ, Passaro E , Jr. The gastrinoma triangle: operative implications. *Am J Surg* 1984; **147**: 25–31.

19. Norton JA, Kivlen M, Li M, Schneider D, Chuter T, Jensen RT. Morbidity and mortality of aggressive resection in patients with advanced neuroendocrine tumors. *Arch Surg* 2003; **138**: 859–66.

20. Solorzano CC, Lee JE, Pisters PW, et al. Nonfunctioning islet cell carcinoma of the pancreas: survival results in a contemporary series of 163 patients. *Surgery* 2001; **130**: 1078–85.

21. Kazanjian KK, Reber HA, Hines OJ. Resection of pancreatic neuroendocrine tumors: results of 70 cases. *Arch Surg* 2006; **141**: 765–9; discussion 9–70.

22. Soga J, Yakuwa Y. Somatostatinoma/inhibitory syndrome: a statistical evaluation of 173 reported cases as compared to other pancreatic endocrinomas. *J Exp Clin Cancer Res* 1999; **18**: 13–22.

23. Nesi G, Marcucci T, Rubio CA, Brandi ML, Tonelli F. Somatostatinoma: clinico-pathological features of three cases and literature reviewed. *J Gastroenterol Hepatol* 2008; **23**: 521–6.

24. Long RG, Bryant MG, Mitchell SJ, Adrian TE, Polak JM, Bloom SR. Clinicopathological study of pancreatic and ganglioneuroblastoma tumours secreting vasoactive intestinal polypeptide (VIPomas). *BMJ* 1981; **282**: 1767–71.

25. Nicoll JM, Catling SJ. Anaesthetic management of glucagonoma. *Anaesthesia* 1985; **40**: 152–7.

26. Caplin ME, Buscombe JR, Hilson AJ, Jones AL, Watkinson AF, Burroughs AK. Carcinoid tumour. *Lancet* 1998; **352**: 799–805.

27. Modlin IM, Sandor A. An analysis of 8305 cases of carcinoid tumors. *Cancer* 1997; **79**: 813–29.

28. Kinney MA, Warner ME, Nagorney DM, et al. Perianaesthetic risks and outcomes of abdominal surgery for metastatic carcinoid tumours. *Br J Anaesth* 2001; **87**: 447–52.

29. Oberg K, Eriksson B. Nuclear medicine in the detection, staging and treatment of gastrointestinal carcinoid tumours. *Best Pract Res Clin Endocrinol Metab* 2005; **19**: 265–76.

30. Dilger JA, Rho EH, Que FG, Sprung J. Octreotide-induced bradycardia and heart block during surgical resection of a carcinoid tumor. *Anesth Analg* 2004; **98**: 318–20.

31. Weingarten TN, Abel MD, Connolly HM, Schroeder DR, Schaff HV. Intraoperative management of patients with carcinoid heart disease having valvular surgery: a review of one hundred consecutive cases. *Anesth Analg* 2007; **105**: 1192–9.

32. Castillo JG, Filsoufi F, Adams DH, Raikhelkar J, Zaku B, Fischer GW. Management of patients undergoing multivalvular surgery for carcinoid heart disease: the role of the anaesthetist. *Br J Anaesth* 2008; **101**: 618–26.

33. Farling PA, Durairaju AK. Remifentanil and anaesthesia for carcinoid syndrome. *Br J Anaesth* 2004; **92**: 893–5.

34. Rigg JR, Jamrozik K, Myles PS, et al. Epidural anaesthesia and analgesia and outcome of major surgery: a randomised trial. *Lancet* 2002; **359**: 1276–82.

35. Stone MD, Wilson RJ, Cross J, Williams BT. Effect of adding dopexamine to intraoperative volume expansion in patients undergoing major elective abdominal surgery. *Br J Anaesth* 2003; **91**: 619–24.

36. Pearse R, Dawson D, Fawcett J, Rhodes A, Grounds RM, Bennett ED. Early goal-directed therapy after major surgery reduces complications and duration of hospital stay. A randomised, controlled trial [ISRCTN38797445]. *Crit Care* 2005; **9**: R687–93.

Multiple endocrine neoplasia

Saffron Whitehead

Multiple endocrine neoplasia (MEN) is a rare autosomal dominant disorder characterised by primary tumours in at least two different endocrine glands. There are two types of MEN, MEN 1 and MEN 2. Both types are caused by mutations of identified genes which may arise sporadically or may be inherited (familial). The familial form of MEN (more common) is identified as a MEN patient who has one first-degree relative showing at least one of the characteristic endocrine tumours. MEN tumours may be benign or malignant, functional (i.e., capable of synthesising hormones in excess) or non-functional. Thus patients with MEN may present with a diverse range of pathology and symptoms [1].

MEN 1 is characterised by tumours of the parathyroid glands, the endocrine pancreas and the pituitary gland, and most patients have mutations of the menin gene. MEN 2 is subdivided into MEN 2A and MEN 2B. Patients with MEN 2A will typically develop medullary carcinomas of the thyroid gland, phaeochromocytomas and/or tumours of the parathyroid glands. In MEN 2B hyperparathyroidism is typically absent but tumours include medullary thyroid carcinomas, phaeochromocytomas and tumours of nerve cells and nerve fibres (neuromas). Both types of MEN 2 are caused by mutations of the *RET* (REarranged during Transfection) gene. Mutations of the same gene also cause familial medullary thyroid carcinoma [1].

MEN 1: incidence, clinical features and diagnosis

In the early twentieth century, a syndrome that involved the concurrence of tumours of the parathyroid glands, the pancreatic islets and the anterior pituitary gland was first described. But it was not until 1954 that Werner described such a syndrome in a family in which the father and four of nine siblings were affected [2]. He called the syndrome multiple endocrine adenomatosis

although it has subsequently been renamed as MEN 1 or is more rarely referred to as Werner's syndrome. The incidence is about one in 30 000 patients of whom 90% have inherited MEN 1 mutations and about 10% have arisen *de novo* [3].

Typically, the first clinical manifestation of MEN 1 is primary hyperparathyroidism (Chapter 3) and over 95% patients with MEN 1 initially present with hyperparathyroidism (Figure 6.1; Table 6.1). There are, however, differences in the hyperparathyroidism of the MEN 1 syndrome and sporadic cases of primary hyperparathyroidism that occur in the population as a whole. Primary hyperparathyroidism in MEN 1 usually occurs at an earlier age (average 20–25 years) compared with sporadic primary hyperparathyroidism (typically 55–60 years) and has an equal male to female ratio compared with sporadic cases in which the male to female ratio is 1:3. It also involves all four parathyroid glands (more if there are supernumerary glands) compared with a single gland characteristic of sporadic primary hyperparathyroidism. MEN 1 accounts for only 2–4% cases of primary hyperparathyroidism in the general population [1].

Since parathyroid hormone (PTH) stimulates bone resorption and increases calcium reabsorption in the kidney tubule, biochemical diagnosis is made by elevated serum PTH and hypercalcaemia. Although patients are often asymptomatic and may be for a long period of time, they may present with clinical symptoms of primary hyperparathyroidism such as fatigue, polydipsia, polyuria, myalgias or abdominal pain. Typical clinical signs of primary hyperparathyroidism are renal calculi or osteitis fibrosa cystica, resulting from excess PTH and hypercalcaemia.

Surgery for hyperparathyroidism in MEN 1 is the preferred option and this may involve subtotal parathyroidectomy (three parathyroid glands and half of the fourth one) or total parathyroidectomy with

Core Topics in Endocrinology in Anaesthesia and Critical Care, eds. George M. Hall, Jennifer M. Hunter and Mark S. Cooper. Published by Cambridge University Press. © Cambridge University Press 2010.

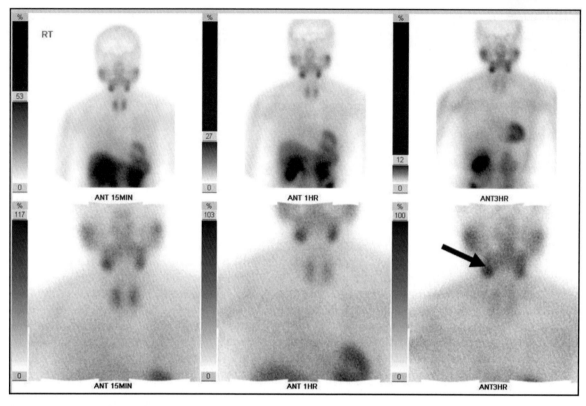

Fig. 6.1 Tc-99m Sestamibi scan of a patient with multiple endocrine neoplasia (MEN) type 1. The black arrow indicates a large parathyroid adenoma identified by retention of the radioactivity after three hours. Hyperplasia of the other three glands was only identified at surgery.

Table 6.1 Tumours associated with multiple endocrine neoplasia type 1 (MEN 1) and their penetrance.

Localisation	~ Penetrance (%)	Other common non-endocrine manifestations
Parathyroid	90	Facial angiofibromas
Enteropancreatic		Collagenomas
Gastrinoma	40	Lipomas
Insulinoma	20	Leiomyomas
Non-functioning	20	
Pituitary		
Prolactinoma	15	
Other	20	
Adrenal		
Non-functioning cortex	20	
Phaeochromocytoma	< 1	
Foregut (carcinoids)		
Gastric	5	
Thymic	2	
Bronchial	2	

an autologous parathyroid graft of the 'most normal-appearing' tissue into the non-dominant forearm. There is no general consensus which is the preferred option, although late recurrence of hyperparathyroidism may occur with subtotal parathyroidectomy and may affect up to 50% cases by 8–12 years after surgery [4]. Recently, calcium-sensing receptor agonists that stimulate the unique G-protein coupled calcium receptor on chief cells of the parathyroid glands have been shown to decrease PTH release (Chapter 3). They may also decrease parathyroid tumour growth and thus become an important therapy in the treatment of MEN 1 primary hyperparathyroidism [5].

The second most common manifestation of MEN 1 is neoplasia of the pancreatic islets, although these tumours can also arise at other sites such as the duodenal wall and stomach – hence the term gastro-entero-pancreatic (GEP) tumours (Chapter 5). These tumours of the upper gastrointestinal tract occur in 30–80% of patients with MEN 1 (Table 6.1). They may be either benign or malignant and are usually multiple and develop at a young age [6]. Tumours that secrete excess gastrin, gastrinomas, account for about 40–50% of GEP tumours associated with MEN 1. They are typically malignant and have metastasised before they are detected. The production of excess gastrin which, via histamine, stimulates the secretion of gastric acid from the stomach, is called Zollinger–Ellison syndrome. This usually occurs by itself but when it is associated with MEN 1 the onset is at an earlier age. Poor prognosis is associated with pancreatic primary gastrinomas, which are larger and more aggressive than duodenal gastrinomas and they account for the major morbidity and mortality associated with MEN 1. They induce peptic ulcers, diarrhoea, cachexia and abdominal pain. Mortality is associated with metastasis of the tumours, notably to the liver. Diagnosis is made by elevated fasting serum gastrin concentrations and an increased output of basal gastric acid [7].

Treatment of gastrinomas can involve both drugs and surgery. The effects of hypersecretion of gastric acid can be controlled by histamine H_2 receptor antagonists (histamine being the mediator of gastrin effects) or H^+, K^+-ATPase inhibitors that directly inhibit gastric acid secretion. Surgical intervention is somewhat controversial since its outcome is rarely successful but this will depend on whether or not the tumours can be precisely located, their aggressiveness and the decision of the clinical team [7].

Insulinomas account for 10–30% of all MEN 1-related islet tumours although they rarely co-exist with gastrinomas. Patients will present with symptoms of fasting hypoglycaemia which can be relieved by glucose intake. The diagnosis of insulinoma is made with a prolonged fast and serial measurements of plasma glucose and insulin at the time of hypoglycaemia. There are inappropriately elevated serum concentrations of insulin, pro-insulin and the redundant cleaved sequence of the pro-insulin molecule, the C peptide, despite hypoglycaemia. These lesions are usually benign and surgery is curative. Intraoperative monitoring of glucose and insulin is helpful to verify removal of the tumour(s) [8].

Rarer GEP tumours include glucagonomas, VIP (vasoactive intestinal polypeptide)-omas, PP (pancreatic polypeptide)-omas and somatostatinomas as well as non-functioning tumours. These generally present as large neoplasms. The patients also tend to have necrotising skin lesions, cachexia, new onset diabetes and profound watery diarrhoea. Pancreatic surgery for asymptomatic patients may be considered when the size of the tumour exceeds 2 cm. Since somatostatin has a paracrine inhibitory role on pancreatic secretions, the long-acting somatostatin analogue, octreotide, is considered to be the drug of choice for treating glucagonomas and VIPomas [9].

The third type of tumour associated with MEN 1 are the tumours of the anterior pituitary gland and their occurrence ranges from 10 to about 70% depending on the series of patients. The most common form is benign non-functioning macroadenomas (≥ 1 cm) of the chromophobes. These usually present with bitemporal hemianopia, due to compression of the optic chiasm, and hypopituitarism. Only 10–15% of anterior pituitary tumours are functioning and these can secrete excessive prolactin, growth hormone or adrenocorticotrophin (ACTH) [10]. These excess secretions can cause amenorrhoea, infertility and galactorrhoea in women (impotence in men), acromegaly or Cushing's disease respectively. Thus symptoms of MEN 1 pituitary tumours depend very much on tumour volume and hormonal secretion. In general, treatment for these tumours is the same as that for sporadic pituitary tumours, i.e., medical, radiation and/or surgical (Chapter 1). Transphenoidal surgery is the treatment of choice for non-functioning pituitary adenomas, acromegaly and Cushing's disease, whilst drugs that inhibit the secretion of prolactin, i.e., dopamine agonists are the preferred treatment for prolactin secreting tumours. Somatostatin analogues are second line treatment for acromegaly.

Other tumours associated with MEN 1 are carcinoids, tumours of the adrenal gland and non-endocrine tumours such as lipomas [1]. Carcinoid tumours are seen in approximately 5% of patients with MEN 1 and are usually located in the bronchi, gastrointestinal tract or thymus. MEN 1 bronchial carcinoids are more usually found in women (male to female ratio of 1:4) and they are usually benign though they have the potential for 'mass' effects, with metastases or recurrence after surgery. Some secrete ACTH and thus patients may present with Cushing's syndrome. This is in contrast to carcinoids of the thymus gland which occur more frequently in men and tend to be aggressive. In both cases, surgery remains the primary treatment option.

Primary adrenocortical tumours are common in MEN 1 and affect 5–40% of patients [1]. They are typically bilateral, hyperplastic and non-functional, although occasionally some secrete excess cortisol or aldosterone. Tumours of the adrenal medulla, phaeochromocytomas, affect < 1% of MEN 1 patients and, though rare, they are important to identify prior to any surgery to avoid severe hypertension during surgery (Chapter 4).

A variety of non-endocrine tumours can affect MEN 1 patients and these include tumours of adipose tissue and the skin [1]. The incidence of benign lipomas in MEN 1 is about 20–30% and these are usually multiple, may be large or small, and most frequently occur in visceral fat. They rarely recur after surgery. Facial angiofibromas, benign tumours of blood vessels and connective tissue, have been observed in 40–85% of MEN 1 patients, and over 50% of MEN 1 patients have five or more angiofibromas over their faces. Multiple cutaneous nodules, collagenomas, also arise frequently in MEN 1 patients and these are typically symmetrically arranged on the trunk, neck and upper limbs. They are roundish and can range from a few millimetres to several centimetres in diameter. They are typically asymptomatic.

MEN 1, the *MEN 1* gene and its protein, menin.

The gene that codes for menin is located on chromosome 11q12–13 and transcribes an mRNA consisting of 10 exons which encodes the 610 amino acid protein, menin [11]. It is widely expressed from an early stage in development. Despite intensive investigation, the exact role of the *MEN 1* gene is unknown, although it is generally considered to be a tumour suppressive gene with menin regulating the cell cycle via several mechanisms [12]. Menin is mainly located in the nucleus and most menin interacting proteins suggest that menin plays an important role in gene expression with downstream effects on critical genes regulating normal and tumour processes (Figure 6.2).

Over a thousand mutations of the *MEN 1* gene have been reported through the entire coding region but unfortunately there is no correlation between these mutations with the clinical phenotype of MEN 1 [13]. Most MEN 1 mutations are inactivating resulting in the transcription of a truncated inactive protein. Less common (10–15%) are missense mutations that potentially alter the interaction of menin with other proteins that play a role in the physiological regulation of the cell cycle and/or favour the rapid degradation of menin.

Since mutations of the *MEN 1* gene do not correlate with the development of specific tumours associated with MEN 1, there is currently no rationale guiding therapeutic intervention in patients diagnosed with *MEN 1* mutations, which is in stark contrast to patients with MEN 2 syndromes (see below). Patients with identified mutations of *MEN 1* should be closely monitored for evidence of tumours associated with this syndrome and then treated when there is clinical or biochemical evidence characteristic of this disease. Annual screening for a parathyroid adenoma includes serum calcium and PTH measurements. If these are elevated, a Sestamibi scan should be done. Similarly, for gastrinoma screening, fasting serum gastrin and gastric acid output should be measured and an octreotide scan ordered if they are raised. For insulinomas, fasting glucose and insulin should be estimated; for other enteropancreatic tumours, chromogranin-A, glucagon and proinsulin are measured and if elevated an octreotide, CT or MRI scan performed. For anterior pituitary tumours, serum measurement of prolactin, insulin-like growth factor-1 (IGF-1) and an MRI scan are necessary; and for carcinoid a CT scan [6].

MEN 2: incidence, clinical features and diagnosis

MEN 2 is a rare disorder with an estimated prevalence of one in 20 000 and, like MEN 1, is an autosomal dominant syndrome [1, 14]. MEN 2 exists as one of two distinct clinical subtypes, MEN 2A or MEN 2B and both

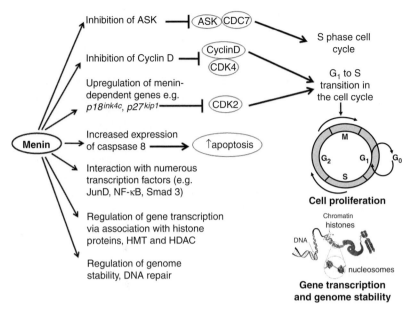

Fig. 6.2 A highly simplified diagram showing some of the ways in which menin may regulate gene transcription, cell proliferation, apoptosis and genome stability. Menin represses cell division by inhibiting activator of S-phase kinase (ASK) which, in complex with CDC7 protein kinase, serves as a regulator of the S phase of the cell cycle. Menin inhibits cell proliferation by repressing the expression of Cyclin D1 and D3 which forms an active kinase with cyclin-dependent kinase (CDK) and stimulates the G_1 to S transition in the cell cycle. Menin also inhibits the G_0/G_1 to S by increasing the expression of $p18^{ink4c}$ and $p27^{kip1}$ which represses CDK2 activity. Menin induces the expression of caspase 8 which is an essential component in receptor-related apoptotic pathways. Menin is known to interact with various transcription factors and may also regulate gene expression by altering chromatin structure through recruitment of histone methyltransferases (HMT) that upregulate gene expression or through recruitment of histone deacetylases (HDAC) that repress gene expression. It is not, however, clear whether these tumour suppressing functions of menin in culture are crucial for the development of MEN 1. Phases of the cell cycle: M, mitosis; G_1, cell growth; G_0, quiescent phase (variable); S, DNA synthesis, G_2, preparation for mitosis

Table 6.2 Tumours associated with multiple endocrine neoplasia (MEN) type 2A, MEN 2B and familial medullary thyroid carcinoma (FMTC) and their penetrance.

Tumour	~Penetrance (%)	Other non-endocrine manifestations
MEN 2A		
Medullary thyroid carcinoma	100	
Phaeochromocytoma	50	Multigland parathyroid tumours
Hyperparathyroidism	30	
MEN 2B		
Medullary thyroid carcinoma	100	Marfanoid habitus, mucosal neuromas, intestinal ganglioneuromas
Phaeochromocytoma	50	
FMTC		
Medullary thyroid carcinoma	100	None

are caused by a mutation of the *RET* gene. Familial medullary thyroid carcinoma (FMTC) is related to MEN 2 and caused by mutations of the same gene. MEN 2A accounts for about 80% cases, MEN 2B for 5% and FMTC 15% [15].

Medullary thyroid carcinoma (MTC) occurs in all MEN 2 patients (Table 6.2) and is usually the first clinical manifestation of this disorder [1, 6]. Such tumours are frequently multifocal and bilateral. MTC tumours of the calcitonin-secreting parafollicular C cells derived from neural crest cells as opposed to the follicular cells of the thyroid gland as is the case with differentiated thyroid carcinomas. Thus patients with MTC usually have increased concentrations of circulating calcitonin and this provides a good plasma tumour marker for MEN 2 and FMTC [6]. In MEN 2A patients, MTC occurs between the ages of 5 and 25 years with diarrhoea being the most common systemic symptom in association with raised plasma concentrations of calcitonin (> 10 ng ml^{-1}). If untreated, these tumours can manifest with a neck lump or neck pain [1]. In MEN 2B patients, MTC is more aggressive and symptoms generally develop about a decade earlier. Medullary thyroid carcinoma is the most common endocrine-related cause of death in patients with MEN 2A, MEN 2B and FMTC.

Early detection of MTC is important. This can be done by tests to evaluate calcitonin secretion in response to stimulation with secretagogues such as pentagastrin or calcium [6]. These tests, however, may be inaccurate and do not always allow for early detection of tumours. Commercial *RET* mutation tests are now available and can identify 97% of patients with MEN 2 [16, 17]. Thus prophylactic treatment can be given before the age of possible progression of the malignancy and/or its metastasis [18]. Fine needle aspiration biopsy of a lump in the neck may also establish the diagnosis of MTC, and CT or MRI is useful in identifying locally advanced or metastatic disease. Treatment is by total thyroidectomy with lymph node dissection. Sometimes external beam radiotherapy is used to treat for metastatic disease. Raised calcitonin levels after surgery can be a sign of persistent, recurrent or generalised MTC.

Secondary to *RET* mutations are phaeochromocytomas which develop on the background of adrenomedullary hyperplasia of the chromaffin cells (Figure 6.3). Like follicular C cells of the thyroid gland, adrenomedullary cells are also of neural crest origin but instead of secreting excess calcitonin they secrete excess catecholamines into the circulation. The phaeochromocytomas associated with MEN are almost always benign and tend to be bilateral in up to 50–80% cases [1, 14]. The clinical features are typical of excess catecholamines and include paroxysmal hypertension, palpitations, nervousness, episodic headaches and sweating. In about 25% of cases of MEN 2A, these are the first clinical signs and symptoms of the syndrome. In approximately 35% of MEN 2 cases, phaeochromocytomas are diagnosed at the same time as MTC whilst in the remainder, MTC occurs prior to the onset of phaeochromocytoma. The peak age of onset is approximately 40 years (although children as young as 10 years old have been reported) and about 50% of patients with MEN 2A develop it (Table 6.2). It should, however, be

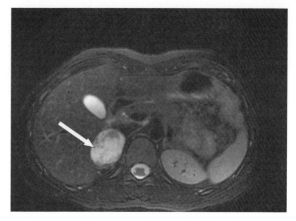

Fig. 6.3 Large phaeochromocytoma (white arrow) seen on a post-contrast MRI scan in a multiple endocrine neoplasia (MEN) type 2A patient.

noted that most cases of MTC or phaeochromocytoma are sporadic and only about 10% of all cases are related to MEN 2.

The presence of a phaeochromocytoma can be assessed by measurement of plasma or 24-hour urinary concentrations of catecholamines and/or their metabolites along with a MIBG scan. Either CT or MR imaging is useful to know the extent of the tumour [1, 6]. Treatment is surgical removal either by laparoscopic excision if less than 6 cm in size or by open surgery. Surgery is only done after proper alpha- followed usually by beta-adrenergic blockade (Chapter 4). It is important to diagnose a functioning phaeochromocytoma prior to any surgery to avoid severe hypertension during the operation and hypotension after removal of the tumour.

Hyperparathyroidism occurs in 20–30% patients with MEN 2A (although it is usually asymptomatic) and recommended treatment for this tumour associated with MEN 2A is excision of enlarged glands only [15, 19]. Hyperparathyroidism does not occur in MEN 2B patients, but 40% of patients with this syndrome suffer from multiple mucosal neuromas (Figure 6.4), and/or diffuse ganglioneuromatosis of the gastrointestinal tract which can cause colic, abdominal distension, diarrhoea or constipation. MEN 2B patients may also manifest developmental abnormalities such as a Marfanoid phenotype (Figure 6.4), decreased upper/lower body ratio and skeletal deformations. Rare variants of MEN 2A include cutaneous lichen amyloidosis and Hirschsprung's disease (a congenital disorder of the colon). Thus there are similarities and differences between MEN 2A and MEN 2B although morbidity and mortality are greater for MEN 2B than MEN 2A.

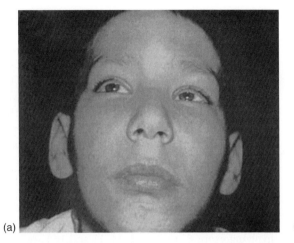
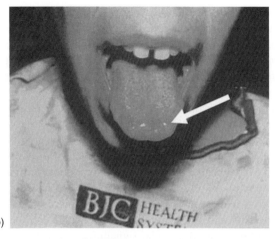

Fig. 6.4 Typical facial features of multiple endocrine neoplasia (MEN) type 2B patients. (a) Marfanoid features. (b) Mucosal neuromas on the tongue (white arrow).

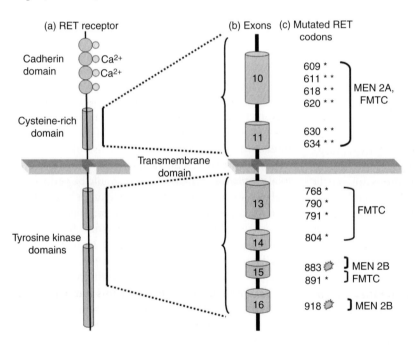

Fig. 6.5 (a) Diagram of the RET receptor showing the different domains of the receptor protein. (b) The structure of the RET mRNA in which germline mutations have been identified and the location of mutated codons. (c) Genotype-phenotye correlations of MEN 2A and MEN 2B. Hirschsprung's disease is associated with germline mutations at 609, 611, 618, 620 and loss of function mutations all over the gene. *low risk; **high risk and ✿ highest risk of developing aggressive MTC and will determine the timing of total thyroidectomy and lymph node dissection (see text).

The *Ret* gene and MEN type 2

The *RET* protooncogene, located on chromosome 10q11.2, transcribes an mRNA consisting of 21 exons. This encodes the RET receptor which is a single membrane spanning protein containing four Ca^{2+}-dependent cell adhesion (Cadherin)-like domains; a cysteine-rich domain in the extracellular part of the receptor; and two tyrosine kinase domains in the intracellular component (Figure 6.5). The RET receptor, of which there are several isoforms, is expressed by cells

of neural crest origin: the parafollicular C-cells of the thyroid gland, adrenal medullary cells, parathyroid cells and enteric autonomic ganglion cells [17, 19].

Normally RET is activated by a complex of ligands and coreceptors. The ligands belong to the glial cell line-derived neurotrophic factor (GDNF) family of proteins and include neurturin, artemin and persephin. These do not bind directly to the RET receptor but to one of the four glycosyl-phosphatidylinositol-anchored (GDNF)-family of α receptors (GFRαs). These receptors are normally bound to the plasma membrane within the lipid rafts and when a GDNF ligand binds to a GFRα it induces dimerisation of two RET receptors and subsequently autophosphorylation of the tyrosine residues on the intracellular domain of the RET receptor. Although GFRαs are normally bound to the plasma membrane, soluble forms also exist and these can also cause dimerisation and activation of the RET receptor upon binding of a GDNF ligand [17].

The signal transduction pathways of the activated RET receptor are complex but they play an important role in regulating cell survival, differentiation, proliferation, migration and chemotaxis. Different phosphorylated tyrosines on the RET receptor serve as docking sites for different adaptor proteins which then activate different intracellular signalling pathways. These include activation of phospholipase C and subsequently protein kinase C, and activation of mitogen activated protein kinase (MAPK), extracellular regulated kinase (ERK) and the PI3-kinase/AKT pathway [17].

Mutations in the extracellular domain, notably in the codons for the cysteine residues in exons 8, 10 and 11, can paradoxically exert dual effects (Figure 6.5). Firstly, gain of function mutations which are due to aberrant disulphide bonding between cysteine residues of two mutant RET receptors occurs. This leads to ligand-independent dimerisation of two receptors with constitutive activation of the down-stream MAPK. These gains of function mutations are mostly seen in MEN 2A, MEN 2B and FMTC. Secondly, loss of function mutations, which result in decreased RET levels at the cell surface, occurs. These mutations are associated with Hirschsprung's disease [15, 17].

Mutations in the intracellular catalytic domain affect adenosine triphosphate (ATP) binding and autophosphorylation of the two distinct tyrosine kinase domains within the receptor – in which there are at least 12 autophosphorylation sites. Thus constitutive activation (phosphorylation) of the tyrosine kinases in the absence of a ligand induces aberrant activity of intracellular signalling proteins thereby inducing uncontrolled cell proliferation.

Unlike MEN 1, MEN 2 syndrome shows a strong genotype–phenotype correlation. Missense mutations in the cysteine-rich codons in exon 10 and 11 (the extracellular domain) are responsible for the majority (93–98%) of MEN 2A cases and the majority (80–96%) of FMTC cases (Figure 6.5). Interestingly, a specific mutation at codon 634 in exon 11 is present in 85% patients with MEN 2A syndrome and is strongly associated with the occurrence of phaeochromocytoma and/or hyperparathyroidism.

In contrast, only 30% of patients with FMTC have codon 634 mutations in exon 11 [1, 15].

While rare cases of MEN 2A and FMTC have been associated with missense mutations in exons 13, 14 and 15 that code for part of the intracellular domain of the RET receptors, most MEN 2B cases are associated with mutations of this domain. Ninety-five per cent of MEN 2B patients bear the M918 mutation at exon 16 whilst about 5% MEN 2B patients have a A883F mutation at exon 15 (Figure 6.2) [6, 15].

Screening and surveillance of MEN 2

Molecular information has revolutionised the understanding and treatment of MEN 2. Since mutations involving exons 8, 10, 11, 13, 14, 15 and 16 have been identified in patients with MEN 2A, MEN 2B and FMTC (Figure 6.5), these exons are routinely screened for *RET* mutations to ascertain carrier status within a family and to determine the risk of developing MTC, phaeochromocytoma and hyperparathyroidism. Medullary thyroid carcinoma is the principal endocrine cause of mortality in patients with MEN 2A, MEN 2B and FMTC and there appears to be a relationship between the precise codon mutation and the aggressiveness of MTC [6, 15, 20]. For example, in MEN 2B patients with mutations in codon 918 or 883 the risk of developing MTC, particularly at an early age, is highest and thus total prophylactic thyroidectomy should be performed, preferably within the first few months after birth. Other mutations, described above, show varying degrees of disease risk although total thyroidectomy by five years is recommended for high-risk MEN 2A patients with specific mutations in the codons of the extracellular domain of the receptor, i.e., codons 611, 618, 620 and 634. The risk of developing MTC is lower with other mutations and there is, as yet, no consensus about the age at which prophylactic treatment should be given in patients with mutations of codons 609, 768, 790, 791, 804 and 891. Total thyroidectomy may be the treatment of choice by 5–10 years. Alternatively, these patients can be screened to detect any biochemical abnormalities that may arise, such as the calcitonin response to secretagogues and biochemical tests for phaeochromocytoma and hyperparathyroidism.

Summary

The discovery of the *Men* gene and the *RET* gene in 1997 and 1993 respectively, opened up a new era in our understanding of the pathogenesis of MEN 1 and MEN 2 syndromes and the early recognition and clinical management of affected individuals at risk [21]. While the menin protein has been shown to control phases of the cell cycle, apoptosis, gene expression and genome stability in *in vitro* studies, it is not yet known precisely how mutated *Men* genes cause endocrine neoplasias in MEN 1 patients. Although hundreds of *Men* mutations have been identified, there is no genotype which correlates with the clinical phenotype of this syndrome. This contrasts with mutations of the *Ret* gene in which there are clear genotype/clinical phenotype correlations depending on the location of the mutations within the receptor protein. Thus MEN 2A patients have mutations in the extracellular domain and MEN 2B in the intracellular domain and prediction of the development of different endocrine tumours and their potential aggressiveness can be made by identifying the precise codon location of the mutations.

The increasing knowledge of the molecular mechanisms of MEN coupled with the clinical outcome and the availability of genetic testing has greatly reduced its morbidity and mortality. All identified MEN patients should receive routine biochemical and image screening to detect and treat early onset of the disease prior to the development of symptoms. Very early surgical intervention is required for MEN 2B patients at high or very high risk of developing FMTC. However, more studies are required to elucidate the precise molecular pathways underlying the tumourigenesis associated with MEN so that new targeted therapeutic strategies can be designed.

Acknowledgements

I would like to thank Dr Gul Bano for her help during the preparation of this chapter and for the imaging pictures. I also thank Dr V. Murday for the photograph of the MEN 2 patient.

References

1. Falchetti A, Marini F, Luz E, et al. Multiple endocrine neoplasms. *Best Pract Res Clin Rheumatol* 2008; **22**: 149–63.

2. Werner P. Genetic aspects of adenomatosis of endocrine glands. *Am J Med 1954;* **16**: 363–71.

3. Agarwal SK, Lee Burns A, Sukhodolets KE, et al. Molecular pathology of the MEN1 gene. *Ann N Y Acad Sci* 2004; **1014**: 189–98.

4. Burgess JR, David R, Parameswaran V, et al. The outcome of subtotal parathyroidectomy for the treatment of hyperparathyroidism in multiple endocrine neoplasia type 1. *Arch Surg* 1998; **133**: 126–9.

5. Peacock M, Bilezikian JP, Klassen PS, et al. Clinacalet hydrochloride maintains long-term normocalcemia in patients with primary hyperparathyroidism. *J Clin Endocrinol Metab* 2005; **90**: 135–41.

6. Brandi ML, Gagel RF, Angeli A, et al. Guidelines for diagnosis and therapy of MEN type 1 and type 2. *J Clin Endocrinol Metab* 2001; **86**: 5658–71.

7. Piecha G, Chudek J, Wiecek A . Multiple endocrine neoplasia type 1. *Eur J Intern Med* 2008; **19**: 99–103.

8. Oberg K, Eriksson B. Endocrine tumours of the pancreas. *Best Pract Res Clin Gastroenterol* 2005; **19**: 753–81.

9. Doherty GM. Rare endocrine tumours of the GI tract. *Best Pract Res Clin Gastroenterol* 2005; **19**: 807–17.

10. Vergès B, Boureille F, Goudet P, et al. Pituitary disease in MEN type 1 (MEN1): data from the France–Belgium MEN1 multicenter study. *J Clin Endocrinol Metab* 2002; **87**: 457–65.

11. Balogh K, Rácz K, Patócs A, et al. Menin and its interacting proteins: elucidation of menin function. *Trends Endocrinol Metab* 2006; **17**: 357–64.

12. Yang Y, Hua X. In search of tumor suppressing function of menin. *Mol Cell Endocrinol* 2007; **265–266**: 34–41.

13. Lemos MC, Thakker RV. Multiple endocrine neoplasia type 1 (MEN1): analysis of 1336 mutations reported in the first decade following identification of the gene. *Hum Mutat* 2008; **29**: 22–32.

14. Raue F, Frank-Raue K. Multiple endocrine neoplasia type 2: 2007 update. *Horm Res* 2007; **68** Suppl 5: 101–4.

15. Lakhani VT, You YN, Wells SA. The multiple endocrine neoplasia syndromes. *Annu Rev Med* 2007; **58**: 253–65.

16. Lips CJ, Landsvater RM, Höppener JW, et al. Clinical screening as compared with DNA analysis in families with multiple endocrine neoplasia type 2A patients. *N Engl J Med* 1994; **331**: 828–35.

17. De Groot JW, Links TP, Plukker JTM, et al. RET as a diagnostic and therapeutic target in sporadic and hereditary endocrine tumors. *Endocr Rev* 2006; **27**: 535–60.

18. Machens A, Dralle H. Genotype-phenotype based surgical concept of hereditary medullary thyroid carcinoma. *World J Surg* 2007; **31** 957–68.

19. Stålberg P, Carling T. Familial parathyroid tumors: diagnosis and management. *World J Surg* 2009, 1 Feb. [Epub ahead of print].

20. Machens A, Dralle H. Multiple endocrine neoplasia type 2 and the RET protooncogene: From bedside to bench to bedside. *Mol Cell Endocrinol 2006*; **247**: 34–40.

21. Lewis CE, Yeh, MW. Inherited endocrinopathies: an update. *Mol Genet Metab* 2008; **94**: 271–8.

Perioperative care of the patient with diabetes mellitus
Diabetes: aetiology and pathophysiology

George M. Hall

The International Diabetes Federation estimated that in 2008 there were 246 million adults worldwide with diabetes mellitus (DM) and the prevalence is expected to reach at least 380 million by 2025 [1]. In developed societies the prevalence is already at least 6%, and among obese white adolescents 4% had DM and 25% had abnormal glucose tolerance [2]. About 90% of individuals with DM have type 2 (non-insulin-dependent) diabetes although only about 10% of these can be accounted for by monogenic forms such as maturity-onset diabetes of the young (MODY) and mitochondrial diabetes which is characterised by β-cell dysfunction. Most cases of diabetes can be ascribed to 'common' type 2 diabetes which has a multifactorial pathogenesis. Only 5–10% of all diabetic patients have type 1 DM (insulin-dependent), which starts earlier in life than type 2 diabetes and is a serious chronic disorder.

The burdens of DM are medical, economic and social, and are caused mainly by the resultant complications, particularly microvascular and macrovascular. Patients with DM are a great financial burden on healthcare systems so public health measures to decrease the incidence of type 2 diabetes are being undertaken with great urgency in many countries.

Diagnosis of diabetes mellitus

Diabetes is diagnosed on the basis of criteria agreed by the World Health Organization (WHO) in 1999 (Table 7.1). The criteria incorporated fasting plasma venous glucose concentrations and plasma glucose values after a 75 g oral glucose load [3]. Thus it became possible to diagnose DM on the basis of fasting circulating glucose concentrations alone. The oral glucose tolerance test (OGTT) was considered inappropriate for routine diagnostic purposes because of its inconvenience, greater cost and poor reproducibility. However, the OGTT is still used when the diagnostic category

is unclear. The conditions of impaired fasting glucose and impaired glucose tolerance are of clinical importance as about 7% of individuals with these conditions progress to overt DM each year [4]. Also impaired glucose tolerance itself is associated with an increased risk of microvascular disease. There are a few practical points to consider if the fasting plasma glucose value is used as a diagnostic criterion. Firstly, the duration of fasting must be at least 8 hours, secondly an increased glucose concentration must be found on at least two occasions and lastly, plasma glucose values are about 7–10% greater than the more commonly measured blood glucose concentration after fasting.

Type 1 diabetes

Destruction of the pancreatic β-cells is characteristic of type 1 DM and usually results in an absolute deficiency of insulin. Two forms have been described: type 1A that results from a cell-mediated autoimmune attack on β-cells; type 1B that has no known cause, is infrequent and occurs mostly in Asian individuals who have varying amounts of insulin deficiency.

Causation of type 1 diabetes

The current model for the development of the immune form of type 1 diabetes was developed over 20 years ago but the basic concepts remain valid [5]. This model proposes that every individual is born with a degree of susceptibility to develop type 1 diabetes and that this susceptibility varies greatly between individuals. Susceptibility is mostly inherited, predominantly in the HLA genotypes DR and DQ and to a lesser extent in a large number of other genetic loci called IDDM (insulin-dependent diabetes mellitus) susceptibility genes. The HLA locus confers about 50% of genetic susceptibility. The next stage is exposure to one or more triggers thereby starting β-cell destruction. Supposed triggers include viruses, environmental toxins and

Core Topics in Endocrinology in Anaesthesia and Critical Care, eds. George M. Hall, Jennifer M. Hunter and Mark S. Cooper. Published by Cambridge University Press. © Cambridge University Press 2010.

Table 7.1 Diagnostic criteria for diabetes mellitus (glucose 75 g orally if used).

Category	Plasma venous glucose (mmol l^{-1})
Impaired fasting glucose	Fasting ≥ 6.1 and < 7.0 2 h post-glucose load < 7.8
Impaired glucose tolerance	Fasting < 7.0 2 h post-glucose load > 7.8 and < 11.1
Diabetes mellitus	Fasting ≥ 7.0 2 h post-glucose load ≥ 11.1

foods, but there is little agreement on a single causative factor. Activation of the T-cell-mediated response results in 'insulitis' within the β-cell as well as a B-cell response with production of autoantibodies to β-cell antigens such as glutamic acid decarboxylase (GAD) and protein tyrosine phosphatase IA2 (IA-2AA). The presence of antibodies in the serum may precede the clinical onset of type 1 diabetes by many years. The continuing destruction of β-cells leads to a progressive loss of secretory reserve. Initially, this is shown by the loss of the first phase insulin response to a glucose load, followed by clinical diabetes and finally, in most type 1 diabetics, by absolute insulin deficiency.

Support for the autoimmune pathogenesis of type 1 diabetes is provided by the susceptibility of these individuals to other autoimmune diseases such as Hashimoto's thyroiditis, Graves' disease, Addison's disease, coeliac disease and myasthenia gravis. However, there is no unifying theory of causation and two other hypotheses have been proposed; the hygiene hypothesis and the accelerator hypothesis. In brief, the hygiene hypothesis suggests that the failure to expose children to infection or immune challenges leads to the loss of protective immunological influences and a propensity to develop atopic disorders [6]. The accelerator hypothesis proposes that diabetes is a single disease and not two distinct entities, type 1 and type 2 [7]. The only differences between the two types of diabetes are the rate of β-cell destruction and the responsible accelerators. In type 2 diabetes the accelerators are the inherent high rate of β-cell apoptosis and insulin resistance, whereas in type 1 diabetes there is an additional accelerator – a genetic predisposition to β-cell autoimmunity. Both these alternative hypotheses have yet to receive widespread support.

Presentation of type 1 diabetes

Type 1 diabetes is often considered to be a disease of childhood and adolescents with an acute presentation, such as diabetic ketoacidosis. Recently it has been suggested that only about half of those with type 1 diabetes

are younger than 16–18 years at onset and that there is a low incidence throughout adult life [8]. The epidemiology of type 1 diabetes in children younger than 15–18 years has been studied extensively in many countries and several conclusions can be drawn [9]. First, the incidence has been increasing at about 2–5% per year worldwide. Second, there is a large geographical variation in incidence, almost 100-fold between the lowest (China) and highest values (Finland). Third, there is a trend towards a lower age of presentation, suggesting either a greater exposure to environmental triggers or an effect due to the increasing weight of children. Finally, migrants acquire the incidence rates of their new countries within a few years, again suggesting a large contribution of environmental factors to causation.

Management of type 1 diabetes

The principles of management of type 1 DM are based on the detailed observations made in two major trials; the Diabetes Control and Complications Trial (DCCT) [10] and the subsequent Epidemiology of Diabetes Interventions and Complications study (EDIC) [11]. It was shown that there was a close association between the adequacy of glycaemic control, as measured by glycosylated haemoglobin concentrations (HbA$_{1c}$), over a long period and the onset and progression of microvascular complications. The relationship of long-term HbA$_{1c}$ with macrovascular complications was less convincing. In addition to glycaemic control, factors such as smoking, obesity, hypertension and hyperlipidaemia were also implicated in the development of complications. The importance of early intensive treatment of type 1 diabetes was emphasised by the observation that these patients continued to have greater protection from the development of complications than those treated conventionally in the early stages of the disease. This protection persisted even when glycaemic control was similar after the early intervention, indicating the presence of a glycaemic or metabolic 'memory' [12]. Predictably intensive insulin therapy was associated with an increased risk of severe hypoglycaemic episodes [13]. Thus the benefits of early intensive treatment with the maintenance of tight glycaemic control must be weighed against the risks of hypoglycaemia.

Target values for circulating glucose concentrations and HbA$_{1c}$ values in type 1 diabetes vary with the age of the patient and individual risk factors. The National Institute for Clinical Excellence (NICE) has recommended that the blood glucose concentration should be 4–8 mmol l^{-1} before meals in children and 4–7 mmol l^{-1} before meals in adults with type 1 and type 2 diabetes [14]. Glycosylated haemoglobin values of ≤ 8.0% and ≤ 7.0% have been suggested target concentrations in children and adults respectively [15]. There remains, however, a considerable discrepancy between the targets recommended and the values achieved clinically; few patients attain ideal glycaemic control.

There are various approaches to the provision of insulin for type 1 diabetics. Traditionally, isophane or ultralente insulin was given once or twice daily as the basal insulin with regular boluses of fast-acting insulin before meals. The development of long-acting and rapid-acting analogues of insulin has permitted the introduction of basal-bolus routines with multiple daily injections; for example, insulin glargine (basal) with insulin lispro (bolus). Insulin pumps use fast-acting insulin continuously with bolus doses before meals (see Chapter 8 for description of commonly used insulins). Although the basal-bolus insulin regimen is rational physiologically, few studies have shown significant improvements in glycaemic control, assessed by HbA$_{1c}$, compared with traditional regimens [16]. Monitoring of blood glucose is fundamental to the management of all diabetics and it has been shown that frequent monitoring helps glycaemic control, the avoidance of hypoglycaemia and the flexibility of changes in daily life such as exercise and diet.

Long-term control of blood glucose is usually assessed by the measurement of HbA$_{1c}$ concentrations which reflect the overall glucose concentrations in the previous 90–120 days. There have been difficulties in providing universal standards for the assay of HbA$_{1c}$ [17]. Current HbA$_{1c}$ measurements are aligned to the assay used in the DCCT but the International Federation of Clinical Chemistry and Laboratory Medicine (IFCC) have prepared a new standard for HbA$_{1c}$. This will enable global standardisation of measurements. Glycosylated haemoglobin results will be expressed as mmol per mol of unglycated haemoglobin. Initially, results in the UK will be provided

Table 7.2 Severity of hypoglycaemia.

Mild	Autonomic symptoms occur
	palpitations
	sweating
	trembling
	anxiety
	nausea
Moderate	Autonomic and neuroglycopenic* symptoms occur
	*confusion
	weakness
	drowsiness
	dizziness
	blurred vision
Severe	Confusion, convulsions or coma requires glucose i.v. or glucagon s.c.

as both DCCT-aligned units (the customary %) and IFFC-standardised units (mmol/mol). From 2011 it is expected that results will be reported only in the new IFCC units.

Hypoglycaemia

Hypoglycaemia is a major concern for many type 1 diabetic patients and is usually described as mild, moderate or severe (Table 7.2). Fear of hypoglycaemia often deters patients from trying to attain near normal blood glucose concentrations. The occurrence of neuroglycopaenia without the early warning adrenergic symptoms, such as sweating, palpitations and trembling, can occur in patients with long-standing type 1 diabetes. Furthermore, an episode of severe hypoglycaemia predisposes an individual to further episodes probably as the result of a decrease in counter regulatory responses [18]. Consequences of severe or repetitive hypoglycaemia include mild cognitive impairment in adolescents and adults with long-standing disease. Intensive insulin therapy in type 1 diabetics was associated with a 3.3-fold increased risk of severe hypoglycaemia compared with conventionally treated patients [19].

Complications of diabetes mellitus

Most of the increased morbidity and mortality associated with DM is the result of the micro- and macrovascular complications. Factors predisposing to the development of complications of DM are shown in Table 7.3.

Microvascular complications

Diabetic nephropathy is now the most common cause of renal failure in developed countries. It progresses through several well-defined stages: sub-clinical disease, microalbuminuria (albumin excretion rate > $20 < 200$ µg day^{-1}), overt nephropathy or macroalbuminuria (>200 µg day^{-1}) with renal dysfunction, and finally end-stage renal disease [20]. Persistent albuminuria should be treated aggressively with the emphasis on good glycaemic control and the management of hyperlipidaemia and hypertension, if present. Angiotensin-converting enzyme (ACE) inhibitors or angiotensin-receptor-blocking agents are particularly effective in slowing the progression of renal disease [21]. Diabetic patients who develop end-stage renal disease have worse outcomes on dialysis and transplantation programmes than non-diabetic patients and also have excessive cardiovascular morbidity and mortality [22].

Diabetic retinopathy is now the commonest cause of acquired blindness in the developed world. Like diabetic nephropathy it progresses through well-defined stages: early non-proliferative changes – so-called background retinopathy, preproliferative retinopathy, proliferative retinopathy with the risk of retinal detachment and vitreous haemorrhage and macular oedema [23]. Diabetic retinopathy and nephropathy are closely associated.

Diabetic neuropathy includes focal and generalised changes. The most common generalised neuropathy is a mixed sensory and motor polyneuropathy, which usually presents as a peripheral sensory neuropathy alone. The combination of peripheral vascular disease and a sensory neuropathy often results in skin ulceration, poor healing and eventually gangrene in the feet and legs that require amputation [24]. A diabetic autonomic neuropathy is common in patients with long-standing type 1 diabetes, and cardiac dysfunction and gastroparesis are of particular concern to anaesthetists [25]. Focal neuropathies include carpal tunnel syndrome, third cranial nerve palsies and diabetic amyotrophy.

Macrovascular

Cardiovascular disease accounts for about 75% of all deaths in type 2 diabetics, but the association with type 1 diabetes is less clear. Risk factors for cardiovascular disease in type 1 diabetics include the presence of nephropathy, autonomic neuropathy, hypertension, hyperlipidaemia and perhaps microvascular cardiac disease. The

Table 7.3 Risk factors for complications of diabetes.

Early onset and long duration of diabetes
Poor glycaemic control
Obesity
Smoking
Hypertension
Hyperlipidaemia
Sedentary lifestyle

benefits of good glycaemic control in preventing macrovascular disease are unclear, but a systematic review has suggested that intensive insulin treatment may stabilise disease and prevent progression [26]. The reduction of risk of vascular disease is based on lifestyle changes such as weight control and exercise, cessation of smoking, optimum blood pressure and lipid control as well as good glycaemic control (Table 7.3). Weight control is important as increasing rates of obesity in type 1 diabetics are associated with the development of characteristics of type 2 diabetes, insulin resistance with enhanced cardiovascular risk, the so-called 'double diabetes'.

Type 2 diabetes

Genetic factors are involved in the pathogenesis of type 2 diabetes in addition to the well-known triggers of obesity and lifestyle. A positive family history confers a 2.4-fold increased risk of type 2 diabetes. It has been estimated that if both parents are affected the prevalence in the offspring is about 60% by the age of 60 years [27]. In view of this hereditary component there has been a detailed search to identify candidate genes. Polymorphisms in the peroxisome-proliferator-activated receptor gamma (PPARγ) gene, the ATP-sensitive K channel subunit KIR6.2 (KCNJ11) gene, the hepatocyte nuclear factor-1 beta (HNF 1B) gene, and the wolframin (WFS 1) gene are the most prevalent [28]. The encoded proteins are involved with adipose tissue insulin resistance, β-cell dysfunction, and β-cell dysfunction and β-cell apoptosis respectively. Genome-wide studies have identified other genetic susceptibility loci, including ones near the transcription factor-7-like 2 (TCF7L2) gene and solute carrier family 30, member 8 (SLC30A8) gene [29]. Other candidate genes may be identified by combining bioinformatics with genome-wide association studies.

Hyperglycaemia in type 2 diabetes

Circulating blood glucose concentrations are maintained within a narrow range of about 3–6 mmol l^{-1} in

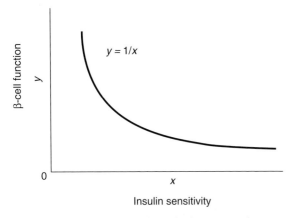

$y = 1/x$

β-cell function / y

Insulin sensitivity

0   x

Fig. 7.1 The normal curvilinear relationship between insulin sensitivity and β-cell function

non-diabetic individuals even after prolonged starvation or 'cafeteria' feeding. Insulin is the key hormone for the regulation of blood glucose and there is normally a balance between insulin secretion and activity. A decrease in insulin activity is accompanied by an up-regulation in secretion and vice versa; the relationship between normal β-cell function and insulin sensitivity is curvilinear (Fig 7.1). Deviation from this hyperbolic relationship occurs in type 2 diabetes when β-cell function is inadequate for a defined amount of insulin sensitivity. Consequently, β-cell dysfunction is considered a component of the pathogenesis of type 2 diabetes and this has been confirmed clinically [30].

Insulin resistance in type 2 diabetes

Insulin resistance occurs when the biological effects of insulin are less than expected for a given concentration in terms of glucose disposal peripherally and suppression of endogenous glucose production in the liver. Endogenous glucose production is enhanced in patients with impaired fasting glucose and type 2 diabetes. This increase occurs in the presence of raised circulating insulin concentrations, in the early stages of the disease, indicating that hepatic insulin resistance is a key factor in the causation of hyperglycaemia in type 2 diabetes [31].

Insulin resistance is strongly associated with obesity and physical inactivity. Increased stored triglyceride, particularly in visceral adipose depots, results in large adipocytes that are resistant to the effects of insulin in suppressing lipolysis [32]. The resultant increased release of non-esterified fatty acids (NEFA) and glycerol enhances insulin resistance in the liver and skeletal

muscle. A close association between intrahepatic lipids and hepatic insulin resistance has also been found [33]. In addition to NEFA, inflammatory cytokines such as interleukin-6 and several adipokines are also released in visceral obesity and inhibit the activity of insulin.

Insulin receptor knockout models have been developed in the mouse to try to understand the contributions from insulin resistance in a particular tissue to glucose regulation. Glucose intolerance did not develop in knockout models specific for muscle and fat cells, but only in those animals with liver and β-cell specific knockouts [34]. These observations support the notion of a key role for hepatic insulin resistance in the development of type 2 diabetes and the necessity of an adequate insulin signal in the β-cell. It was notable that the mice lacking the insulin receptor in adipose tissue were lean and had an extended lifespan.

Insulin signalling

Insulin elicits its metabolic effects by binding to and activating a specific receptor on the cell membrane that has tyrosine kinase activity. The insulin receptor substrate (IRS) proteins are tyrosine phosphorylated at several sites, which permits binding of a variety of adaptor proteins with a downstream signalling cascade [35]. Insulin activates enzymes linked to the translocation of glucose transporters to the cell surface, the synthesis of glycogen, protein, mRNAs and nuclear DNA with cell proliferation. In insulin resistance various molecular mechanisms that block insulin signalling are likely to be involved. A possible factor is the widely expressed phosphotyrosine phosphatase 1B (PTP 1B), which has an important part to play in the negative regulation of insulin signalling [36]. It acts by dephosphorylation of the tyrosine side chains of the IRS proteins.

Adiponectin, an adipose specific protein, also has a beneficial effect on glucose metabolism [37]. It acts through adenosine monophosphate (AMP) kinase, not the insulin signalling pathway, to suppress hepatic gluconeogenesis and inhibit lipolysis. AMP kinase has been implicated in the mechanism of action of metformin and the thiazolidinediones (Chapter 8). Circulating concentrations of adiponectin are decreased in visceral obesity.

In addition to their effects on insulin signalling, circulating factors derived from adipose tissue activate inflammatory cells that adversely affect atherogenesis and vascular endothelial function. Thus, the increased risk of vascular disease in patients with type 2 diabetes is closely linked with insulin resistance.

Table 7.4 Site of action of drugs used to treat type 2 diabetes.

Tissue	Drug
Gastrointestinal tract	α-Glucosidase inhibitors
β-cell pancreas	Sulphonylureas Meglitinides GLP-1 mimetics/DDP-4 inhibitors
Liver	Metformin
Muscle	Thiazolidinediones
Fat	Thiazolidinediones

DPP-4, dipeptidyl peptidase-4; GLP-1, glucagon-like peptide-1.

β-cell dysfunction

Abnormalities in insulin secretion are present in type 2 diabetics although they are not as obvious as in type 1 disease. In the early stages of the disease hyperinsulinaemia is often present, presumably as a response to the raised circulating blood glucose values found in both the fed and fasted states. It has been shown experimentally with glucose clamp studies that insulin secretion is markedly impaired in type 2 diabetes compared with non-diabetic individuals of similar adiposity [38]. Furthermore, secretory defects have been shown in individuals with impaired glucose tolerance and impaired fasting glucose, and normoglycaemic offspring of type 2 diabetics have decreased insulin secretion [38]. The insulin defect is probably inherited and obesity and ageing may exacerbate the problem leading to overt diabetes.

Insulin secretion

Glucose is taken up by the β-cell of the pancreas by the glucose transporter 2 (GLUT 2) and is then phosphorylated by glucokinase which is the rate limited step. Oxidative metabolism proceeds with the formation of adenosine triphosphate (ATP) in the mitochondria. A change in the cellular adenosine triphosphate/adenosine diphosphate (ATP/ADP) ratio activates the sulphonylurea receptor 1 (SUR 1) which results in the closure of the adjacent potassium inward rectifier (KIR) 6.2 channel. Closure of the potassium channel alters the membrane potential, calcium channels open and preformed insulin-containing granules are released. This exocytosis is also an ATP-dependent process.

Hyperglycaemia itself can decrease insulin secretion and deterioration of β-cell function over time is common in type 2 diabetics. This has lead to the concept of glucose toxicity which implies the development of irreversible damage to the β-cell [39]. The mechanism by which glucose toxicity is mediated is unclear but may involve the excessive production of reactive oxygen species with damage to cellular components such as pancreas duodenum homeobox 1 (PDX 1), which is a regulator of insulin promoter activity.

In addition to the concept of glucose toxicity, the idea of lipotoxicity of the β-cells has also been proposed [40]. Circulating NEFA values are increased in type 2 diabetes as a result of enhanced lipolysis in adipocytes. Oxidation of NEFA in the β-cell of the pancreas leads to the formation of long-chain acyl coenzyme A, which at high concentrations is thought to have several deleterious effects on insulin secretion. These include opening the KIR 6.2 channel, increased expression of uncoupling protein-2 with a decline in the intracellular ATP/ADP ratio and enhanced apoptosis of the β-cells.

Islet amyloid polypeptide, amylin, is co-secreted with insulin but at a much slower rate [41]. The physiological role of this compound is unclear and it may inhibit insulin and glucagon secretion. Deposits of amyloid are found in the pancreas of many type 2 diabetics but their role, if any, in the pathophysiology remains unknown.

Management of type 2 diabetes

The primary aim of treatment is to delay the onset and progression of the cardiovascular complications of the disease. In addition to drug treatment, interventions to improve insulin sensitivity such as weight loss and exercise are an integral part of management. Drugs used to treat type 2 diabetes target various tissues involved with the regulation of blood glucose; gastrointestinal tract, β-cell of pancreas, liver, muscle and adipose tissue (Table 7.4). Insulin is increasingly used in type 2 diabetics to enhance the effects of insulin sensitisers such as metformin (Chapter 8).

Management of cardiovascular complications

Coronary artery disease, cerebrovascular disease and hypertension occur more frequently in type 2 diabetics than matched controls [42]. The benefits of antihypertensive therapy have been shown in a large prospective study and many type 2 diabetics take several antihypertensive drugs to attain the target blood pressure of less than 130/80 mm Hg. The HOPE (Heart Outcomes Prevention Evaluation) study demonstrated that the use of an ACE inhibitor was associated with a significantly decreased risk of death, myocardial infarction and stroke in diabetic patients [43]. The use of lipid-lowering drugs, such as statins, has a similar beneficial effect on mortality [44].

Patients with type 2 diabetes and microalbuminuria who were treated with an intensive regimen of tight glucose control, ACE inhibitor or angiotensin-receptor-blocking drug, lipid-lowering agent and aspirin had half the risk of vascular complications compared with conventionally treated patients [45]. This risk reduction was maintained in a 5-year follow-up in spite of similar treatments; decrease of 59% in non-fatal cardiovascular events and a decrease in all-cause mortality of 57%. This important study emphasises the necessity of early vigorous treatment, not only of glucose, but also cardiovascular disease in improving survival in type 2 diabetics.

Prevention of type 2 diabetes in individuals at high risk is obviously preferable to treating the overt disease. Several studies have shown that an intensive diet and exercise programme, sometimes with the addition of drugs such as acarbose, metformin or the thiazolidinediones, results in a significant risk reduction of 25–50% in developing diabetes [4, 46]. The improvement of only one factor involved in the pathogenesis of type 2 diabetes, insulin resistance, β-cell dysfunction and fluctuations in circulating glucose values, is sufficient to delay the onset. Clinically, the prevention of obesity remains the key factor in decreasing the prevalence of type 2 diabetes.

References

1. Editorial. The global challenge of diabetes. *Lancet* 2008; **371**: 1723.

2. Sinha R, Fisch G, Teague B, et al. Prevalence of impaired glucose tolerance among children and young adolescents with marked obesity. *N Engl J Med* 2002; **346**: 802–10.

3. World Health Organization Expert Committee . Definition, diagnosis and classification of diabetes mellitus and its complications. Report of a WHO consultation, part 1: diagnosis and classification of diabetes mellitus. Geneva, World Health Organization, 1999.

4. Diabetes Prevention Program Research Group . Reduction in the incidence of type 2 diabetes with lifestyle intervention or metformin. *N Engl J Med* 2002; **346**: 393–403.

5. Eisenbarth GS. Type 1 diabetes mellitus. A chronic autoimmune disease. *N Engl J Med* 1986; **314**: 1360–8.

6. Gale EAM. A missing link in the hygiene hypothesis. *Diabetologia* 2002; **45**: 588–94.

7. Wilkin TJ. The accelerator hypothesis: weight gain as the missing link between type 1 and type 2 diabetes. *Diabetologia* 2001; **44**: 914–22.

8. Devendra D, Liv E, Eisenbarth GS. Type 1 diabetes: recent developments. *BMJ* 2004; **328**: 750–4.

9. Daneman D. Type 1 diabetes. *Lancet* 2006; **367**: 847–58.

10. Diabetes Control and Complications Trial Research Group . Effect of intensive treatment of diabetes on the development and progression of long-term complications in insulin-dependent diabetes mellitus. *N Engl J Med* 1993; **329**: 977–86.

11. Diabetes Control and Complications Trial/ Epidemiology of Diabetes Interventions and Complications Research Group . Retinopathy and nephropathy in patients with type 1 diabetes four years after a trial of intensive therapy. *N Engl J Med* 2000; **342**: 381–9.

12. Diabetes Control and Complications Trial/ Epidemiology of Diabetes Interventions and Complications Research Group . Effect of intensive therapy on the microvascular complications of type 1 diabetes mellitus. *JAMA* 2002; **287**: 2563–9.

13. The Diabetes Control and Complications Trial Research Group . Hypoglycemia in the diabetes control and complications trial research group. *Diabetes* 1997; **46**: 271–86.

14. National Institute for Health and Clinical Excellence (NICE). *Clinical guidelines CG15 type 1 diabetes and CG66 diabetes-type 2 (update)*. http://www.nice.org.uk.

15. Canadian Diabetes Association. Clinical practice guidelines for the prevention and management of diabetes in Canada. *Can J Diab* 2003; **27**: S21–3.

16. Ratner RE, Hirsh IB, Neifing JL, Mecca TE, Wilson CA. Less hypoglycaemia with insulin glargine in intensive insulin therapy for type 1 diabetes. *Diabetes Care* 2000; **23**: 639–43.

17. Sacks DB. ADA/EASD/IDF working group of the HbA1c assay. Global harmonization of haemoglobin A1c. *Clin Chem* 2005; **51**: 681–3.

18. Cryer PE. Diverse causes of hypoglycaemia-associated autonomic failure in diabetes. *N Engl J Med* 2004; **350**: 2272–9.

19. Danne T, Mortensen HB, Hougaard P, et al. Persistent differences among centers over 3 years in glycemic control and hypoglycaemia in a study of 3,805 children and adolescents with type 1 diabetes from the Hvidore Study Group. *Diabetes Care* 2001; **24**: 1342–7.

20. Mogensen CE, Christensen CK. Predicting diabetic nephropathy in insulin-dependent patients. *N Engl J Med* 1984; **311**: 83–93.

21. Lovell HG. Angiotensin converting enzyme inhibitors in normotensive diabetic patients with microalbuminuria. *Cochrane Database Syst Rev* 2001; **1**: CD 002183.

22. Finne P, Reunanen A, Stenman S, Groop PH, Gronhagen-Riska C. Incidence of end-stage renal disease in patients with type 1 diabetes. *JAMA* 2005; **294**: 1782–7.

23. Fong DS, Aiello LP, Ferris FL, Klein R. Diabetic retinopathy. *Diabetes Care* 2004; **27**: 2540–53.

24. McAnulty GR, Robertshaw HJ, Hall GM. Anaesthetic management of patients with diabetes mellitus. *Br J Anaesth* 2000; **85**: 80–90.

25. Robertshaw HJ, Hall GM. Diabetes mellitus: anaesthetic management. *Anaesthesia* 2006; **61**: 1187–90.

26. Lawson ML, Gerstein HC, Tsui E, Zinman B. Effect of intensive therapy on early macrovascular disease in young individuals with type 1 diabetes. A systematic review and meta-analysis. *Diabetes Care* 1999; **22**: B35–9.

27. Tattersal RB, Fajans SS. Prevalence of diabetes and glucose intolerance in 199 offspring of thirty-seven conjugal diabetic parents. *Diabetes* 1975; **24**: 452–62.

28. Stumvoll M, Goldstein BJ, van Haeften TW. Type 2 diabetes: principles of pathogenesis and therapy. *Lancet* 2005; **365**: 1333–46.

29. Stumvoll M, Goldstein BJ, van Haeften TW. Type 2 diabetes: pathogenesis and treatment. *Lancet* 2008; **371**: 2153–6.

30. Weyer C, Bogardus C, Mott DM, Pratley RE. The natural history of insulin secretory dysfunction and insulin resistance in the pathogenesis of type 2 diabetes mellitus. *J Clin Invest* 1999; **104**: 787–94.

31. Meyer C, Stumvoll M, Nadkarni V, Dostov J, Mitrakou A, Gerich J. Abnormal renal and hepatic glucose metabolism in type 2 diabetes mellitus. *J Clin Invest* 1998; **102**: 619–24.

32. Boden G. Role of fatty acids in the pathogenesis of insulin resistance and NIDMM. *Diabetes* 1997; **46**: 3–10.

33. Seppala-Lindrous A, Vehkavarra S, Hakkinen AM, et al. Fat accumulation in the liver is associated with defects in insulin suppression of glucose production and serum free fatty acids independent of obesity in normal men. *J Clin Endocrinol Metab* 2002; **87**: 3023–8.

34. Michael MD, Kulkarni RN, Postic C, et al. Loss of insulin signalling in hepatocytes leads to severe insulin resistance and progressive hepatic dysfunction. *Mol Cell* 2000; **6**: 87–97.

35. White MF. IRS proteins and the common path to diabetes. *Am J Physiol Endocrinol Metab* 2002; **283**: E413–22.

36. Zick Y. Insulin resistance: a phosphorylation-based uncoupling of insulin signaling. *Trends Cell Biol* 2001; **11**: 437–41.

37. Yamauchi T, Kamon J, Minokoshi Y, et al. Adiponectin stimulates glucose utilisation and fatty-acid oxidation by activating AMP-activated protein kinase. *Nat Med* 2002; **8**: 1288–95.

38. Gerrich JE. The genetic basis of type 2 diabetes mellitus; impaired insulin secretion versus impaired insulin sensivitity. *Endocr Rev* 1998; **19**: 491–503.

39. Yki-Järvinen H. Glucose toxicity. *Endocr Rev* 1992; **13**: 415–31.

40. Robertson RP, Harmon J, Tran PO, Poitout V. Beta-cell glucose toxicity, lipotoxicity and chronic oxidative stress in type 2 diabetes. *Diabetes* 2004; **53**: S119–24.

41. Hull RL, Westermark GT, Westermark P, Kahn SE. Islet amyloid: a critical entity in the pathogenesis of type 2 diabetes. *J Clin Endocrinol Metab* 2004; **89**: 3629–43.

42. Beckman JA, Creager MA, Libby P. Diabetes and atherosclerosis: epidemiology, pathophysiology and management. *JAMA* 2002; **287**: 2750–81.

43. HOPE Study Group . Effects of ramipril on cardiovascular and microvascular outcomes in people with diabetes mellitus: results of the HOPE study and MICRO-HOPE substudy. Heart Outcomes Prevention Evaluation Study Investigators. *Lancet* 2000; **355**: 253–9.

44. Heart Protection Study Collaborative Group . MRC/BHF Heart Protection Study of cholesterol lowering with simvastatin in 20536 high-risk individuals: a randomised placebo-controlled trial. *Lancet* 2002; **360**: 7–22.

45. Gaede P, Lund-Andersen H, Parving HH, Pedersen O. Effect of a multifactorial intervention on mortality in type 2 diabetes. *N Engl J Med* 2008; **358**: 580–91.

46. Tuomilehto J, Lindstrom J, Eriksson JG, et al. Prevention of type 2 diabetes mellitus by changes in lifestyle among subjects with impaired glucose tolerance. *N Engl J Med* 2001; **344**: 1343–50.

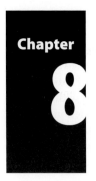

Drugs used in diabetes mellitus

Grainne Nicholson

Diabetes mellitus (DM) is characterised by an absolute (type 1) or relative (type 2) deficiency of insulin. Type 2 DM, which is the most common form, is characterised by insulin resistance, abnormal hepatic glucose production and progressive worsening of pancreatic β-cell function over time [1]. The prevalence of DM is increasing exponentially and this increase is not merely confined to developed countries. Moreover complications of DM contribute significantly to healthcare costs. Improved glycaemic control has been shown to reduce the risk for development of microvascular complications and may also reduce the risk for macrovascular complications such as myocardial infarction and stroke, although development of cardiovascular disease is obviously multifactorial. Greater understanding of the pathophysiology of DM has contributed to the development of new pharmacological approaches to the management of the condition. There are currently eight different pharmacological classes of antidiabetic agents; these include agents that increase insulin secretion, improve insulin action and delay carbohydrate absorption. Newer treatments, such as incretin therapy, have multiple glucoregulatory effects including enhancement of insulin secretion, reduction of glucagon secretion, reduction of food intake and slowing of gastric emptying.

The currently available classes of antidiabetic agents are sulphonylureas (first and second generation), meglitinides, biguanides, thiazolidinediones (glitazones), α-glucosidase inhibitors, GLP-1 (glucagon-like peptide-1) receptor agonists, DPP-4 (dipeptidyl peptidase-4) inhibitors and synthetic amylin analogues (Table 8.1). In addition, endocannabinoid antagonists acting at the CB 1 receptor show promise for affecting food intake and improving glucose homeostasis. Finally, insulin treatment itself particularly with the release of newer rapid-acting and long-acting analogues is becoming increasingly acceptable for type 2 diabetics.

Sulphonylureas

Sulphonylureas are known as insulin secretagogues as their major mechanism of action is to increase insulin secretion. They have been used since the 1950s and their efficacy is well established. However, several questions have been raised over their safety profile but these have recently been addressed (see below).

Sulphonylureas work by stimulating insulin release from the beta cells of the pancreas. This is achieved by binding to a specific receptor resulting in closure of an adenosine triphosphate (ATP) -dependent K$^+$ channel, leading to depolarisation of the membrane and an influx of Ca^{2+} ions, thereby increasing insulin secretion. They may also improve insulin resistance in peripheral target tissues such as muscle and fat. Sulphonylureas are divided into first and second generation agents. These drugs have been shown to reduce glycosylated haemoglobin concentrations (HbA$_{1c}$) by 1–2% and fasting blood glucose concentrations by 3.3–3.9 mmol l^{-1} [2–4]. Hypoglycaemia is the most common side effect of these agents and is more common in patients receiving second-generation sulphonylureas than in those receiving metformin or thiazolidinediones. Hypoglycaemia is of concern with agents which are metabolised to an active metabolite with significant renal excretion, such as chlorpropamide and glibenclamide; these should be avoided in patients with renal impairment and in elderly patients. Other well-recognised side effects include an increase in appetite and weight gain and these agents, therefore, may not be the first choice for management of obese patients [5]. Treatment failure may also occur with sulphonylureas and can be divided into primary and secondary categories. In primary failure,

Core Topics in Endocrinology in Anaesthesia and Critical Care, eds. George M. Hall, Jennifer M. Hunter and Mark S. Cooper. Published by Cambridge University Press. © Cambridge University Press 2010.

Table 8.1 Current pharmacological treatments for type 2 diabetes mellitus.

Sulphonylureas
First generation
chlorpropamide
tolbutamide
Second generation
glibenclamide
gliclazide
Third generation
glimepiride
Meglitinides
Repaglinide
Biguanides
Metformin
Thiazolidinediones
Rosiglitazone
Pioglitazone
a-Glucosidase inhibitors
Acarbose
GLP-1 receptor agonists
Exenatide
DPP-4 inhibitors
Sitagliptin
Vildagliptin
Synthetic amylin analogues
Pramlintide
Insulin

DPP-4, dipeptidyl peptidase-4; GLP-1, glucagon-like peptide-1.

From Cefalu [1] with permission.

the patient exhibits a poor initial response to therapy with inadequate reduction in fasting blood glucose (< 1.1 mmol l^{-1}). This is observed in 20–25% of patients commenced on sulphonylurea treatment. In secondary failure, which occurs in 5–10% of patients per year, an initial response (a decrease in fasting blood glucose of > 1.7 mmol l^{-1}) is followed by a failure to maintain adequate blood glucose concentrations.

Several controversies have also existed regarding the perceived cardiovascular risk associated with use of these agents. The University Group Diabetes Program suggested that sulphonylurea use was associated with an increased risk for cardiovascular events [6–8]. However two high profile randomised trials have addressed these concerns. The UKPDS (UK Prospective Diabetes Study) and ADOPT (A Diabetes

Outcome Progression Trial) have suggested a reduced cardiovascular risk which approached statistical significance and a lower incidence of cardiovascular events, using glibenclamide, compared with rosiglitazone or metformin [9, 10]. The introduction of newer agents for the management of type 2 DM has obviously had an impact on the use of sulphonylureas but this class of drugs is effective, cost-effective and has a good safety record.

Meglitinides

The glinides are newer insulin secretagogues that include the meglitinide, repaglinide, a benzoic acid derivative, and the amino acid (D-phenylalanine) derivative, nateglinide [11]. These agents stimulate rapid insulin production by the pancreas and have been shown to reduce postprandial blood glucose and to reduce HbA$_{1c}$ by 0.5–2.0% [12]. Early insulin release may suppress hepatic glucose production more rapidly and hence reduce the need for additional insulin secretion. They have a faster onset and shorter duration of action than the sulphonylureas [13]. They are also associated with a reduced risk of hypoglycaemia and cause less weight gain. They are useful in patients with erratic meal schedules but should only be taken immediately before meals or will result in hypoglycaemia. They are metabolised and excreted hepatically so can be used in patients with impaired renal function.

Biguanides

Metformin and phenformin were introduced for the therapy of DM in the 1950s. Phenformin was withdrawn from clinical use in the 1970s because of its strong association with lactic acidosis, and metformin is the sole agent in clinical use in this class. Metformin is considered an insulin sensitiser and decreases hepatic gluconeogenesis, inhibits glycogenolysis and improves insulin sensitivity especially in skeletal muscle. Other beneficial effects include a reduction in plasma triglyceride and low-density lipoprotein (LDL) concentrations. The exact mechanism of action of metformin is not known but may be via adenosine monophosphate protein kinase (AMPK). Activation of AMPK in the liver leads to the stimulation of fatty acid oxidation and inhibition of lipogenesis, glucose production and protein synthesis [14]. Metformin, before the introduction of newer agents (see below), was the only available agent which improved glycaemia and was associated with a lack of weight gain and even weight loss in some patients. This makes it an ideal first-line agent particularly in overweight patients. Metformin may also improve other cardiovascular risk factors; the UKPDS group studies suggest that metformin used as monotherapy in obese patients reduced the rate of myocardial infarction and all-cause mortality [15]. The 10-year follow up of UKPDS again emphasised the benefits of long-term glycaemic control on all causes of death, micro- and macrovascular complications [16].

Metformin has a mostly favourable side effect profile. Because it does not affect insulin secretion, it is not associated with hypoglycaemia when used as monotherapy but can do so when used in combination with sulphonylureas or insulin. Gastrointestinal side effects such as metallic taste, nausea, abdominal pain and diarrhoea occur to varying degrees in up to 30% of patients. Most of these are transient and occur when the drug is introduced or the dose increased rapidly. Taking the drug with meals may also lessen the severity.

Lactic acidosis is also a potential concern with metformin. Phenformin was withdrawn from clinical use in the 1970s because of its clear association with lactic acidosis. This occurs because phenformin has to be hydroxylated prior to renal excretion and this process is genetically defective in 10% of whites. The incidence is 10–20 times lower with metformin as this is excreted unmetabolised. Indeed, the evidence for metformin-induced lactic acidosis stems from about 300 case reports [17]. Underlying medical conditions, such as chronic renal disease or myocardial infarction, are well-established risk factors for lactic acidosis and attributing lactic acidosis to metformin versus an underlying condition is often difficult. The reported frequency of metformin-induced lactic acidosis is 3 cases per 100 000 patient years [17]. However, metformin is not recommended in patients with renal disease (creatinine clearance < 60 ml min^{-1}, serum creatinine > 120 μmol l^{-1} in women or > 130 μmol l^{-1} in men), hepatic disease, cardiac (New York Heart Association [NYHA] class III or IV), chronic pulmonary disease, severe infection, alcohol abuse, history of lactic acidosis, pregnancy or use of intravenous radiographic contrast medium [1, 14]. Despite these concerns, metformin remains one of the mainstays of diabetic management. Stumvoll et al. has highlighted the lack of good evidence to support the contraindications to metformin and suggested that this drug can be safely used in elderly patients, and those with stable heart failure, moderate renal impairment (using a reduced dose), or mild liver impairment (which is often due to fatty liver and which improves with metformin) [18, 19].

Thiazolidinediones

Thiazolidinediones (TZDs), like metformin, belong to the class of drugs known as insulin sensitisers. Metformin acts mainly on the hepatocyte and muscle, while TZDs act predominantly on muscle and the adipocyte. These agents enhance insulin sensitivity by increasing the efficiency of glucose transporters, lower HbA$_{1C}$ by 1–2% and reduce both fasting and postprandial glucose concentrations [13]. They do not cause hypoglycaemia when used as a single agent but can do so when used in combination with other agents. Troglitazone was the first TZD approved to treat type 2 DM in 1997, but was withdrawn from clinical practice in 2000 because of rare idiosyncratic hepatotoxicity, a side effect not observed with the other TZDs, rosiglitazone and pioglitazone. Thiazolidinediones activate peroxisome proliferators-activated gamma nuclear receptors (PPAR-γ) throughout the body, exerting their main insulin sensitisation in muscle and fat. This in turn results in altered gene transcription in adipocytes, a modulation of fatty acid metabolism and a reduction in circulating free fatty acids by 20–40% [20, 21].

A decrease in circulating free fatty acids is postulated to enhance insulin-receptor signalling in skeletal muscle, resulting in increased insulin sensitivity throughout the body. A further benefit may be favourable effects on pancreatic β-cell function by reducing exposure of β-cells to lipotoxicity which may contribute to β-cell death [20, 22]. This proposed improvement in β-cell function may account for the lower risk of monotherapy failure after 5 years for rosiglitazone versus metformin (32% lower) or rosiglitazone versus glyburide (glibenclamide) (63% lower) [10].

Thiazolidinediones can cause oedema and weight gain and are contraindicated in patients with liver disease and in those with NYHA class III or IV cardiac status [8]. Thiazolidinediones increase weight because of differentiation of adipocytes and expansion of adipocyte mass [23]. However, activation of PPAR-γ stimulates differentiation to insulin-sensitive, smaller adipocytes and redistributes fat from visceral to subcutaneous deposits, a pattern which is associated with a lower risk for cardiovascular disease [24]. Both rosiglitazone and pioglitazone increase high-density lipoprotein cholesterol (HDL-c) and low-density lipoprotein cholesterol (LDL-c) resulting in larger more buoyant particles with little change in LDL particle concentration [25]; pioglitazone also decreases triglyceride concentrations. Other benefits associated with TZD use include anti-inflammatory effects [26, 27], improved peripheral and coronary vascular endothelial function and a modest improvement in hypertension [28–30].

New or worsening peripheral oedema is common with TZD use with the incidence ranging from 2.5–16.2%. The risk is enhanced age, increasing drug dose, female sex, impaired renal function and concomitant insulin use. One of the likely mechanisms for this is increased renal resorption of sodium and plasma volume expansion. A greater concern, however, is the potential for worsening of heart failure with these drugs. Although relatively uncommon, the annual increment in heart failure is 0.25–0.45% per year. Thus, these drugs are contraindicated in patients with NYHA class III or IV cardiac status and should be used with caution in those with class II disease [31].

Thiazolidinediones have also been associated with an increased incidence of myocardial infarction (MI). A meta-analysis by Nissen and Wolski evaluated the cardiovascular effects of rosiglitazone versus placebo or active controls from 42 trials and concluded that rosiglitazone was associated with a significant 43% relative increased odds for MI and a trend towards a 64% increased odds for cardiovascular death [32]. However, none of these studies were designed to assess cardiovascular effects and had extremely low cardiovascular event rates. A US Food and Drug Administration (FDA) enquiry concluded in 2007 that the evidence against rosiglitazone was insufficient to recommend that it be withdrawn [33].

Thiazolidinediones, therefore, have a number of effects on the cardiovascular system apart from their effects on glucose metabolism. One important study, the PROactive study (Prospective Pioglitazone Clinical Trial in Macrovascular Events), has demonstrated a non-statistically significant 10% reduction in the hazard ratio and a reduction in all-cause mortality, non-fatal MI and stroke in high-risk patients with type 2 DM randomised to pioglitazone or placebo [34]. Furthermore there may exist differences between the two available agents. In an observational study of almost 30 000 patients with a 1.2 year follow-up, pioglitazone was associated with a 22% lower rate of MI compared with rosiglitazone and a 15% decrease in MI and coronary revascularisation [35].

In January 2008, both the American Diabetes Association (ADA) and European Association for the Study of Diabetes (EASD) recommended TZDs as second line treatment for type 2 diabetes after lifestyle intervention and metformin. In 2008 the ACCORD (Action to

Control Cardiovascular Risk in Diabetes) trial was terminated early when it was shown that patients in the intensive treatment arm, 91% of whom received rosiglitazone, were at significantly increased risk of death from cardiovascular disease [36]. Further analysis showed that the use of intensive therapy to achieve normal glycosylated haemoglobin values for 3.5 years increased mortality, attributed mostly to hypoglycaemia, and did not significantly reduce major cardiovascular events. There was no evidence to show that any one drug class was directly responsible [37]. Nevertheless, in October 2008 both the ADA and the EASD issued guidelines that explicitly advised against the use of rosiglitazone for the treatment of type 2 diabetes. Current consensus relegates pioglitazone to third line treatment and explicitly states that rosiglitazone is not recommended [38]. However, Woo has re-emphasised the differences in clinical practice guidelines between Canada, America and Europe and the lack of evidence from long-term studies regarding the risk association between rosiglitazone and MI [39]. The results of the RECORD (Rosiglitazone Evaluated for Cardiac Outcomes and Regulation of glycaemia in Diabetes) study, which is designed to prospectively assess the cardiac outcomes of rosiglitazone, are awaited with interest [40].

Alpha-glucosidase inhibitors

Alpha-glucosidase inhibitors block the enzyme α-glucosidase in the brush border of the small intestine, which delays absorption of glucose, thereby decreasing meal-related blood glucose increases, which in turn decreases the required insulin response [11, 13]. They competitively inhibit binding of oligosaccharides to α-glucosidase, which prevents their cleavage into monosaccharides that can then be absorbed. Currently available drugs include acarbose and miglitol. They are taken before carbohydrate-containing meals and should not be taken when meals are missed. However, they do not cause weight gain or hypoglycaemia. Treatment with acarbose has been associated with elevations in serum transaminase concentrations and these also increase with renal impairment. Hence their use is contraindicated in patients with hepatic or renal impairment (serum creatinine > 180μmol l^{-1}). Other contraindications include inflammatory bowel disease or a history of bowel obstruction [2]. Side effects include bloating, flatulence, abdominal cramps and diarrhoea, limit their clinical use and do not address pancreatic β-cell α-glucosidase inhibitors dysfunction. When compared with other oral hypoglycaemic agents, they are less effective in reducing fasting blood glucose and HbA_{1c} and they are probably of greatest use in patients with mild fasting hyperglycaemia or those who are already on combination oral therapy but require an additional agent. However, some studies have suggested that their use is associated with a reduction in cardiovascular events and a favourable effect on lipid metabolism. Chaisson et al. found that treating patients with impaired glucose tolerance with acarbose significantly reduced the risk of cardiovascular disease and hypertension [41]. Kado et al. suggested that acarbose may also benefit postprandial hyperlipidaemia as well as hyperglycaemia [42].

Incretins/GLP-1 mimetics

Incretins are gut-derived peptides secreted in response to meals, specifically the presence and absorption of nutrients in the intestinal lumen. The incretin effect refers to the augmented release of insulin from oral ingestion of glucose compared with an intravenous glucose challenge. The two major incretins are glucagon-like peptide-1 (GLP-1), which is produced by the neuroendocrine L cells of the ileum and colon, and glucose-dependent insulinotropic peptide (GIP), which is produced by the K cells of the duodenum and jejunum. Both are released rapidly after a meal and their cardinal role appears to be attenuation of postprandial glucose excursions [43]. Incretins stimulate insulin production from pancreatic β-cells and GLP-1 also decreases glucagon secretion, slows gastric emptying and suppresses appetite. GLP-1 may reduce β-cell apoptosis and promote β-cell proliferation [44, 45]. Patients with diabetes demonstrate a blunted rise in GLP-1 concentrations following food intake [46]. Intravenous GLP-1 infusion will increase insulin release and reduce fasting blood glucose concentrations, even in patients with longstanding type 2 diabetes [1]. One of the major clinical concerns about the use of GLP-1 is its limited availability due to its rapid enzymatic degradation by dipeptidyl peptidase-4 (DPP-4), which requires that it is administered by continuous intravenous or subcutaneous infusion. To counteract this, agents that are resistant to DPP-4 degradation, such as exenatide or liraglutide, have been developed. Another approach is the development of specific DPP-4 inhibitors (see below).

There is currently only one commercially available GLP-1 agonist, exenatide; liraglutide is in phase 3 testing. Exenatide is derived from the naturally occurring peptide, exendin-4, which was isolated from the salivary secretions of the lizard *Heloderma suspectum* (Gila monster). This lizard eats once a month and the function of exendin-4 is to rapidly increase the production of insulin in response to nutrients entering the gut [11]. Exenatide is a complete agonist at the GLP-1 receptor, is resistant to DPP-4 degradation and is cleared by the kidneys. It is usually administered by a twice daily injection and appears to provide adequate GLP-1 replacement for the day. Exenatide is approved for the treatment of type 2 diabetes in patients receiving concurrent metformin or sulphonylurea treatment, although the dose of sulphonylurea may need to be reduced to avoid hypoglycaemia. Clinical trials have demonstrated a reduction in both fasting and postprandial glucose concentrations, a 1–2% reduction in HbA_{1c} concentrations and moderate weight loss of 2–5 kg with its use [47–49]. Side effects of exenatide include nausea and, less commonly, vomiting or diarrhoea, particularly when starting therapy, and rarely pancreatitis. It is recommended that treatment is initiated with a dose of 5 µg twice daily which may be increased to 10 µg twice daily approximately 1 month later.

Liraglutide, currently in phase 3 testing, is administered once daily, is not excreted by the kidneys and is not subject to DPP-4 degradation; it may be a promising alternative [50]. More recently studies of once weekly dosing using a sustained release formulation of exenatide have demonstrated greater improvements in glycaemic control, no increased risk of hypoglycaemia and similar reductions in body weight [51].

In summary, incretin therapy appears to offer an effective alternative to currently available hypoglycaemic agents, although continued evaluation and further long-term studies are required to determine its clinical role [52] .

Dipeptidyl peptidase-4 inhibitors

Glucagon-like peptide 1 (GLP-1) and glucose-dependent insulinotropic peptide (GIP), so-called incretins, stimulate insulin release, suppress glucagon concentrations, delay gastric emptying and increase satiety. Their actions, however, are short-lived because of rapid degradation and inactivation by the enzyme DPP-4. This enzyme is widely expressed throughout the body and circulates in a soluble form. Its acts by cleavage of the two NH_2-terminal amino acids of bioactive peptides, provided the second amino acid is alanine or proline. Cleavage is rapid and endogenous GLP-1 has a short half-life (< 2 min). To overcome this problem, GLP-1 receptor agonists that are not degraded by DPP-4 have been developed (see above), but another therapeutic approach is to inhibit the activity of DPP-4. The rationale for this latter option is to prevent the inactivation of GLP-1 and prolong the activity of the endogenously released hormone [53]. In contrast to GLP-1 receptor agonists, these drugs are available orally and have a longer duration of action, requiring only once daily dosing. The drugs currently available are sitagliptin and vildagliptin (approved for use in Europe and awaiting FDA approval). Both are effective at controlling hyperglycaemia, reduce HbA_{1c} concentrations by ~1%, improve pancreatic β-cell function and can be used as monotherapy or in combination with other agents. They are safe and well tolerated with a low risk of hypoglycaemia. They do not appear to cause gastrointestinal disturbance, but do not reduce appetite or cause weight loss like GLP-1 agonists [54]. One potential concern, however, relates to the ability of DPP-4 to cleave other bioactive peptides, including neuropeptide Y, gastrin-releasing peptide, substance P and various chemokines [53]. This may, in turn, cause adverse events such as increased blood pressure, neurogenic inflammation and immunological reactions. No such effects have been reported in animal or human studies to date, but further long-term trials are needed.

Synthetic amylin analogues

Amylin is a peptide neurohormone which is manufactured and secreted by the β-cells of the pancreas with insulin. Patients lacking functional β-cells, i.e., patients with type 1 diabetes or advanced type 2 diabetes, are deficient in both insulin and amylin. Amylin secretion, like GLP-1, is stimulated by the presence of food in the gut and its 24-h profile resembles that of insulin with low baseline values and a rapid increase in response to meals. The physiological effects of amylin are also similar to those of GLP-1 but it is not an incretin hormone. Amylin suppresses glucagon secretion, delays gastric emptying and acts centrally in the area postrema of the hindbrain to induce satiety. By suppressing glucagon secretion and delaying gastric emptying, amylin slows the passage of glucose into the bloodstream while insulin stimulates cellular uptake of glucose to reduce blood glucose concentrations [55, 56].

Efforts have been made to treat diabetic patients with human amylin but it has a tendency to self-aggregate and form fibrils making formulation difficult. To overcome this, synthetic analogues of amylin have been developed. Pramlintide is a stable, bioactive analogue that differs from human amylin by three amino acid substitutions [57]. These structural changes improve solubility. It is given as a subcutaneous injection two to three times daily and it is administered before meals. It has a rapid onset of action (typically 20 min) and a duration of action of 2–4 hours. It is currently approved for use in patients with type 1 diabetes and those patients with type 2 diabetes using mealtime insulin or insulin in combination with a sulphonylurea or metformin [58]. The most common side effect of pramlintide is nausea and it is therefore recommended that the drug dose is increased gradually from 15 μg in patients with type 1 DM to 30–60 μg over 3 days; for patients with type 2 DM, the initial starting dose is 60 μg, which may be increased to 120 μg. Another side effect that can occur is hypoglycaemia, particularly in the first four weeks of treatment. Reducing the dose of pre-meal insulin by 50% when starting therapy will avoid this. Pramlintide also causes some weight loss, typically 1–2 kg [59, 60], reduces HbA_{1c} by 0.3–0.6% and significantly lowers postprandial glucose [58].

The role of pramlintide in the treatment of type 2 DM is unclear but it may be of some benefit to those patients already on intensive insulin regimens.

Insulin therapy

Type 1 DM is caused by autoimmune destruction of the pancreas and patients require insulin therapy from the outset of their illness. Type 2 diabetes is characterised by β-cell dysfunction and inadequate insulin secretion and insulin resistance. However, type 2 DM is a progressive disease and with advancing β-cell failure, individuals may require insulin therapy. The blood glucose lowering potency of individual agents is limited but insulin therapy is the most effective at decreasing blood glucose [61]. Insulin therapy is no longer seen as a therapeutic 'last resort' after long-term oral agent combinations have failed, but rather as a therapeutic tool for earlier use in achieving glycaemic targets. Starting insulin therapy with low doses in combination with oral agents is effective at achieving glycaemic targets and maintaining HbA_{1c} values [62]. Furthermore, insulin therapy can improve insulin resistance [61] and may have potential cardiovascular benefits. The DIGAMI (Diabetes Insulin-Glucose Infusion in Acute Myocardial Infarction) study showed that insulin infusion during acute MI, followed by intensive multiple dose insulin therapy reduced the relative mortality by 28% compared to conventional therapy after an average follow up of 3.4 years [63]. Interestingly, the same investigators were unable to reproduce these benefits in the later DIGAMI 2 study as the use of insulin had become standard practice [64]. Moreover concerns

Table 8.2 Pharmacokinetics of human insulin and analogues.

Treatment	Onset of action (h)	Peak (h)	Duration (h)
Rapid acting			
Lispro	5–15 min	60 min	4–5
Aspart	5–15 min	60 min	4–5
Glulisine	5–15 min	60 min	4–5
Short acting			
Regular	30–60 min	2–4	6–8
Intermediate acting			
Isophane	2–4	4–6	12–16
Insulin zinc suspension	2–4	6–12	12–20
Basal			
Glargine	2	Flat	~24
Detemir	2	Flat	~24
From Cefalu [1] with permission.			

that insulin therapy would worsen weight gain, obesity and accelerate coronary artery disease have not been realised.

The goal for insulin therapy is to mimic as closely as possible the physiological pattern of insulin secretion seen in non-diabetic patients. Normally, insulin secretion in response to a meal consists of a first- and second-phase response and type 2 DM is characterised by a defect in first-stage or acute glucose-induced insulin secretion. The goal of administering insulin therapy is to address both basal and postprandial insulin requirements, the *basal-bolus concept* (Table 8.2) [1]. This requires basal insulin to suppress glucose production between meals and overnight and bolus insulin to limit postprandial hyperglycaemia. Bolus insulin may comprise up to 10–20% of total daily insulin at each meal. When used in this way, insulin should demonstrate an immediate rise and a sharp peak to effectively control glucose excursions. This is made feasible by the development of newer fast-acting and basal insulin formulations. Short-acting or regular insulin has been the mainstay of insulin therapy for many years, but newer rapidly acting insulin analogues, such as lispro, have a more rapid onset and shorter duration of action making it easier to titrate insulin therapy to control prandial glucose concentrations. The three short-acting insulin analogues are insulin lispro, insulin aspart and insulin glulisine. Changes in their amino acid structure reduce their tendency to aggregate into dimers thus speeding their absorption after subcutaneous injection. They have a rapid onset of action (typically 5–15

min), peak activity 1 hour after injection and their effect has almost disappeared after 4–5 hours. This matches normal mealtime peaks of plasma insulin more closely than human regular insulin and in turn results in less immediate postprandial hyperglycaemia and less late postprandial hypoglycaemia [61]. They are not used for intravenous administration.

Intermediate-acting insulins such as isophane insulin and insulin zinc suspension have been used twice daily to provide 24-hour basal insulin but are limited in that their peaks and troughs of insulin concentrations are not representative of normal endogenous basal insulin release. Peak effects are usually between 4–8 hours with a total duration of action of 10–16 hours, but there is significant day to day variability which can result in unpredictable glucose concentrations and potential hypoglycaemia.

Newer long-acting insulin formulations, such as glargine, appear to provide better glycaemic control than before without the risk of hypoglycaemia. Insulin glargine results from two modifications of human insulin, substitution of glycine at position A21 and addition of two arginine molecules at the C terminal of the B chain. These substitutions reduce its solubility at physiological pH and stabilise it. It is released very gradually from the injection site and its duration of action is prolonged allowing a relatively constant basal insulin supply which approaches 24 hours. Insulin detemir has a similar duration of action.

The need to inject insulin remains an obstacle to patient acceptance and compliance. Pen delivery devices have improved this considerably, in addition to infusion pumps providing continuous subcutaneous delivery systems.

References

1. Cefalu WT. Pharmacotherapy for the treatment of patients with type 2 diabetes mellitus: rationale and specific agents. *Clin Pharmacol Ther* 2007; **81**: 636–49.

2. Luna B, Feinglos MN. Oral agents in the management of type 2 diabetes mellitus. *Am Fam Physician* 2001; **63**: 1747–56.

3. Feinglos MN, Bethel MA. Treatment of type 2 diabetes mellitus. *Med Clin North Am* 1998; **82**: 757–90.

4. Luna B, Hughes AT, Feinglos MN. The use of insulin secretagogues in the treatment of type 2 diabetes. *Prim Care* 1999; **26**: 895–915.

5. Kelley DE. Effects of weight loss on glucose homeostasis in NIDDM. *Diabetes Rev* 1995; **3**: 366–77.

6. Meinert CL, Knatterud GL, Prout TE, Klimt CR. A study of the effect of hypoglycaemic agents on vascular complications in patients with adult-onset diabetes. II. Mortality results. *Diabetes* 1970; **19** Suppl: 789–830.

7. Feinglos MN, Bethel MA. Therapy of type 2 diabetes, cardiovascular death, and the UGDP. *Am Heart J* 1999; **138**: 346–52.

8. Sheehan MT. Current therapeutic opinion in type 2 diabetes mellitus: a practical approach. *Clin Med Res* 2003; **1**: 189–200.

9. UK Prospective Diabetes Study (UKPDS) Group . Intensive blood glucose control with sulfonylureas or insulin compared with conventional treatment and risk of complications in patients with type 2 diabetes (UKPDS 33). *Lancet* 1998; **352**: 837–53.

10. Kahn SE, Haffner SM, Heise MA, et al. ADOPT Study Group. Glycaemic durability of rosiglitazone, metformin or glyburide monotherapy. *N Engl J Med* 2006; **355**: 2427–43.

11. McDonnell ME. Combination therapy with new targets in type 2 diabetes mellitus: a review of available agents with a focus on pre-exercise adjustment. *J Cardiopulm Rehabil Prev* 2007; **27**: 193–201.

12. Black C, Donnelly P, McIntyre L, Royle PL, Shepherd JP, Thomas S. Meglitinide analogues for type 2 diabetes mellitus. *Cochrane Database Syst Rev* 2007; **18**: CD004654.

13. Fonseca VA, Kulkarni KD. Management of type 2 diabetes: oral agents, insulin and injectables. *J Am Diet Assoc* 2008; **108**: S29–33.

14. Stumvoll M, Häring H-U, Matthaei S. Metformin Pathogenesis of type 2 diabetes. *Endocr Res* 2007; **32**: 39–57.

15. UK Prospective Diabetes Study (UKPDS) Group . Effect of intensive blood glucose control with metformin on complications in overweight patients with type 2 diabetes (UKPDS 34). *Lancet* 1998; **352**: 854–65.

16. Holman RR, Paul SK, Bethel MA, Matthews DR, Neil HA. Ten-year follow-up of intensive glucose control in type 2 diabetes. *N Engl J Med* 2008; **359**: 1577–89.

17. Bolen S, Feldman L, Vassy J, et al. Systematic review: comparative effectiveness and safety of oral medications for type 2 diabetes mellitus. *Ann Intern Med* 2007; **147**: 386–99.

18. Stumvoll M, Nurjhan N, Perriello G, Dailey G, Gerich JE. The metabolic effects of metformin in non-insulin-dependent diabetes mellitus. *N Engl J Med* 1995; **333**: 550–4.

19. Holstein A, Stumvoll M. Contraindications can damage your health – is metformin a case in point? *Diabetologia* 2005; **48**: 2454–9.

20. Fonseca V, Rosenstock J, Patwardhan R, Salzman A. Effect of metformin and rosiglitazone combination therapy in patients with type 2 diabetes mellitus: a randomized controlled trial. *JAMA* 2000; **283**: 1695–702.

21. Phillips LS, Grunberger G, Miller E, et al. Once- and twice-daily dosing with rosiglitazone improves glycemic control in patients with type 2 diabetes. *Diabetes Care* 2001; **24**: 308–15.

22. Bell DS, Ovalle F. Tissue triglyceride levels in type 2 diabetes and the role of thiazolidinediones in reversing the effects of tissue hypertriglyceridemia: review of the evidence in animals and humans. *Endocr Pract* 2001; **7**: 135–8.

23. Okuno A, Tamemoto H, Tobe K, et al. Troglitazone increases the number of small adipocytes without the change of white adipose tissue mass in obese Zucker rats. *J Clin Invest* 1998; **101**: 1354–61.

24. Adams M, Montague CT, Prins JB, et al. Activators of peroxisome proliferator-activated receptor gamma have depot-specific effects on human preadipocyte differentiation. *J Clin Invest* 1997; **100**: 3149–53.

25. McGuire DK, Inzucchi SE. New drugs for the treatment of diabetes mellitus: Part I: thiazolidinediones and their evolving cardiovascular implications. *Circulation* 2008; **117**: 440–9.

26. Haffner SM, Greenberg AS, Weston WM, Chen H, Williams K, Freed MI. Effect of rosiglitazone treatment on nontraditional markers of cardiovascular disease in patients with type 2 diabetes mellitus. *Circulation* 2002; **106**: 679–84.

27. Marx N, Imhof A, Froehlich J, et al. Effect of rosiglitazone treatment on soluble CD40L in patients with type 2 diabetes and coronary artery disease. *Circulation* 2003; **107**: 1954–7.

28. Caballero AE, Saouaf R, Lim SC, et al. The effects of troglitazone, an insulin-sensitizing agent, on the endothelial function in early and late type 2 diabetes: a

placebo-controlled randomized clinical trial. *Metabolism* 2003; **52**: 173–80.

29. Forst T, Lubben G, Hohberg C, et al. Influence of glucose control and improvement of insulin resistance on microvascular blood flow and endothelial function in patients with diabetes mellitus type 2. *Microcirculation* 2005; **12**: 543–50.

30. Chiquette E, Ramirez G, Defronzo R. A meta-analysis comparing the effect of thiazolidinediones on cardiovascular risk factors. *Arch Intern Med* 2004; **164**: 2097–104.

31. Nesto RW, Bell D, Bonow RO, et al. Thiazolidinedione use, fluid retention, and congestive heart failure: a consensus statement from the American Heart Association and American Diabetes Association. *Circulation* 2003; **108**: 2941–8.

32. Nissen SE, Wolski K. Effect of rosiglitazone on the risk of myocardial infarction and death from cardiovascular causes. *N Engl J Med* 2007; **356**: 2457–71.

33. Misbin RI. Lessons from the Avandia controversy: a new paradigm for the development of drugs to treat type 2 diabetes mellitus. *Diabetes Care* 2007; **30**: 3141–4.

34. Dormandy JA, Charbonnel B, Eckland DJ, et al. Secondary prevention of macrovascular events in patients with type 2 diabetes in the PROactive Study (Prospective Pioglitazone Clinical Trial in Macrovascular Events): a randomised controlled trial. *Lancet* 2005; **366**: 1279–89.

35. McAfee AT, Koro C, Landon J, Ziyadeh N, Walker AM. Coronary heart disease outcomes in patients receiving antidiabetic agents. *Pharmacoepidemiol Drug Saf* 2007; **16**: 711–25.

36. Buse JB and the ACCORD Study Group . Action to control cardiovascular risk in diabetes (ACCORD) trial. Design and methods. *Am J Cardiol* 2007; **99**: S21–33.

37. Gerstein HC, Miller ME, Byington RP, et al. Effects of intensive glucose lowering in type 2 diabetes. *N Engl J Med* 2008; **358**: 2545–59.

38. Nathan DM, Buse JB, Davidson MB, et al. Medical management of hyperglycemia in type 2 diabetes: a consensus algorithm for the initiation and adjustment of therapy. *Diabetes Care* 2009; **32**: 193–203.

39. Woo V. Important differences; Canadian Diabetes Association 2008 clinical practice guidelines and the consensus statement of the American Diabetes Association and the European Association for the Study of Diabetes. *Diabetologia* 2009; **52**: S52–3.

40. Home PD, Jones NP, Pocock SJ, et al. for the RECORD Study Group. Rosiglitazone RECORD study: glucose control outcomes at 18 months. *Diabet Med* 2007; **24**: 626–34.

41. Chaisson JL, Josse RG, Gomis R, et al. Acarbose treatment and the risk of cardiovascular disease and hypertension in patients with impaired glucose tolerance: the STOP-NIDDM trial. *JAMA* 2003; **290**, 486–94.

42. Kado S, Murakami T, Aoki A, et al. Effect of acarbose on postprandial lipid metabolism in type 2 diabetes mellitus. *Diabetes Res Clin Pract* 1998; **41**: 49–55.

43. Inzucchi SE, McGuire DK. New drugs for the treatment of diabetes mellitus: Part II: incretin-based therapy and beyond. *Circulation* 2008; **117**: 574–84.

44. Drucker DJ. The biology of incretin hormones. *Cell Metab* 2006; **3**: 153–65.

45. Wong VS, Brubaker PL. From cradle to grave: pancreatic beta-cell mass and glucagon-like peptide-1. *Minerva Endocrinol* 2006; **31**: 107–24.

46. Nathan DM, Schreiber E, Fogel H, et al. Insulinotropic action of glucagon-like peptide-1-(7–37) in diabetic and nondiabetic subjects. *Diabetes Care* 1992; **15**: 270–6.

47. Buse JB, Henry RR, Han J, et al. Effects of exenatide (exendin-1) on glycaemic control over 30 weeks in sulfonylurea-treated patients with type 2 diabetes. *Diabetes Care* 2004; **27**: 2628–35.

48. Defronzo RA, Ratner RE, Han J, et al. Effects of exenatide (exendin-4) on glycaemic control and weight over 30 weeks in metformin-treated patients with type 2 diabetes. *Diabetes Care* 2005; **28**: 1092–100.

49. Kendall DM, Riddle MC, Rosenstock J, et al. Effects of exenatide (exendin-4) on glycaemic control over 30 weeks in patients with type 2 diabetes treated with metformin and a sulfonylurea. *Diabetes Care* 2005; **28**: 1083–91.

50. Vilsboll T. Liraglutide: a once daily GLP-1 analogue for the treatment of type 2 diabetes mellitus. *Expert Opin Investig Drugs* 2007; **16**: 231–7.

51. Drucker DJ, Buse JB, Taylor K, et al. Exenatide once weekly versus twice daily for the treatment of type 2 diabetes: a randomised, open-label, non-inferiority study. *Lancet* 2008; **372**: 1240–50.

52. Amori RE, Lau J, Pittas AG. Efficacy and safety of incretin therapy in type 2 diabetes. *JAMA* 2007; **298**: 194–206.

53. Ahrén B. Dipeptidyl peptidase-4 inhibitors. *Diabetes Care* 2007; **30**: 1344–50.

54. Pratley RE, Salsali A. Inhibition of DPP-4: a new therapeutic approach for the treatment of type 2 diabetes. *Curr Med Res Opin* 2007; **23**: 919–31.

55. Kruger DF, Gloster MA. Pramlintide for the treatment of insulin-requiring diabetes mellitus: rationale and review of clinical data. *Drugs* 2004; **64**: 1419–32.

56. Schmitz O, Brock B, Rungby J. Amylin agonists: a novel approach in the treatment of diabetes. *Diabetes* 2004; **53**: S233–8.

57. Samsom M, Szarka LA, Camilleri M, et al. Pramlintide, an amylin analog, selectively delays gastric

emptying: potential role of vagal inhibition. *Am J Physiol Gastrointest Liver Physiol* 2000; **278:** G946–51.

58. Ryan GJ, Jobe LJ, Martin R. Pramlintide in the treatment of type 1and type 2 diabetes mellitus. *Clin Ther* 2005; **27**: 1500–12.

59. Ratner RE, Dickey R, Fineman M, et al. Amylin replacement with pramlintide as an adjunct to insulin therapy improves long-term glycaemic and weight control in type 1 diabetes mellitus. *Diabet Med* 2004; **21**: 1204–12.

60. Hollander P, Maggs DG, Ruggles JA, et al. Effect of pramlintide on weight in overweight and obese insulin-treated type 2 diabetes patients. *Obes Res* 2004; **12**: 661–8.

61. Wyne KL, Mora PF. Insulin therapy in type 2 diabetes. *Endocr Res* 2007; **32**: 71–107.

62. GarberAJ, Wahlen J, Wahl T, et al. Attainment of glycaemic goals in type 2 diabetes with once-, twice-, or thrice-daily dosing with biphasic insulin aspart 70/30 (The 1-2-3 study). *Diabetes Obes Metab* 2006; **8**: 58–66.

63. Malmberg K, Norhammar A, Wedel H, Rydén L. Glycometabolic state at admission: important risk marker of mortality in conventionally treated patients with diabetes mellitus and acute myocardial infarction: long-term results from the Diabetes and Insulin-Glucose Infusion in Acute Myocardial Infarction (DIGAMI) study. *Circulation* 1999; **99**: 2626–32.

64. Malmberg K, Rydén L, Wedel H, et al. Intense metabolic control by means of insulin in patients with diabetes mellitus and acute myocardial infarction (DIGAMI 2): effects on mortality and morbidity. *Eur Heart J* 2005; **26**: 650–61.

Management of diabetes in surgical inpatients

George M. Hall

Since the prevalence of diabetes mellitus (DM) is increasing, it is inevitable that the number of diabetic patients presenting for surgery also increases. Surgery may be undertaken for the complications of DM, such as coronary artery disease, peripheral vascular disease and renal failure, or the diabetes may be unrelated to the surgical procedure. A recent survey of diabetic surgical patients found that the duration of hospital stay was greater than for non-diabetic patients, in particular following plastic and orthopaedic surgery, although the cause(s) of the difference was not investigated [1]. There is increasing economic pressure to minimise the duration of hospital stay and in diabetic patients it is expected that improved perioperative glycaemic control will result in fewer postoperative complications, particularly wound infections, and hence expedite discharge from hospital. Many cardiac surgical studies have also shown that diabetic patients have a greater mortality and morbidity than non-diabetic patients and that good glycaemic control in both groups of patients decreases postoperative wound infections [2–4]. There are very few studies, however, of diabetic patients undergoing general surgery to guide clinical decisions. The perioperative management of diabetic patients is based, at present, more on an understanding of the pathophysiology of DM, the metabolic and endocrine response to surgery and the mode of action of drugs used in diabetes than on the current literature.

Preoperative assessment

The preoperative assessment of diabetic patients must be meticulous and, in addition to the usual medical history and examination, the following points should be emphasised (Table 9.1). The type, duration and current treatment of diabetes must be established. This basic information will indicate whether the patient is, for example, a long-standing type 1 diabetic with the likelihood of having developed micro- and macrovascular complications, or a recently diagnosed type 2 diabetic controlled by metformin and diet. The total daily insulin dose is helpful in predicting whether glycaemic control is likely to be difficult in the perioperative period, for example a total dose of 80–100 U/24 h indicates a state of insulin resistance before the added physiological insult of surgery, whereas a total dose of 24–30 U/24 h suggests that the patient will respond to the usual doses of perioperative insulin. Recent HbA_{1c} values are helpful as they indicate the adequacy of the glycaemic control in the preceding 2–3 months; high values > 8% show that current treatment is inadequate, or the patient non-compliant, and that higher doses of insulin than predicted are likely to be needed perioperatively.

Overt cardiovascular disease is common in diabetic patients: coronary artery disease; peripheral vascular disease; hypertension and cerebrovascular disease. These should be investigated as appropriate for each patient and current therapy carefully noted. Even if basic cardiological investigations suggest that there is minimal coronary artery disease in long-standing diabetics, it is prudent to manage these patients as if they are at high risk of perioperative myocardial ischaemia.

A diabetic nephropathy is of particular relevance to anaesthetists because of the renal route for excretion of many drugs. The microvascular complications of DM often occur simultaneously and if a retinopathy is present there is usually also a nephropathy. The presence of albuminuria, and the amount excreted per 24 hours, will confirm the presence and severity of a diabetic nephropathy (Chapter 7). Circulating creatinine concentrations should be measured preoperatively in all diabetic patients.

The presence and extent of a peripheral neuropathy should be established in all diabetic patients in whom

Core Topics in Endocrinology in Anaesthesia and Critical Care, eds. George M. Hall, Jennifer M. Hunter and Mark S. Cooper. Published by Cambridge University Press. © Cambridge University Press 2010.

Table 9.1 Basic preoperative evaluation of diabetic surgical patients.

Diabetes
type
duration
treatment
Cardiovascular disease
coronary artery disease
peripheral vascular disease
hypertension
cerebrovascular disease
Drugs and allergies
Renal disease
Peripheral neuropathy
Metabolic control HbA$_{1c}$
Airway, cervical spine, stiff joint syndrome

Table 9.2 Basic preoperative investigations.

Blood glucose (fasting and 2 h postprandial, if possible)
Urinalysis (albumin and ketones)
Blood urea, creatinine and electrolytes
Haemoglobin
ECG

regional anaesthesia is used. There is no evidence that the neuropathy is exacerbated by central neuraxial blockade but recent investigations have suggested that the peripheral nerves may be more susceptible to trauma and local anaesthetic toxicity in diabetic patients (see below).

While all patients have their airway assessed preoperatively, this is particularly important in diabetic patients. Type 1 diabetic patients can develop the stiff joint syndrome (SJS) with limited mobility of the upper cervical spine [5]. This results in a poor view on direct laryngoscopy and may make tracheal intubation difficult. Since these patients may also have a diabetic autonomic neuropathy (DAN) with gastroparesis they are at particular risk of regurgitation and aspiration. The diagnosis of the SJS can be made preoperatively by asking the patient to pray by pressing the palmar surfaces of their hands together [6]. Stiffness of the interphalangeal joints is shown by the failure to oppose the fingers and palms – the positive prayer sign. A positive prayer sign should alert the anaesthetist to the possibility of a difficult laryngoscopy and intubation.

Autonomic dysfunction is detectable in up to 50% of type 1 and 20% of type 2 diabetic patients [7]. Many patients with DAN are asymptomatic but symptoms such as diarrhoea, gustatory sweating, impotence and postural hypotension are strongly suggestive of an autonomic neuropathy. Testing for DAN preoperatively is not undertaken routinely. It is usually assessed by determining heart rate variability; variability is lost with DAN [8]. The severe impairment of heart rate variability in patients with end-stage diabetic nephropathy probably results from DAN and coexisting cardiac disease and may be a major risk factor for ventricular arrhythmias and sudden death in these patients [9]. Diabetic autonomic neuropathy has been implicated in the unexpected occurrence of bradycardia and hypotension in the perioperative period, particularly in cardiac and vascular surgery.

Preoperative investigations in the diabetic patient are determined by the findings of the history and examination. In diabetic patients with severe cardiovascular disease an intensive cardiological assessment may be essential including exercise stress testing. However, the following investigations should be undertaken preoperatively in all diabetic patients: blood glucose concentration (ideally fasting and two hours after a meal but this is usually not possible), urinalysis for ketones and albumin, blood urea, electrolyte and creatinine concentrations, haemoglobin and ECG (Table 9.2).

Metabolic challenge of surgery

The control of blood glucose in the diabetic patient is complicated by several factors (Table 9.3). Preoperative starvation should be minimised and it has been traditional to operate on diabetic patients as early in the day as possible. However many diabetic patients are now admitted on the day of surgery even for major procedures. In these circumstances it is often prudent to delay surgery for a few hours to obtain stable blood glucose values. Anaesthetists strive to shorten the period of preoperative starvation but in diabetic patients postoperative starvation is of greater importance as it prolongs the need for a glucose-insulin-potassium (GIK) infusion. The early resumption of oral intake enables the diabetic patient to return to their usual treatment regimen. Therefore, the prevention of postoperative nausea and vomiting, and the prompt treatment of this complication if it occurs, is an important part of perioperative care.

The endocrine and metabolic response to surgery further complicates glucose control in the diabetic

Table 9.3 Factors complicating glucose control perioperatively.

| Starvation |
| preoperative |
| postoperative |
| Endocrine and metabolic response to surgery |
| Anaesthetic technique |
| Postoperative immobilisation |

Table 9.4 Aims of metabolic management.

| Avoid hypoglycaemia |
| Prevent hyperglycaemia (≤ 10 mmol l^{-1}) |
| Minimise lipolysis and proteolysis |
| Prevent electrolyte loss (K, Mg, P$_i$) |

Table 9.5 Deleterious effects of hyperglycaemia.

| Impaired reactive endothelial nitric oxide generation |
| Decreased complement activity |
| Increased expression of leucocyte and endothelial adhesion molecules |
| Increased cytokine synthesis |
| Impaired neutrophil chemotaxis and phagocytosis |

patient. In brief, in non-diabetic patients surgery evokes an increase in catabolic hormone secretion (catecholamines, cortisol, growth hormone) with a decrease in anabolic hormone secretion (insulin). The catabolic hormones stimulate hepatic glycogenolysis and gluconeogenesis which result in an increased blood glucose concentration. There is a failure of insulin secretion to respond to the glycaemic stimulus, possibly due to the α_2 inhibitory effects of the circulating catecholamines [10]. In the postoperative period, insulin secretion is restored but functionally it is relatively ineffective – insulin resistance is present [11]. Thus in non-diabetic patients undergoing surgery the intra- and postoperative period is characterised by a state of functional insulin deficiency. In type 1 diabetic patients with no endogenous insulin secretion and type 2 diabetics with insulin resistance and impaired β-cell function there are no hormonal constraints on the hyperglycaemic effects of enhanced catabolic hormone secretion.

Anaesthetic techniques and drugs may modify the endocrine and metabolic response to surgery. For example, regional anaesthesia can decrease catabolic hormone secretion, which will reduce the glycaemic response to surgery in non-diabetic patients [10]. High doses of opioids and benzodiazepines inhibit hypothalamic-pituitary hormone secretion and should benefit metabolic control (see below for details of anaesthetic management).

Aims of metabolic management

The aims of metabolic management perioperatively are to avoid hypoglycaemia, excessive hyperglycaemia, and minimise lipolysis and proteolysis by the provision of exogenous glucose and insulin (Table 9.4). For many years the fear of undetected hypoglycaemia during general anaesthesia was the major influence in determining blood glucose concentrations in diabetic patients. High glucose values were tolerated on the basis that 'permissive hyperglycaemia' was safer than rigorous control of blood glucose with the risk

of hypoglycaemia. However, in cardiac surgery there is evidence to suggest that intraoperative and postoperative insulin therapy in non-diabetics and diabetics improves morbidity, particularly the incidence of postoperative wound infections [12, 13]. Many of these cardiac surgical studies were based on the extrapolation of results obtained in critically ill patients and were observational, non-randomised investigations, with a wide range of target blood glucose concentrations (upper limit from 6.1 to < 11.1 mmol l^{-1}) [14]. A recent randomised controlled trial with blinded assessment compared 'tight' glucose control (4.4–5.6 mmol l^{-1}) with routine control (glucose < 11.1 mmol l^{-1}) intraoperatively in 400 cardiac surgical patients and concluded that outcome was not improved in non-diabetic or diabetic patients with 'tight' control [15].

At present there are few studies examining the effects of glucose control in diabetic patients undergoing non-cardiac surgery. No data are available on intraoperative glucose control and only two studies have investigated postoperative intensive insulin therapy. A retrospective cohort study found that increased postoperative glucose values were an independent risk factor for patients undergoing peripheral vascular surgery [16]. A small randomised pilot study compared conventional blood glucose treatment (< 12 mmol l^{-1}) with insulin therapy (< 6.6 mmol l^{-1}) in neurosurgery and found a decreased infection rate but no difference in mortality and outcome [17].

It is notable that in most trials in which 'strict' glucose control was implemented, typically < 6.1 mmol l^{-1}, hypoglycaemia occurred with an incidence of 9–17% [15]. Thus the anaesthetist is left trying to decide on safe upper limits of blood glucose with no clinical evidence to guide this decision for most surgical patients.

In contrast to the limited clinical data, there is considerable *in vitro* work to show the deleterious effects of hyperglycaemia. High glucose concentrations have been shown to impair reactive endothelial NO generation, increase expression of leucocyte and endothelial adhesion molecules, decrease complement function, impair neutrophil chemotaxis and phagocytosis, and enhance the synthesis of inflammatory cytokines [18] (Table 9.5). The overall effect of these glucose-induced changes is to enhance inflammation and increase vulnerability to infection. The concentration of glucose at which these deleterious effects can be shown is surprisingly uniform, usually > 9 or 10 mmol l^{-1}, which is similar to the values at which clinical infections become more common.

Target glucose concentration perioperatively

In the virtual absence of clinical studies in general surgery, and considering the basic biological data on the harmful effects of hyperglycaemia, it is reasonable to recommend that blood glucose should be maintained in the range of 6–10 mmol l^{-1} [19]. This is concordant with the position statement of the American College of Endocrinology in 2004 and represents a range which would minimise the risks from hyperglycaemia and of hypoglycaemia [20]. Furthermore, it has been suggested that marked variability in glucose values is more harmful than absolute values and the former is more common with attempts to maintain 'strict' glucose control (< 6.1 mmol l^{-1}) [21].

Perioperative glucose control

There is general agreement that all type 1 diabetic patients should be managed with an intravenous GIK infusion for inpatient surgery (see Chapter 12 for ambulatory surgery). It has been suggested that patients on a basal-bolus regimen may continue on their long-acting insulin and that additional glucose/insulin can be given if necessary. There is an obvious risk of hypoglycaemia with the continuation of basal insulin and this regimen lacks the flexibility of a GIK infusion [22]. The GIK regimen should be started as soon as possible after admission on the morning of surgery and continued for at least two hours after the first meal. If it is terminated before feeding rebound hyperglycaemia can occur.

Type 2 diabetics undergoing major surgery are also managed with a GIK regimen, whereas those undergoing minor surgery only need to have the oral hypoglycaemic drug omitted on the day of surgery. The management of type 2 diabetics undergoing 'moderate surgery' is contentious. It has been suggested that the imposition of a GIK regimen in these patients results in greater metabolic disturbance than careful monitoring with glucose/insulin as required [23]. A major problem is deciding what is 'moderate surgery' and this will vary between hospitals and surgeons. Some anaesthetists treat all type 2 diabetics with a GIK infusion to allow for flexibility in the scheduling of operating lists. Type 2 diabetics undergoing minor surgery may need insulin subcutaneously postoperatively for a short time to regain glucose control.

The first GIK regimen for diabetics was proposed by Alberti and Thomas 30 years ago [24]. In this regimen insulin and potassium were added to a 500 ml bag of glucose 10% so that the patient received all three components simultaneously. A typical infusion given at 100 ml h^{-1} for a patient with a blood glucose of about 10 mmol l^{-1} would be 500 ml 10% glucose + 15 U soluble insulin + 10 mmol potassium. This regimen is inherently safe as regardless of the rate of intravenous infusion the patient always receives glucose, insulin and potassium. However, it lacks flexibility and if the dose of insulin or potassium needs to be changed then a new infusion bag has to be prepared. The Alberti regimen has largely been superceded by the sliding scale regimen which consists of separate infusions of insulin (typically soluble insulin 50 U in 50 ml) and glucose 5% or 10% with potassium at 100 ml h^{-1}. The infusions must join before the intravenous cannula and a non-return valve must be used. The sliding scale regimen is flexible as the rate of insulin infusion can be varied to achieve the target glucose concentration. It does not have the intrinsic safety of the Alberti regimen and infusion pumps have failed with disastrous consequences. Alberti proposed that at least 180 g of glucose should be infused per 24 h and this usually necessitates the use of 10% glucose solution [24]. Most hospitals have guidelines for sliding scale regimens with infusion rates of insulin for each range of blood glucose values. It is important that these are interpreted intelligently. The insulin requirements of a stable diabetic with a daily dose < 30 U day^{-1} will be far less than an unstable, insulin-resistant, critically ill diabetic with a daily dose of 80–100 U day^{-1} at the same blood glucose concentration.

Anaesthesia

Regional anaesthesia

Although there is no evidence in diabetic patients that regional anaesthesia (RA) improves mortality and morbidity after major surgery compared with general anaesthesia (GA), there are several potential advantages (Table 9.6). In an awake patient hypoglycaemia is easily detected and the avoidance of tracheal intubation obviates the problem of the SJS and gastroparesis. Regional anaesthesia may decrease the catabolic hormonal response to surgery reducing insulin requirements. Recovery after surgery is often better after RA than GA, with decreased opioid usage and hence less postoperative nausea and vomiting with the early resumption of feeding.

There are potential disadvantages of RA in diabetic patients. An extensive sympathetic blockade with epidural or spinal analgesia in the presence of an autonomic neuropathy can result in severe hypotension. If there is also severe blood loss then maintenance of an adequate arterial pressure is particularly difficult. There is an increased risk of infection with neuraxial blockade, meningitis and epidural abscess, so that a scrupulous aseptic technique is essential when undertaking epidural and spinal analgesia in diabetic patients [25, 26]. Because of the problems associated with neuraxial blockade, peripheral nerve blocks have become more common. Many diabetic patients have a peripheral polyneuropathy and concerns have been expressed recently about the safety of RA [27]. It has been suggested that local anaesthetic drugs may be more toxic in diabetic patients (although this may reflect the severity of the associated cardiac disease), that the dose given should be decreased, and that the nerves are more susceptible to needle damage with an exacerbation in the rate of neuronal failure. Although, there is little evidence to support these concerns, RA must be considered on a risk-benefit basis for each patient.

General anaesthesia

All volatile anaesthetic agents, *in vitro*, inhibit the insulin response to glucose at clinical concentrations in a dose-dependent and reversible manner [28]. Clinically, a similar effect has been shown with isoflurane in non-diabetic patients [29]. The effect of inhalational agents on type 2 diabetics with residual insulin secretion has not been investigated but it is probable that insulin release is inhibited. This mechanism also

Table 9.6 Regional anaesthesia for diabetic patients.

Advantages
Awake patient
Avoids tracheal intubation
Decreases catabolic hormone response
Good postoperative analgesia
Disadvantages
Neuraxial block
increased cardiovascular instability
increased risk of infection
Peripheral block
exacerbation of neuropathy by direct damage
increased local anaesthetic toxicity

provides a plausible explanation for the initial failure of insulin secretion in response to the glycaemic stimulus of surgery (see above). The potential deleterious effects of the volatile agents may be avoided by the use of total intravenous anaesthesia (TIVA). However, the effects of propofol on insulin secretion have not been investigated and diabetic patients have been found to have a decreased ability to clear lipids from the circulation so the benefits of TIVA may be illusory [30].

Intravenous fluids

It is common practice to administer the glucose infusion in the GIK regimen at 100–125 ml h^{-1}. The prolonged use of this regimen is associated with the development of hyponatraemia as the glucose is metabolised to leave excess free water. The failure to emphasise the need for sodium in diabetic patients is surprising but probably arose, in part, as a consequence of the recommendation 30 years ago to avoid the use of lactate-containing solutions such as Hartmann's solution (Na$^+$ 131 mmol l^{-1}) because they were considered to exacerbate hyperglycaemia [31]. The clinical data to support the notion were very weak and simple calculations of the gluconeogenic potential of lactate demonstrate that the infusion of Hartmann's solution at rates commonly used intra- and postoperatively would have little effect on circulating glucose [32].

Additional intravenous fluids in diabetic patients can be either 0.9% sodium chloride solution or Hartmann's solution, but in elderly patients receiving 100–125 ml h^{-1} GIK regimen there is a risk of fluid overload. The infusion of 50% glucose rather than 10% or 5% glucose decreases the volume of glucose solution

97

but this concentrated solution must be given slowly into a central vein to decrease the risk of thrombophlebitis. Currently there is not an ideal single crystalloid solution for infusion in diabetic patients undergoing surgery. In the USA 5% glucose with 0.45% sodium chloride and 20 mmol l⁻¹ potassium chloride is available and has been recommended but this contains insufficient substrate if infused at conventional rates and the potassium concentration may have to be varied [33].

Red cell concentrates for transfusion are stored in SAGM (saline-adenine-glucose-mannitol) with a glucose concentration of 0.9% (50 mmol l⁻¹). If several packs of red cells are transfused then this additional glucose load must be considered; an increased rate of insulin infusion is often necessary to maintain the target glucose range.

Monitoring of metabolism

The key to managing diabetic patients in the perioperative period is frequent measurement of blood glucose with appropriate changes in insulin and/or glucose administration as necessary (Table 9.7). When point-of-care (POC) glucose strip assays are used to determine glucose concentration it is preferable to use whole blood rather than capillary blood as accuracy is slightly better (7% of whole blood samples deviated by more than 20% from laboratory value compared with 15% of capillary blood samples) [34]. The POC techniques, assay strips and arterial blood gas analysis, tend to overestimate glucose values at low concentrations with the risk of missing hypoglycaemia [35]. Other factors that affect POC measurement of blood glucose include peripheral hypoperfusion, anaemia, increased circulating bilirubin and uric acid, mannitol, dopamine, dextran and paracetamol [36].

During and immediately after major surgery blood glucose should be measured hourly. The comparative inaccuracy of POC measurements of glucose should be considered before altering infusion regimens. For example, a decrease from 10 to 8 mmol l⁻¹ glucose could be within the limits of accuracy of the method of measurement. When stable blood glucose concentrations have been achieved postoperatively the interval between testing can be increased to two and then four hours.

Plasma potassium concentrations should be measured on alternate glucose samples. Arterial gas analysis is useful and can often be undertaken on the same sample used for glucose and potassium estimation. Measurement of pH, plasma bicarbonate and

Table 9.7 Monitoring of diabetic patients perioperatively.

Frequent blood glucose estimations (hourly during major surgery)
Plasma potassium
Arterial blood gas analysis
Urinary ketones (acetoacetate)
Blood β-hydroxybutyrate

blood lactate will show whether the patient is acidotic. Circulating lactate values are often increased slightly in patients with raised blood glucose. The presence of an acidosis with a normal or high normal lactate should alert the anaesthetist to the possibility of ketoacidosis. If possible the urine should be tested for ketones but the reagent strips only measure acetoacetate and not β hydroxybutyrate. Measurement of blood β hydroxybutyrate concentration by POC strip assays has been used to guide treatment in diabetic ketoacidosis (Chapter 16) but has not been used at present with surgery [37].

Postoperative care

Anaesthetists are not usually involved with the postoperative care of diabetic patients after they have left the recovery area in theatre. Before discharge to the ward, analgesia, treatment for nausea and vomiting and appropriate intravenous fluids should be prescribed. Good postoperative analgesia, particularly RA, decreases catabolic hormone secretion. Non-steroidal anti-inflammatory drugs (NSAIDs) must be used with great caution as they may further impair renal function in patients with a nephropathy. Prophylaxis against nausea and vomiting should have been undertaken intraoperatively but must be treated vigorously if it occurs. In addition to the GIK regimen other sodium-containing intravenous fluids may be required. Urine output may be misleading as a sign of adequacy of hydration if glycosuria is present with an osmotic diuresis.

The anaesthetist should ensure that the blood glucose is stable within the target range, that the plasma potassium is normal and that an appropriate sliding scale has been prescribed before the patient leaves the theatre area.

Conclusion

The management of diabetic surgical inpatients is not currently evidence based. Instead, it is based on an understanding of the pathophysiology of diabetes, the physiological effects of insulin and the intensive monitoring of blood glucose. The anaesthetic quest for physiological normality may be inappropriate for diabetic patients.

References

1. NHS Institute for Innovation and Improvement. Focus on: inpatient care for people with diabetes. http://www.institute.nhs.uk/quality_and_value/high_volume_care/focus_on:_diabetes.html, 2008.

2. Risum O, Abdelnoor M, Svennevig JL, et al. Diabetes mellitus and morbidity and mortality risks after coronary artery bypass surgery. *Scand J Thorac Cardiovasc Surg* 1996; **30**: 71–5.

3. Zacharias AZ, Habib RH. Factors predisposing to median sternotomy complications. *Chest* 1996; **110**: 1173–8.

4. Thourani VH, Weintraub WS, Stein B, et al. Influence of diabetes on early and late outcome after coronary artery bypass grafting. *Ann Thorac Surg* 1999; **67**: 1045–52.

5. Salzarulo HH, Taylor LA. Diabetic 'stiff joint syndrome' as a cause of difficult intubation. *Anesthesiology* 1986; **64**: 366–8.

6. Nadal JLY, Fernandez BG, Escobar IC, Black M, Rosenblatt WH. The palm print as a sensitive predictor of difficult laryngoscopy in diabetics. *Acta Anaesthesiol Scand* 1998; **42**: 199–203.

7. Flynn MD, O' Brien IA, Corrall RJ. The prevalence of autonomic and peripheral neuropathy in insulin-treated diabetic subjects. *Diabet Med* 1995; **12**: 310–13.

8. Stys A, Stys T. Current clinical applications of heart rate variability. *Clin Cardiol* 1998; **21**: 719–24.

9. Kirvela M, Salmela K, Toivonen L, Koivusalo A-M, Lindgren L. Heart rate variability in diabetic and non-diabetic renal transplant patients. *Acta Anaesthesiol Scand* 1996; **40**: 804–8.

10. Hall GM. The anesthetic modification of the endocrine and metabolic response to surgery. *Ann R Coll Surg Engl* 1985; **67**: 25–9.

11. Desborough JP. The stress response to trauma and surgery. *Br J Anaesth* 2000; **85**: 109–12.

12. Van Den Bergh G, Wouters P, Weekers F, et al. Intensive insulin therapy in critically ill patients. *N Engl J Med* 2001; **345**: 1359–67.

13. Gandhi GY, Nuttal GA, Abel MD, et al. Intraoperative hyperglycemia and perioperative outcomes in cardiac surgery patients. *Mayo Clin Proc* 2005; **80**: 862–6.

14. Lipshutz AKM, Gropper MA. Perioperative glycemic control. An evidence-based review. *Anesthesiology* 2009; **110**: 408–21.

15. Gandhi GY, Nuttal GA, Abel MD, et al. Intensive intraoperative insulin therapy versus conventional glucose management during cardiac surgery. *Ann Intern Med* 2007; **146**: 233–43.

16. Vriesendorp TM, Morelis QJ, Devries JH, Legemate DA, Hoekstra JB. Early postoperative glucose levels are an independent risk factor for infection after peripheral vascular surgery. A retrospective study. *Eur J Vasc Endovasc Surg* 2004; **28**: 520–5.

17. Bilotta F, Spinelli A, Giovannini F, Doronzio A, Delfini R, Rosa G. The effect of intensive insulin therapy on infection rate, vasospasm, neurologic outcome and mortality in neurointensive care unit after intracranial aneurysm clipping in patients with subarachnoid hemorrhage. A randomized prospect pilot trial. *J Neurosurg Anesthesiol* 2007; **19**: 156–60.

18. Langouche L, Vanhorebeek I, Vlasselaers D, et al. Intensive insulin therapy protects the endothelium of critically ill patients. *J Clin Invest* 2005; **115**: 2277–86.

19. Martinez EA, Williams KA, Pronovost PJ. Thinking like a pancreas: perioperative glycemic control. *Anesth Analg* 2007; **104**: 4–6.

20. Garber AJ, Moghissi ES, Bransome ED, et al. American College of Endocrinology Task Force on Inpatient Diabetes Metabolic Control. American College of Endocrinology position statement on inpatient diabetes and metabolic control. *Endocr Pract* 2004; **10** Suppl 12: 4–9.

21. Monnier L, Mas E, Ginet C, et al. Activation of oxidative stress by acute glucose fluctuations compared with sustained hyperglycemia in patients with type 2 diabetes. *JAMA* 2006; **295**: 1681–7.

22. Olson RP, Bethel MA, Lien LL. Preoperative hypoglycaemia in patient on detemir insulin. *Anesth Analg* 2009; **108**: 1836–8.

23. McAnulty GR, Robertshaw HJ, Hall GM. Anaesthetic management of patients with diabetes mellitus. *Br J Anaesth* 2000; **85**: 80–90.

24. Alberti KEMM, Thomas DJB . The management of diabetes during surgery. *Br J Anaesth* 1979; **51**: 693–710.

25. Nikolasjen L, Ilkjaer S, Christensen JH, Krøner K, Jensen TS. Randomised trial of epidural bupivacaine and morphine in prevention of stump and phantom limb pain in lower limb amputation. *Lancet* 1997; **350**: 135–7.

26. Kindler CH, Seeberger MD, Staender SE. Epidural abscess complicating epidural anaesthesia and analgesia. An analysis of the literature. *Acta Anaesthesiol Scand* 1998; **42**: 614–20.

27. Williams BA, Murinson BB. Diabetes mellitus and subclinical neuropathy. *Anesthesiology* 2008; **109**: 361–2.

28. Desborough JP, Jones PM, Persaud SJ, Landon MJ, Howell SL. Isoflurane inhibits insulin secretion in isolated rat pancreatic islets of Langerhans. *Br J Anaesth* 1993; **71**: 873–6.

29. Desborough JP, Knowles MG, Hall GM. Effects of isoflurane-nitrous oxide anaesthesia on insulin

secretion in female patients. *Br J Anaesth* 1998; **80**: 250–2.

30. Wicklmayr M, Rett K, Dietz G, Mehnert H. Comparison of metabolic clearance rates of MCT/LCT and LCT emulsions in diabetics. *JPEN J Parenteral Enteral Nutr* 1988; **12**: 68–71.

31. Thomas DJ, Alberti KG. Hyperglycaemic effects of Hartmann's solution during surgery in patients with maturity onset diabetes. *Br J Anaesth* 1978; **50**: 185–8.

32. Simpson AK, Levy N, Hall GM. Peri-operative iv fluids in diabetic patients – don't forget the salt. *Anaesthesia* 2008; **63**: 1043–5.

33. Schiff RL, Emanuele MA. The surgical patient with diabetes mellitus: guidelines for management. *J Gen Intern Med* 1995; **10**: 154–61.

34. Desachy A, Vuagnat AC, Ghazali AD, et al. Accuracy of beside glucometry in critically ill patients: Influence of clinical characteristics and perfusion index. *Mayo Clin Proc* 2008; **83**: 400–5.

35. Kanji S, Buffie J, Hutton B, et al. Reliability of point-of-care testing for glucose measurement in critically ill adults. *Crit Care Med* 2005; **33**: 2778–85.

36. Fahy BG, Coursin DB. Critical glucose control. The devil is in the details. *Mayo Clin Proc* 2008; **83**: 394–7.

37. Wiggam MI, O' Kane MJ, Harper R, et al. Treatment of diabetic ketoacidosis using normalization of blood 3-hydroxybutyrate concentration as the endpoint of emergency management. *Diabetes Care* 1997; **20**: 1347–52.

Chapter 10

Management of diabetes in obstetric patients

Neville Robinson and David J. Vaughan

Diabetes is the most common endocrine disorder of pregnancy. In pregnancy, it has considerable cost and care demands and is associated with increased risks to the health of the mother and the outcome of the pregnancy. However, with careful and appropriate screening, multidisciplinary management and a motivated patient these risks can be minimised.

Epidemiology

There are approximately 650 000 births in England and Wales each year. It is estimated that between 2–5% of women have diabetes in pregnancy [1]. Pre-existing type 1 (0.27%) and type 2 (0.10%) diabetics jointly account for 0.37% of all births. The prevalence of existing diabetes in women of childbearing age is increasing, perhaps due to the increase in certain ethnic minority groups (African, black Caribbean, South Asian, Middle Eastern and Chinese) in the UK. The prevalence of gestational diabetes which may or may not resolve after birth is estimated at 3.5% of pregnant women but varies from region to region depending on the prevalence of the at risk minority groups. It is estimated that, of pregnancies complicated by diabetes, 87.5% are due to gestational diabetes, 7.5% being due to type 1 diabetes and the remaining 5% due to type 2 diabetes [2].

Risks associated with diabetes in pregnancy

Diabetic mothers have an increased risk of obstetric complications. Spontaneous abortion, thromboembolism, polyhydramnios, maternal infection and complications secondary to increased fetal size are all increased in this group.

There are risks to the labouring parturient. There is an increased risk of premature labour – diabetic mothers are 5 times more likely to deliver before 37 weeks.

There is an increased risk of obstructed labour in diabetics; twice as many singleton babies of diabetics are macrosomic (a birth weight of ≥ 4000 g) when compared to the general maternity population. Shoulder dystocia is more common in diabetics with a reported incidence of 8% when compared to the general population incidence of 3% [3]. There is an increased risk of Caesarean section also: the Confidential Enquiry into Maternal and Child Health (CEMACH) reports a 67% Caesarean section rate in diabetic women as compared to 22% in the general maternity population [2].

There is an increased risk of fetal and neonatal complications. A fivefold increased risk of stillbirth or late intrauterine deaths is reported in diabetic mothers. Fetal distress in labour is more commonly reported. There is an increased perinatal mortality with a threefold increased risk of death within the first month of life. A twofold increase in congenital malformations in the newborn is reported with neurological and cardiac abnormalities being the most common. There is also an increased incidence of neonatal hypoglycaemia, respiratory distress syndrome and jaundice in the babies born to diabetics. Babies of women with diabetes are ten times more likely to have Erb's palsy. Many of these risk increases are due to a macrosomic baby who may experience a difficult delivery [4].

There are increased risks of complications in pre-existing diabetics. Almost half of the women in the latest CEMACH report had recurrent hypoglycaemia during pregnancy, although there was no evidence that this was associated with a worsened pregnancy outcome for the baby. There is an increased risk of ketoacidosis. There is progression of the microvascular complications of diabetes. Poor glycaemic control in the first trimester and pregnancy-induced or chronic hypertension are independently associated with the progression of retinopathy. Worsening nephropathy can affect maternal blood pressure, and nephropathy

Core Topics in Endocrinology in Anaesthesia and Critical Care, eds. George M. Hall, Jennifer M. Hunter and Mark S. Cooper. Published by Cambridge University Press. © Cambridge University Press 2010.

with superimposed pre-eclampsia is the most common cause of preterm delivery in women with diabetes [5].

Many maternal factors are associated with an adverse pregnancy outcome. Maternal social deprivation, an unplanned pregnancy, a lack of contraceptive use in the 12 months prior to pregnancy, a lack of preconception folic acid, smoking, sub-optimal glycaemic control, pre-existing diabetic complications and sub-optimal preconception care are all implicated [6].

Preconception management

An essential component of adolescent diabetic education is the avoidance of unplanned pregnancies. The risks with pregnancies increase with the duration of the diabetes [7]. Contraception is advised until good glycaemic control is established. Good glycaemic control for pregnancy is considered to have been achieved when the HbA_{1c} is maintained at less than 6.1%. This reduces the risk of congenital malformations. Women with HbA_{1c} levels above 10% are advised against pregnancy. Monthly monitoring in the preconception period is advised. Patients with a body mass index (BMI) over 27 kg m^2 should be offered dietary advice and patients wishing to become pregnant should take folic acid (5 mg day^{-1}) until 12 weeks gestation to reduce the risk of neonatal neural tube defects. Appropriate referral for renal and retinal assessment needs to be undertaken at this stage [8].

The safety of diabetic medications needs consideration. Oral hypoglycaemic drugs cross the placenta and there is a theoretical risk that increased congenital malformations will occur in the offspring of diabetic mothers using these drugs. The manufacturers and the *British National Formulary* suggest acarbose, repaglinide, nateglinide, pioglitazone and rosiglitazone should be avoided in pregnancy and that insulin should be substituted. Sulphonylureas can cause neonatal hypoglycaemia. If oral hypoglycaemic agents are used then metformin is deemed the safest but it is recommended that informed consent be obtained and documented prior to its use.

Insulin is compatible with pregnancy and is the recommended drug of choice. The rapid-acting insulin analogues (e.g., aspart and lispro) are safe. Women with insulin-treated diabetes should be told that there is insufficient evidence about the safety and use of the long-acting insulin analogues. Isophane insulin is the first choice in pregnancy [9].

Diabetics may be on other drugs. Angiotensin-converting enzyme inhibitors and angiotensin II receptor blockers are used to treat hypertension and to slow the progression of any nephropathy. Major congenital malformations have been reported with this class of drugs and therefore other antihypertensive drugs should be used. For similar reasons, statins should be avoided in diabetic women wishing to become pregnant.

Gestational diabetes

Gestational diabetes is defined as carbohydrate intolerance resulting in hyperglycaemia of variable severity with onset or first recognition during pregnancy [10]. The Pedersen hypothesis suggests that maternal hyperglycaemia results in the excess transfer of glucose to the fetus which results in fetal hyperglycaemia [11]. Insulin production by the fetus which has an additional anabolic action causes increased fetal adipose tissue growth with its attendant risks: neonatal hypoglycaemia, fetal hypoxia with increased risks to the fetus of death, polycythaemia, hyperbilirubinaemia and renal vein thrombosis. There is also an increased long-term risk of diabetes and obesity in the children. Diagnosis and treatment reduces ill health in the mother. It also reduces the progression of type 2 diabetes in the long term and the risk of future pregnancies being complicated by pre-existing or gestational diabetes.

There are independent risk factors for gestational diabetes [12]. These are shown in Table 10.1.

The most common presentation of gestational diabetes in mothers is antenatal glycosuria. Maternal renal plasma flow increases by 25–50% and the glomerular filtration rate rises by about 50% in the first and early second trimester. This results in a massively increased glucose load on the kidney, such that reabsorption in the proximal tubule is overwhelmed and glycosuria occurs. It is generally regarded that an upper limit of loss is set at 140 mg day^{-1}, although levels can exceed 1.5 g day^{-1}.

When glycosuria is detected a random blood glucose should be measured. This is abnormal if the result is > 6.1 mmol l^{-1} in the fasting state or more than 2 hours after food, or > 7.0 mmol l^{-1} within 2 hours of food. The most reliable test is an oral glucose tolerance test (OGTT); diagnosis of gestational diabetes should be made if fasting venous plasma glucose is > 7.0 mmol l^{-1} or fasting venous plasma glucose is < 7.0 mmol l^{-1} but venous plasma glucose is > 7.8 mmol l^{-1} 2 hours after a 75 g glucose load [13].

In most women, gestational diabetes responds to dietary changes (restriction of calorific intake < 25 kcal kg^{-1} day^{-1}) and exercise (> 30 min day^{-1}). Between 10 and 20% require oral hypoglycaemic agents or insulin.

Table 10.1 Maternal risk factors for gestational diabetes mellitus.

Age > 40 years
BMI > 30 kg/m²
Previous baby with macrosomia, birth weight > 4.5 kg
Family history (first degree relative) of diabetes mellitus
Previous gestational diabetes
Family background with a high risk of diabetes mellitus
South Asian
black Caribbean
Middle Eastern
Latin American

Antenatal management

Target ranges for blood glucose have been recommended. There is always a risk of hypoglycaemia but if it is safely achievable women with diabetes should aim to keep their fasting blood glucose between 3.5 and 5.9 mmol l^{-1} and the 1 hour postprandial blood glucose < 7.8 mmol l^{-1} during pregnancy. HbA$_{1c}$ levels are not used routinely in pregnancy. Strict blood glucose monitoring is recommended. Fasting blood glucose and levels one hour after every meal should be undertaken. Insulin-treated diabetics should test their levels prior to going to bed at night and ketone testing is advised if the patient becomes hyperglycaemic or unwell [14]. Hypoglycaemia affects the quality of life and the risk of physical injury; and is aggravated by pregnancy, nausea and vomiting. Hyperemesis gravidarum in pregnant women can lead to ketoacidosis and an associated increased risk of fetal death.

The rapid-acting insulin analogues (aspart and lispro) confer benefits over soluble human insulin in pregnant patients and these include fewer episodes of hypoglycaemia, a reduction in postprandial excursions, improved overall glycaemic control and improved patient satisfaction. Continuous subcutaneous insulin infusions should be considered in women with poor glycaemic control [15].

Regular retinal and renal assessment should occur throughout pregnancy and screening for fetal congenital malformations with a four chamber view of the fetal heart and outflow tracts is recommended at 18–20 weeks. Fetal growth monitoring is important as there is a risk of intrauterine growth restriction in diabetics.

Diabetics are now routinely cared for by appropriately trained specialist obstetricians in combined clinics with diabetologists. Anaesthetists similarly now run antenatal clinics for the identification and management of high-risk patients and unstable diabetics are often referred to these clinics for advice. Patients with a BMI above 35 are routinely referred because of the potential risks of managing regional and general anaesthesia in these at-risk parturients and many of these patients are diabetic [16].

Intrapartum management

Diabetics are high risk and should be delivered in an appropriate hospital environment with consultant-led obstetric care. Department of Health guidelines for the management of diabetics in labour have been issued and reviewed. Regular blood glucose monitoring and ensuring that the blood glucose is within normal range reduces the risk of neonatal hypoglycaemia. In mothers with gestational diabetes, the rate of fetal macrosomia is up to 30% of deliveries and neonatal hypoglycaemia occurs in up to 24% of these babies.

Pregnancy outcomes are improved in diabetics with tight glycaemic control and active management throughout pregnancy. The complication of shoulder dystocia can be decreased by ultrasound monitoring and the elective delivery of those babies weighing over 4250 g. Ultrasound has been found to accurately determine the presence or absence of macrosomia in 87% of women scanned. The aforementioned labour complications mean intense maternal monitoring in pregnancy but this needs to be balanced by the negative maternal experiences of high interventional medical care, labour and delivery. This need not be the case if the mothers are helped to feel in control, are involved in decision making and kept informed and supported within the hospital environment.

Current recommendations for the timing and mode of delivery are that pregnant women with diabetes who have a normally developed fetus should be offered elective birth through induction of labour, or by elective Caesarean section, if indicated after 38 completed weeks. Diabetes is not in itself to be considered a contraindication to attempting vaginal birth after a previous Caesarean section [17].

Glycaemic control in labour

Tight glycaemic control during labour and delivery is important for the well-being of the child. The clinical evidence from the latest CEMACH enquiry surprisingly shows that, overall, suboptimal glycaemic control during pregnancy has little effect on pregnancy outcome – fewer than 50% of women in both groups (poor vs. good pregnancy outcome) had suboptimal first trimester

Table 10.2 A suggested sliding scale regimen for labour.

Fluid infusion: 10% dextrose (1 litre) with 20 mmol of potassium	
Insulin infusion: 50 U of actrapid in 50 ml of 0.9% sodium chloride in a syringe driver	
This may need to be modified in insulin resistant type 2 diabetics, e.g., those needing over 100 U of insulin per day	
Blood glucose level	**Rate/hour**
0–3 mmol l⁻¹	0 U, call doctor immediately
3.1–6 mmol l⁻¹	1 U
6.1–9 mmol l⁻¹	2 U
9.1–12 mmol l⁻¹	3 U
12.1–15 mmol l⁻¹	4 U, repeat after 30 min and call doctor if rising
>15.1 mmol l⁻¹	6 U call doctor immediately

glycaemic control. During labour, however, poor control can have significant effects on neonatal health [18].

Neonatal hypoglycaemia is well recognised as a complication of maternal diabetes of any cause. This is thought to be due to two mechanisms. The more severe form is fetal hyperinsulinaemia secondary to sustained excessive glucose transfer across the placenta leading to severe and sometimes prolonged hypoglycaemia in the neonatal period. This often requires prolonged and careful monitoring and intervention by the neonatal team, and may be associated with increased diabetic and obesity risks in later life. A less severe form of neonatal hypoglycaemia is seen in babies who have not developed hyperinsulinaemia in fetal life, due to good glycaemic control in pregnancy. In this group a sudden response to maternal hyperglycaemia in labour leads to a transient (1–3 hours) inappropriate rise in neonatal insulin levels which may cause hypoglycaemia.

Fetal distress in labour is also clearly associated with maternal hyperglycaemia. This both increases the risk of fetal damage due to asphyxia and increases maternal risk because of an increased rate of emergency Caesarean section in these mothers.

The methods used to maintain labouring diabetics within a normal glucose range (4–7 mmol l⁻¹) vary. Most units now use sliding scale infusions of short-acting insulin with dextrose containing intravenous fluids, titrated against frequent maternal bedside glucose estimations. Some still use mixed bags of insulin and dextrose infused together. There is little clear evidence in the literature as to which is preferable. However, we believe that most doctors and nurses are more familiar with the sliding scale approach, and feel that this approach provides better control as long as close glucose monitoring is available and carried out [19]. A typical regimen is given in Table 10.2, but all obstetric units will have clear policies and these should be adhered to in order to avoid confusion.

Analgesia for labour and vaginal delivery

The stress of labour and birth for women makes diabetes more difficult to control in labour. Any labour interventions need to be considered carefully in terms of the effects on the baby and mother. Relevant factors in terms of the mother with diabetes are: glycaemic control, prevention of metabolic disturbances (acid–base status and ketoacidosis), infection prevention and haemodynamic control (with an emphasis on the avoidance of hypotension as perfusion of the placenta is primarily blood pressure dependent).

Acid–base status

Concerns have been raised regarding the increased susceptibility to infection in diabetics, and thus the concomitant risk of indwelling catheters in these mothers. There is no evidence to support this increased risk of epidural infection, though no firm data exist to support or refute given the enormous numbers that would be required. It is the authors' practice to use the usual criteria as contraindications for epidural analgesia (absolute: refusal, allergy, absence of large bore intravenous access, staffing/equipment issues, coagulopathy, sepsis; relative: haemorrhage, fetal distress, maternal spinal deformity, relapsing neurological conditions). There is little evidence to support the use of antibiotic prophylaxis for non-surgical procedures in diabetics.

Haemodynamic control

Although there is little hard evidence in the literature, most obstetric anesthetists agree that maintenance of normovolaemia is key in labouring diabetics. Avoidance in particular of hypovolaemia and its attendant risk of hypotension leading to placental hypoperfusion is vital. In non-insulin-using parturients, adequate oral fluid intake can usually be achieved by the mother. Provided blood glucose levels are in the normal range and the urine is ketone free, no further active intervention is required, though close monitoring is essential. Those mothers who have been using insulin during pregnancy will need to be started on sliding scale regimens with intravenous fluid support. Careful and frequent titration of insulin dose is standard, but care should also be taken over fluid management to maintain euvolaemia. The presence of an autonomic neuropathy means theoretically that there may be more hypotension in diabetic mothers but this is not borne out in clinical practice.

Neuropathy

The rate of pre-existing neuropathy in diabetic mothers is low, but higher than in the pregnant population as a whole. Epidural anaesthesia is not contraindicated in this group, but the risk of neurological deterioration after epidural is quoted at approximately 0.5%. The most common technical complications are reported as unintentional transient paraesthesia (7%), blood vessel puncture (1.5%) and dural puncture (0.9%).

Obesity

There are no studies on the risks of epidural analgesia in the obese. It is widely accepted that the technique is more challenging as flexion of the lumbar spine may be limited, the space is deeper and identification of landmarks more difficult. This results in an increased rate of failure to site the epidural, and an increased risk of damage to surrounding structures due to inadvertent needle misdirection. Neuraxial blockade may also lead to exaggerated haemodynamic variance, and the presence of a larger than usual uterine mass (macrosomy, polyhydramnios) may cause increased segmental spread leading to a higher block than anticipated.

However, these risks should be weighed against the benefits and metabolic stability provided in labour by good epidural analgesia. Progression to urgent Caesarean section is also not delayed if the epidural is sited early in labour, thus avoiding the greatly increased risks of general anaesthesia.

In summary, epidural analgesia is entirely appropriate in labouring diabetics. As well as providing the best analgesic option, it decreases maternal stress and thus

the risk of hyperglycaemia. Given that diabetic mothers have proportionately larger babies it is likely that vaginal delivery will be more difficult than in the normal population, with a higher rate of instrumentally assisted delivery, episiotomy and conversion to urgent Caesarean section. The presence of a well-established epidural in these cases is very useful.

Anaesthesia for Caesarean section
General principles

It is universally accepted that, in the absence of contraindications, regional analgesia is the preferred form of anaesthetic technique for Caesarean section. Given the risk factors for diabetic mothers discussed above this is particularly true in this group. As in all Caesarean sections, core anaesthetic principles must be adhered to – appropriate staff, preoperative assessment, correct equipment and facilities before commencing the procedure; scrupulous aseptic technique during block insertion; and timely intervention in response to adverse events before, during and after the procedure. It is not within the scope of this chapter to discuss the full management of operative delivery. However, there are several key points relating specifically to the diabetic population.

Specific considerations in diabetics

As with all mothers presenting for Caesarean section, the key to the management of the diabetic patient lies largely in preoperative preparation where possible. Optimisation of glycaemic control is vital over the perioperative period and the use of a short-acting insulin via infusion, titrated against frequent (hourly) plasma glucose measurement is mandatory in all bar the most mild diet-controlled parturients. Preoperative assessment should cover the areas of increased risk in this group (see above: hypertension and pre-eclampsia, sepsis, renal dysfunction) as well as the normal preoperative history, examination and investigations. Regional anaesthesia is positively indicated compared to general, and there is no specific concern related to the spinal over the epidural route. Half-hourly blood glucose monitoring for patients undergoing general anaesthesia is recommended.

It is usual to check neonatal glucose soon after birth as hypoglycaemia is commonly found. Antibiotic and thromboembolic prophylaxis should be meticulous. Each unit should have its own clear policy. We use co-amoxyclav 1.2 g intravenously immediately after delivery, and 5000 IU dalteparin subcutaneously daily post-Caesarean section as well as TED stockings and a calf compression device during the operation.

There should be a low threshold for high dependency care in the first 24 hours following delivery in diabetics to facilitate tight glycaemic control over the period when the mother may still be fasting.

Neonatal management

Neonatal morbidity is increased in those babies born of diabetic mothers, whether gestational or pre-existent. Most of these problems correct themselves within a matter of hours to days, but all still require prompt monitoring and, if necessary, intervention. Cohort and case control studies show attendant problems for the neonate [20]. These are outlined in Table 10.3. Both polycythaemia and hyperviscosity are due to chronic *in utero* hypoxia.

Macrosomia leads to an increase in traumatic birth injuries, principally upper limb and clavicular fracture. Neurovascular damage is also more common, principally brachial plexus injuries but also phrenic and cranial nerve damage. Cerebral contusions and haemorrhages are also increased.

Infant respiratory distress syndrome is associated primarily with prematurity. Other risk factors are also more common in babies from diabetic mothers (birth asphyxia, meconium aspiration) as well as the rare but important cardiac causes, principally left ventricular outflow tract obstruction. Diagnosis is based partly on history and clinical observation and partly on arterial gas and radiological findings (diffuse granular shadowing, cardiomegaly). Treatment is supportive using continuous positive airway pressure or full artificial ventilation as necessary. Intervention with surfactant replacement is now used early in therapy with great success.

Polycythaemia, hypomineralaemia (particularly hypocalcaemia and hypophosphataemia) and hyperbilirubinaemia are all detected via laboratory estimation. These assays should be routinely carried out in all high-risk infants and in those showing clinical evidence of problems – lethargy, irritability, twitching, poor APGAR/neurobehavioural scores or more overt evidence of organ dysfunction.

Neonatal hypoglycaemia

Neonatal hypoglycaemia is defined as a blood glucose value of less than 2.6 mmol l^{-1}. At this concentration

Table 10.3 Neonatal problems for diabetic mothers.

Macrosomia
Birth trauma
Infant respiratory distress syndrome
Hypoglycaemia
Hypomineralaemia
Cardiomyopathy
Polycythaemia
Hyperviscosity
Thrombosis

not all neonates will be symptomatic, but any lower value should be actively treated. This concentration was chosen as there is good evidence to show adverse neurodevelopmental outcome in those whose glucose values fall below it. Characteristically, babies of diabetic mothers are asymptomatic in the presence of hypoglycaemia, which has an early onset after birth (within the first 60 minutes), respond well to intravenous dextrose infusion and, once treated, tend not to relapse [21].

Early feeding is a vital preventative measure in these babies; indeed there is good evidence that the risk of clinically evident hypoglycaemia is almost nil in those who feed well at three hours post-delivery, and rates of measured hypoglycaemia are reduced by 50%. Frequent feeding also reduces the risk of hypoglycaemia. Breastfeeding appears to result in a higher level of ketogenesis in the neonate than formula feeding. This may provide an alternate energy substrate pathway for the baby. There is no clear evidence as to either food having a better hypoglycaemic preventative effect. Blood glucose testing should be carried out using laboratory samples or ward-based glucose electrode meters. Reagent strips have both low sensitivity and specificity for the detection of hypoglycaemia. Testing is best done before a feed [22].

A general guide to intervention is that all babies with risk factors have compromised metabolic adaptation. Early and frequent feeding is to be encouraged. Symptomatic babies or those with very low plasma glucose levels (< 1.4 mmol l^{-1}) should be given intravenous dextrose to raise the glucose level over 2.5 mmol l^{-1}.

Postnatal management
Treatment and follow-up

Women with gestational diabetes are at increased risk of a recurrence in future pregnancies. Quoted incidence of recurrence varies between 30 and 80%, but is 75% in those who have required insulin therapy during pregnancy, and increased in those with a raised BMI [23].

The risk of progression in later life to type 2 diabetes is also increased in gestational diabetics. Systematic reviews indicate that fasting glucose levels taken for OGTTs in pregnancy are indicative of risk; the higher the level, the greater the risk, although no definite limits could be determined. A high BMI and insulin use in pregnancy are also related to increased risk.

Close and continued follow-up is required in all women with gestational diabetes. It is routine for all gestational diabetics to stop pregnancy-related hypoglycaemic therapy immediately post partum pending further review and assessment. Many will return to normal, but all should be tested prior to discharge and referred for diabetic review until normality has been confirmed. Preventative measures are strongly advised in this group. Two main therapeutic approaches are commonly used, ideally simultaneously. Lifestyle education and encouragement in resuming/increasing physical activity is at least as effective in preventing progression as pharmacological intervention (primarily using metformin), though this appears to be less effective in those with lower socio-economic/educational scores, possibly related in part to decreased access to services, support and appropriate facilities [24].

Traditional follow-up screening is with an OGTT at 6-weeks post partum. Recent evidence suggests that fasting plasma glucose levels are as sensitive (100%) and almost as specific (94%), and should be used as a prescreening tool. This should be carried out on a yearly basis. All diabetics should be offered an OGTT in any future pregnancy, and this should be repeated later during the pregnancy if normal. All pre-existing (type 1 or 2) diabetics should be referred back to their previous management team.

Breast or formula feeding

The evidence supporting the benefits to mother and child of breast milk over formula is clearly established, and much effort is taken to ensure this message is passed on to pregnant women. Women with diabetes have, on occasion, been advised not to breastfeed due to the hypoglycaemic risk associated with feeding. In insulin-dependent diabetics who breastfeed a transient dip in mean random glucose levels is seen during the first week after delivery. The only study to look into this reported no increase in hypoglycaemic episodes in breastfeeding mothers on insulin, though glucose values were lowest during feeds. It is recommended that dosages be reduced during this period and that mothers monitor their own glucose levels frequently. Mothers should also be advised to have a snack while feeding their infant [25].

For those on oral hypoglycaemic drugs, only metformin and glibenclamide are regarded as safe for use in breastfeeding by expert consensus, though neither have UK licensing approval for this and documentation of informed consent is advised. There is little clinical evidence to support the safety of other, newer hypoglycaemic agents in breastfeeding diabetics, and the manufacturers of these medicines advise avoidance.

Diabetics are often on other drugs for the treatment or prevention of end-organ disease related to their diabetes. Cholesterol reducing drugs (statins) and obesity drugs are to be avoided in breastfeeding mothers due to manufacturer's advisory notes regarding possible toxicity risks to the infant. Calcium channel blockers are excreted in breast milk, as are angiotensin-converting enzyme inhibitors and angiotensin-II receptor blocking drugs. The levels of these are extremely low and it is thought that their use is worth considering if clinical need demands and maternal informed consent obtained. The *British National Formulary* as well as other drug references contains lists of drugs that are contraindicated in breastfeeding or should be used with care [26].

Conclusions

Diabetes in pregnancy has potential serious adverse effects for both the mother and the neonate. Standardised multidisciplinary care including anaesthetists should be carried out obsessively throughout pregnancy. The provision of continuous safe care to minimise and prevent potential problems will enable a successful outcome to the pregnancy.

References

1. Office for National Statistics. *Key population and vital statistics 2005. Local and Health Authority Areas. No. Series VS, No 32*. Basingstoke, Palgrave Macmillan, 2007.

2. National Institute for Health and Clinical Excellence (NICE). *Type 1 Diabetes: Diagnosis and Management of Type1 Diabetes in Children, Young people and Adults*. London, NICE, 2004.

3. King H. Epidemiology of glucose intolerance and gestational diabetics in women of childbearing age. *Diabetes Care* 1998; **21** Suppl 2: B9–13.

4. Casson IF. Outcomes of pregnancy in insulin dependent diabetic women: results of a 5 year population cohort study. *BMJ* 1997; **315**: 275–8.

5. CEMACH. *Confidential Enquiry into Maternal and Child Health: Pregnancy in Women with Type 1 and Type 2 Diabetes in 2002–03, England, Wales and Northern Ireland.* London, CEMACH, 2007.

6. Hawthorne G. Prospective population based survey of outcome of pregnancy in diabetic women: results of the Northern Diabetic Pregnancy Audit, 1994. *BMJ* 1997; **315**: 279–81.

7. Ricart W, Lopez J, Mozas J, et al. Body mass index has a greater impact on pregnancy outcomes than gestational hyperglycaemia. *Diabetologica Gynecology* 2005; **48**: 1736–42.

8. Steel JM, Johnstone FD, Hepburn DA, et al. Can prepregnancy care of diabetic women reduce the risk of abnormal babies? *BMJ* 1990; **301**: 1070–4.

9. Wyatt JW, Frias JL, Hoyme HE, et al. Congenital anomaly rate in offspring of mothers with diabetes treated with insulin lispro (Humalog). *Diabet Med* 2005; **22**: 803–7.

10. World Health Organization and Department of Noncommunicable Disease Surveillance. *Definition, Diagnosis and Classification of Diabetes Mellitus and its Complications. Report of a WHO Consultation. Part 1: Diagnosis and Classification of Diabetes Mellitus.* Geneva, World Health Organization, 1999.

11. Pedersen J. Weight and length at birth of infants of diabetic mothers. *Acta Endocrinol (Copenh)* 1954; **16**: 330–42.

12. Solomon CG, Willet WC, Carey VJ, et al. A prospective study of pregravid determinants of gestational diabetes mellitus. *JAMA* 1997; **278**: 1078–83.

13. American Diabetes Association. Diagnosis and classification of diabetes mellitus. *Diabetes Care* 2004; **27** Suppl 1: S5–10.

14. Jovanovic L, Druzin M, Peterson CM. Effect of euglycemia on the outcome of pregnancy in insulin-dependent women as compared to normal control subjects. *Am J Med* 1981; **71**: 921–7.

15. National Collaborating Centre for Chronic Conditions. *Type 1 Diabetes in Adults – National Clinical Guideline for Diagnosis and Management in Primary and Secondary Care.* London, Royal College of Physicians, 2004.

16. National Collaborating Centre for Women's and Children's Health. *Diabetes in Pregnancy – Management of Diabetes and its Complications from Preconception to the Postnatal Period.* London, RCOG Press, 2008.

17. Royal College of Obstetricians and Gynaecologists. *Induction of Labour.* London, RCOG Press, 2004.

18. CEMACH. *Confidential Enquiry into Maternal and Child Health. Saving Mothers' Lives: Reviewing Maternal Deaths to Make Motherhood Safer 2003–5.* London, CEMACH, 2007.

19. Lean ME, Pearson DW, Sutherland HW. Insulin management during labour and delivery in mothers with diabetes. *Diabet Med* 1990; **7**: 162–4.

20. Jones CW. Gestational diabetes and its impact on the neonate. *J Neonatal Nurs* 2001; **20**: 10–23.

21. Hod M, Jankovic L, Di Renzo, et al. *Textbook of Diabetes and Pregnancy.* London, Martin Dunitz, 2003.

22. Hawdon JM, Ward Platt MP, Aynsley-Green A. Patterns of metabolic adaption for preterm and term infants in the first neonatal week. *Arch Dis Child* 1992; **67** Suppl 4: 357–65.

23. Lobner K, Knopff A, Baumgarten A, et al. Predictors of postpartum diabetes in women with gestational diabetes mellitus. *Diabetes* 2006; **55**: 792–7.

24. Gillies Cl, Abrams KR, Lambert PC, et al. Pharmacological and lifestyle interventions to prevent or delay type 2 diabetes in people with impaired glucose tolerance: systematic review and meta-analysis. *BMJ* 2007; **334**: 299–302.

25. Saez-de-Ibarra L, Gaspar R, Obesso A, et al. Glycaemic behavior during lactation: post-partum practical guidelines for women with type 1 diabetes. *Practical Diabetes International* 2003; **20**: 271–5.

26. Joint Formulary Committee. *British National Formulary,* 54th edn. London, British Medical Association and Royal Pharmaceutical Society of Great Britain, 2008.

Management of diabetes in paediatric surgery

Ann E. Black and Angus McEwan

Introduction

Diabetes is one of the most common endocrine abnormalities in childhood. Despite the frequency of this condition, little is written on the perioperative management of diabetic children.

There are three main types of diabetes affecting children:

- Type 1 diabetes
- Type 2 diabetes
- Maturity onset diabetes.

Type 1 diabetes

Type 1 diabetes, also known as insulin dependent diabetes mellitus (IDDM), makes up 90–95% of the children with diabetes. This is an autoimmune disease where the insulin producing cells in the pancreas are destroyed. Type 1 diabetes has a peak incidence in the early teens but it does occur in young children. These children are insulin dependent and their management can be difficult. Children may be unable to co-operate with their medical regimen when very young and unwilling, and as they get to their rebellious teenage years, so that the ideal of good diabetic control can be difficult to achieve. In a national audit of diabetic care, only 16% of children achieved a target HbA$_{1c}$ level of less than 7.5%, which is taken as an indicator of good diabetic control [1].

The incidence of type 1 diabetes in children in England and Wales is approximately 17 per 100 000 children per year. The incidence of diabetes varies between geographical areas and over the past 30 years there has been a threefold increase in the number of cases of childhood diabetes [2, 3]. This increase is most pronounced in the younger age groups, particularly those under 5 years. A recent European-wide study investigated the increase in type 1 diabetes and noted that the increase was greatest in the most affluent regions, although the reasons for this remain unclear [4].

Type 2 diabetes

Type 2 diabetes is much less common, making up 2–3% of the paediatric diabetic population. The onset tends to be later, at 12–14 years. Children with type 2 diabetes are often obese and have a family history of type 2 diabetes. The prevalence is increasing as the incidence of childhood obesity rises. Type 2 diabetes makes up 30% of adolescent diabetics over 12 years of age [5]. The cause is either a reduced release of insulin or the development of peripheral resistance to the effects of insulin at cellular level. Children with type 2 diabetes are usually managed with either an insulin regimen or metformin. Metformin acts to decrease glucose production in the liver and to increase the sensitivity of peripheral tissues to insulin. In addition, it is important for affected children to make lifestyle changes, such as increasing their activity and controlling their weight.

Maturity onset diabetes of youth

Maturity onset diabetes of youth (MODY) is a newer diagnosis and reflects an inherited form of non-insulin dependent diabetes.

In addition to these three main groups, diabetes in childhood may also be a result of various congenital and acquired conditions (Table 11.1) [6, 7].

Natural history

Control of diabetes in the young usually requires management with subcutaneous insulin injections. There are many different types of insulin regimens in use, each tailored to the individual needs of the child. This means that the anaesthetist is confronted with a wide range of complex treatment regimens. Most advice for the management of diabetic children admitted for

Core Topics in Endocrinology in Anaesthesia and Critical Care, eds. George M. Hall, Jennifer M. Hunter and Mark S. Cooper. Published by Cambridge University Press. © Cambridge University Press 2010.

Table 11.1 Conditions associated with an increased risk of the development of diabetes.

Congenital	Acquired
Prader–Willi syndrome	Steroids
Down's syndrome	Chemotherapy drugs

Klinefelter's syndrome	Pancreatic failure
	   cystic fibrosis
	   haemosiderosis, e.g., in beta-thalassaemia

Turner's syndrome	Cushing's syndrome
Wolfram's syndrome	Autoimmune polyglandular syndrome
Mitochondrial disorders	

surgery comes from locally devised guidelines and protocols. There is little evidence to guide the management of the diabetic child during anaesthesia. In addition, little is written about the specific effects of anaesthetic agents in diabetic children. It is therefore reasonable to apply our usual anaesthetic strategies while taking into account the specific needs of the diabetic child.

Diabetes is a multisystem, chronic condition. As children grow up they may go through a phase of non-compliance with medication regimens and this does become a practical problem. Good management and control of diabetes early is beneficial and decreases or delays the onset of long-term complications, such as diabetic retinopathy, nephropathy (diabetes is responsible for 25% of patients with end-stage renal failure) and cardiovascular disease.

A National Institute for Health and Clinical Excellence (NICE) guideline [8] recommends the routine screening of diabetic children for the following conditions:

- Coeliac disease – at diagnosis and at least every 3 years thereafter until transfer to adult services.
- Annual screening after 12 years of age for:
  - (a) thyroid disease
  - (b) retinopathy
  - (c) microalbuminuria
  - (d) hypertension.

A number of different regimens are used to administer insulin. While the majority of children will be maintained on a combination of long and rapid-acting insulin injections given two or three times a day, there has been increasing use of continuous subcutaneous rapid-acting insulin delivery systems, particularly in adolescents.

Response to surgery

Children undergoing surgery have a metabolic response to the surgery and anaesthesia. This neuroendocrine stress response results in an increase in catecholamines and cortisol with a decrease in insulin secretion from the pancreas. Hepatic glycogenolysis and enhanced gluconeogenesis result in an increase in blood glucose concentration. Early work by Anand et al. recorded these changes even in the youngest neonates. This work suggested that the hormone response to stress may be associated with a poor outcome following surgery [9]. The idea that there may be an increase in morbidity and mortality in the presence of an exaggerated stress response is controversial. However, in adults, this has been linked to many factors including poor wound healing in the presence of hyperglycaemia. In general, the anaesthetist will aim to avoid any episodes of hypoglycaemia and to also avoid excessive hyperglycaemia throughout the perioperative period.

Preoperative preparation

Children presenting for surgery need careful preparation. This may not always be possible, particularly if surgery is urgent. However, surgery in the child with poorly controlled diabetes is associated with increased morbidity. Factors which will affect their blood glucose level include obesity, physical maturity, co-operation with their medication, co-morbidity, length of preoperative fasting, presence of vomiting, and type and length of operation.

The plan for admission starts at the outpatient clinic. The aim is to maintain the child's insulin regimen and dietary requirements as long as possible. It is now considered appropriate for children who have good diabetic control and are undergoing minor surgery to be treated as day-stay patients. If, however, their control is poor, they are systemically unwell, or have difficulty in complying with preoperative arrangements, it is wise to admit the child the evening before surgery.

All children should be cared for in a paediatric environment with staff expert in the care of children. Liaison with a paediatrician or paediatric endocrinologist should be sought when available. Diabetic children are managed with a variety of insulin regimens and the particular selection of insulins used must be taken into account when arranging the perioperative care.

There are various guidelines available focusing on the perioperative management of diabetes [6, 7, 10]. The development of a preoperative preparation programme using an algorithm for a diabetic child's management is thought to improve care and clarify management [7]. The overall aim of management is to avoid the immediate complications of diabetes, particularly hypoglycaemia and ketoacidosis [10].

General points

- For elective surgery, the child should be on a settled diabetic regimen, so that any recent changes have stabilised and a baseline established.
- A child with diabetes who is fasting preoperatively will still need insulin even though they are not eating.
- A child with diabetes cannot fast without the risk of hypoglycaemia.
- Surgery results in insulin resistance.
- Children with diabetes should be scheduled first on the operating list (am or pm) to avoid a long starvation period [10].

Investigations

In addition to investigations required for the proposed surgery, all diabetic children should have their blood glucose, urea, creatinine and electrolytes measured and these should be within the normal range. The routine urine analysis should show no ketonuria.

A regimen based on assessment of the HbA_{1c} values adjusted for age is routinely used in some institutions [7] (Table 11.2). Although this measurement is not part of the routine workup in many institutions, it does give an indication of the effectiveness of the child's diabetic control over the previous 6–8 weeks.

Management of fasting

Prolonged periods of fasting must be avoided and the diabetic child should be scheduled either first or early on the operating list. For minor surgery, day case care may be appropriate and indeed advantageous, so that the child will rapidly return to their usual diet and medication with their carers who will be expert at managing their day-to-day diabetic regimen.

Table 11.2 Ideal ranges for HbA_{1c} values in children.

Age (years)	HbA_{1c} (%)
5	7–9
5–13	6–8.5
> 13	6–8

Diabetic children should be encouraged to take clear fluids until the preoperative fasting time and so minimise the need for preoperative intravenous fluid use, particularly if the surgery is minor or day case care is planned. Use of routine fasting protocols, i.e., six hours for food and two hours for clear fluids, means that the diabetic child who needs to fast can be at potential risk of hypoglycaemia.

Children with diabetes are usually on a combination of insulins, including ultra short-acting, short-acting and long-acting insulin preparations. Although preoperatively they are not eating, the diabetic child still needs insulin, and how this is managed depends on whether the operation is planned for the morning or afternoon and whether the surgery is major or minor.

Day care

Many diabetic patients can be managed on a day care basis. This must be linked to suitable preoperative assessment, the assumption that the child's condition is stable and that the surgery is unlikely to produce systemic upset sufficient to delay feeding and a rapid return to the child's usual insulin regimen (Table 11.3). In some healthcare systems, preoperative admission is prohibitively expensive and so all patients are managed by admission on the day of surgery. Alternatively, some institutions manage all diabetic children by admitting them on the day prior to surgery. This allows an intravenous regimen to be started preoperatively, if needed, and a period of regular blood glucose monitoring so ensuring metabolic stability. This would be routine practice in a diabetic child having major surgery or needing special preparation, such as for major gastrointestinal surgery.

Peroperative management

There is a small risk of delayed gastric emptying but this is of less clinical significance in children than adults. Large studies of routine paediatric practice have shown that aspiration of gastric contents into the lungs is very rare in paediatric practice and seldom causes respiratory complications [11].

Table 11.3 Important factors in planning day care for diabetic children.

Surgical	Anaesthetic	Medical
Minor surgery		Diabetic control has been good preoperatively No other significant co-morbidity
Morning or afternoon surgery		Avoid excessive fasting
Vomiting unlikely	Early return to oral intake, can take postoperative analgesics. Use antiemetics	
Significant pain unlikely	Anaesthesia block possible	
Anticipated early return to normal function		Parental care adequate Good access to postoperative support and advice
Little anticipated bleeding		No risk factors, coagulation defect or thrombocytopenia.

Many centres classify surgical interventions into those that are minor, and hence day care is planned, those that are more major but elective and planning is possible, and lastly those procedures which are emergency and time for preoperative preparation is restricted. The anaesthetist's aim is to ensure that the child does not develop either hypoglycaemia or hyperglycaemia in the perioperative period. Perioperative hyperglycaemia can be associated with excess diuresis and the risk of dehydration, metabolic disturbance and ketoacidosis. On the other hand, the development of hypoglycaemia during an operation is associated with delayed awakening and the risk of cerebral damage.

General principles for the preparation of all diabetic children are:

- Adjust their insulin regimen and diet to ensure they are prepared and that glucose control has been good.
- Blood glucose and urea and electrolytes are checked on admission.
- The urine is tested for ketones and glucose to ensure that ketoacidosis is not present.
- Blood glucose must be regularly monitored throughout admission:
  - (a) hourly preoperatively
  - (b) half-hourly peroperatively
  - (c) hourly postoperatively.
- Blood glucose is usually maintained at > 4 and < 10 mmol l^{-1}.

Minor surgery

This includes body surface surgery, such as hernia repair, orchidopexy, peripheral orthopaedics, dental extractions, radiology scans or short ear, nose and throat (ENT) procedures.

Morning surgery

If the child receives a dose of long-acting insulin in the evenings then only half their usual dose is given on the evening before surgery. No insulin is given on the morning of surgery. Blood glucose is tested hourly: if > 5 and < 11 mmol l^{-1} this is satisfactory. Provided fasting times have not been prolonged there is no need to start an intravenous infusion preoperatively. Following minor surgery, it is anticipated that the child will be eating and drinking soon after completion of surgery and more complicated arrangements will be unnecessary.

Postoperative care

Blood glucose is checked in the recovery area before transfer to the postoperative ward and hourly thereafter; it should be between 5 and 11 mmol l^{-1}. Once the child can eat and drink then they have their usual short-acting insulin with their breakfast. If recovery is satisfactory, discharge home is appropriate. The child will return to their usual routine of supper and their evening insulin is given. Blood glucose must be checked regularly. If, however, the child is not taking adequate oral fluids then an intravenous infusion will be required and the child will need to be admitted until the discharge criteria are met (Table 11.4).

Afternoon surgery

For minor surgery planned for the afternoon, the initial preoperative preparation and investigation is similar in most respects, but the child will have an early breakfast

Table 11.4 Discharge criteria following day case surgery.

The child should be
Awake
Back to their usual level of activity
Eating and drinking
The child should have
Good pain relief
Absence of postoperative nausea or vomiting (PONV)
Good home circumstances, their carer confident and equipped with relevant contact information
Blood glucose that has remained between 5 and 11 mmol l^{-1} since surgery
Urine that is free of ketones

with their usual morning insulin. However, the lunchtime insulin should be omitted. They should continue to have clear fluids until two hours preoperatively. If surgery is delayed, an intravenous infusion may be required. Preoperative blood glucose values must be checked hourly and then management and the therapeutic goals are the same as with children scheduled for a morning operation. Once the child returns to the ward, feeding is encouraged and a short-acting insulin bolus is given when they have their meal. Postoperatively, the glucose is monitored as described above.

Continuous insulin pumps

Children who are managed with a continuous insulin infusion long term should have this set on a basal delivery regimen for the perioperative period. Then, with regular glucose measurement, any deviations from the limits of 4–10 mmol l^{-1} are managed using the regimen below. Postoperatively, the glucose is measured hourly and once the child is tolerating their food then the infusion is continued at its routine rate. Blood glucose is measured hourly for at least four hours postoperatively and the child may be discharged when the continuous insulin infusion is set at the usual rate and they meet the criteria for recovery.

Major surgery

The general principles related to the perioperative management and careful monitoring of glucose and fluids remain the same as for minor surgery. However, major surgery is associated with greater disruption of glycaemic control.

Preoperative preparation

The child will be admitted on the evening before surgery. Blood glucose, full blood count and urea and electrolytes are measured. The child should have a stable insulin regimen and documented good glycaemic control whenever possible. The urine is checked for glucose and ketones. The child will eat and have their usual short-acting insulin while still eating and drinking. If preoperative fasting is to be more than the routine two to three hours or bowel preparation is to be used then an early intravenous infusion must be commenced. If the child is taking long-acting insulin in the evening, then this is given in half the usual dose on the evening before surgery. On the morning of surgery an intravenous infusion with maintenance fluids and insulin is started and the hourly blood glucose result is used to determine the amount of insulin to be given (Table 11.5).

If there is a tendency to hypoglycaemia, additional glucose must be given orally, if tolerated and the child is not fasting, or, alternatively, intravenously using an initial bolus of 2–5 ml kg^{-1} of 10% dextrose.

An alternative is to use glucagon which can be given intravenously, intramuscularly or subcutaneously.

Hyperglycaemia is managed with a glucose and insulin regimen and a sliding scale of insulin (see below).

Intravenous fluids

A diabetic child who requires intravenous therapy during their perioperative care will need a combination of:

1. Maintenance fluids
2. Insulin
3. Replacement fluids
4. Regular and frequent monitoring of blood glucose, urea and electrolytes and haemoglobin concentration to guide fluid and insulin management.

The fluid used for maintenance is not suitable for replacement of perioperative losses, which are replaced with blood, colloid or isotonic crystalloid as

Table 11.5 Intravenous regimen.

Maintenance fluids	
Glucose 5% and saline 0.45% with potassium chloride 10 mmol per 500 ml	
Volume required	
100 ml kg^{-1} day^{-1} (4 ml kg^{-1} h^{-1}) for the first 10 kg body weight	
50 ml kg^{-1} day^{-1} (2 ml kg^{-1} h^{-1}) for the second 10 kg	
25 ml kg^{-1} day^{-1} (1 ml kg^{-1} h^{-1}) for each kilogram above 20 kg	
With:	
A titrated sliding scale of insulin using	
50 ml syringe with 1 U soluble insulin per ml (e.g., 50 ml 0.9% saline with 50 U soluble insulin)	
Volume required	
Blood glucose concentration (mmol l^{-1})	**Insulin dose infusion rate (U kg^{-1} h^{-1})**
4.0–6.9	0.02
7.0–8.9	0.03
9–12	0.04
> 12	0.05
The delivery of insulin is adjusted to result in a glucose level between 5 and 11 mmol l^{-1}. The rate of infusion is 0.02–0.05 U insulin kg^{-1} h^{-1} adjusted using the sliding scale	
The glucose is checked at least half hourly during surgery and hourly before and after surgery	

From the North Central London Paediatric Diabetic Network [10].

required. During surgery there may be considerable fluctuations in the blood glucose. The stress response to surgery and the fluid shifts will necessitate careful insulin control and this is best achieved with a sliding scale. There are many different regimens for administering glucose and insulin perioperatively. However, the principles are similar and the aim is for close glucose control [6, 7].

If the glucose falls below 4 mmol^{-1}, recommendations for treatment vary. Some endocrinologists believe it is important not to completely stop the insulin infusion, which is continued at 0.01 U per kilogram insulin per hour while also increasing the amount of glucose either by giving a bolus or by increasing the infusion rate. Others recommend stopping the insulin if the blood glucose decreases to 3 mmol l^{-1} and managing the hypoglycaemia with glucose, as before [6].

This combination of maintenance fluid and a sliding scale of insulin is continued postoperatively guided by hourly glucose values and a measurement of the urea and electrolytes immediately postoperatively and then four to six hourly depending on the surgical losses and clinical situation. Nasogastric losses and blood loss are managed by replacement with saline 0.9% and blood products respectively. Once the child can take food and fluids orally then they can be gradually restarted on

their usual insulin regimen with frequent biochemical assessment.

Most diabetic children will not need any additional monitoring apart from that indicated for anaesthesia for the particular surgery. An arterial line will be useful in major cases for cardiovascular monitoring and regular blood sampling for arterial blood gases, haemoglobin and blood glucose.

Emergency surgery in the diabetic child

When diabetic children present for urgent surgery their diabetic control is frequently disrupted by the illness. Routine urinalysis and tests of renal function should be checked. Wherever possible, glucose and electrolyte balance should be corrected preoperatively. Diabetic ketoacidosis (DKA) is associated with increased morbidity and mortality when emergency surgery is required (Chapter 16).

Newly diagnosed diabetes may present as an acute illness in a child. For example, DKA can present as abdominal pain with the signs of an acute abdomen and then the paediatric team must organise the urgent management of the DKA as this is a high-risk situation requiring specialist care. If DKA is present, surgery should be postponed if possible. This is because the physiological changes are difficult to manage even in expert hands and the outcome is often poor [12]. Cerebral oedema is one of the commonest causes of diabetes-related death in children. Development of cerebral oedema during an episode of DKA is associated with a mortality of 24% [13]. To try and avoid it, the metabolic changes of DKA must be corrected slowly and with careful control in the paediatric intensive care unit or a high dependency setting. Fluid resuscitation and correction of the hyperglycaemia will take more than 36 hours. Surgery should ideally be postponed until this has been achieved.

Additional postoperative issues

Antiemetics

Early return to a normal diet and avoidance of vomiting is particularly important in the diabetic child. Postoperative nausea and vomiting (PONV) becomes more important as children get older [14]. There are a number of factors that affect the frequency and severity of PONV. These include a past history of PONV, prolonged surgery, squint surgery, adenotonsillectomy and gastrointestinal surgery as well as the use of volatile agents [15]. Good practice guidelines have been explored for the management of PONV in children. Ondansetron 0.1 mg kg^{-1} has been shown to be effective given at any time perioperatively [16]. Dexamethasone 0.15 mg kg^{-1} is particularly of use in preventing PONV following adenotonsillectomy. There have been concerns that in adults a single dose of dexamethasone may result in increased blood glucose in type 2 diabetic patients [17]. However, this has not been clearly established and the increase in glucose peroperatively is likely to be multifactorial: there is no evidence of the same phenomenon in children.

Analgesia

Good multimodal analgesia is indicated and there are no particular contraindications to all common pain management strategies.

Summary

The management of diabetes in children is complex and there are a wide variety of insulin and non-insulin regimens available. The overall goal of perioperative management is to avoid both hypoglycaemia and hyperglycaemia with ketoacidosis. It is important that local guidelines are developed and followed. If possible, paediatricians with a special interest in diabetes or endocrinologists should be involved in the perioperative care of these patients. If local guidelines are not available the authors suggest the protocol adopted by the North Central London Paediatric Diabetic Network [10].

References

1 The Healthcare Commission. *National Diabetes Audit*. London, Office for Official Statistics, 2004.

2 Gardner SG, Bingley PJ, Sawtell PA, Weeks S, Gale EA. Rising incidence of insulin dependent diabetes in children aged under 5 years in the Oxford region: time trend analysis. The Bart's-Oxford Study Group. *BMJ* 1997; **315**: 713–17.

3 Onkamo P, Vaananen S, Karvonen M, Tuomilehto J. Worldwide increase in incidence of type I diabetes – the analysis of the data on published incidence trends. *Diabetologia* 1999; **42**: 1395–403.

4 Harjutsalo V, Sjoberg L, Tuomilehto J. Time trends in the incidence of type 1 diabetes in Finnish children: a cohort study. *Lancet* 2008; **371**: 1777–82.

5 Fagot-Campagna A, Saaddine JB, Flegal KM, Beckles GL. Diabetes, impaired fasting glucose, and elevated HbA$_{1c}$ in US adolescents: the Third National Health and Nutrition Examination Survey. *Diabetes Care* 2001; **24**: 834–7.

6 Chadwick V, Wilkinson KA. Diabetes mellitus and the pediatric anesthetist. *Paediatr Anaesth* 2004; **14**: 716–23.

7 Rhodes ET, Ferrari LR, Wolfsdorf JI. Perioperative management of pediatric surgical patients with diabetes mellitus. *Anesth Analg* 2005; **101**: 986–99.

8 National Institute for Health and Clinical Excellence (NICE). *NICE and Diabetes: A Summary of Relevant Guidelines*. London, NICE, 2006.

9 Anand KJ, Sippell WG, Aynsley-Green A. Randomised trial of fentanyl anaesthesia in preterm babies undergoing surgery: effects on the stress response. *Lancet* 1987; **1**: 62–6.

10 North Central London Paediatric Diabetic Network. Diabetic children undergoing surgery. http://www.ich.ucl.ac.uk/clinical_information/clinical_guidelines/cmg_guideline_00000, accessed 31 July 2007

11 Flick RP, Schears GJ, Warner MA. Aspiration in pediatric anesthesia: is there a higher incidence compared with adults? *Curr Opin Anaesthesiol* 2002; **15**: 323–7.

12 Basu A, Close CF, Jenkins D, Krentz AJ, Nattrass M, Wright AD. Persisting mortality in diabetic ketoacidosis. *Diabet Med* 1993; **10**: 282–4.

13 Edge JA, Hawkins MM, Winter DL, Dunger DB. The risk and outcome of cerebral oedema developing during diabetic ketoacidosis. *Arch Dis Child* 2001; **85**: 16–22.

14 Eberhart LH, Geldner G, Kranke P, et al. The development and validation of a risk score to predict the probability of postoperative vomiting in pediatric patients. *Anesth Analg* 2004; **99**: 1630–7.

15 Sneyd JR, Carr A, Byrom WD, Bilski AJ. A meta-analysis of nausea and vomiting following maintenance of anaesthesia with propofol or inhalational agents. *Eur J Anaesthesiol* 1998; **15**: 433–45.

16 Madan R, Perumal T, Subramaniam K, Shende D, Sadhasivam S, Garg S. Effect of timing of ondansetron administration on incidence of postoperative vomiting in paediatric strabismus surgery. *Anaesth Intensive Care* 2000; **28**: 27–30.

17 Hans P, Vanthuyne A, Dewandre PY, Brichant JF, Bonhomme V. Blood glucose concentration profile after 10 mg dexamethasone in non-diabetic and type 2 diabetic patients undergoing abdominal surgery. *Br J Anaesth* 2006; **97**: 164–70.

Chapter 12

Management of diabetes in ambulatory surgery

Heidi J. Robertshaw

The number of cases performed in ambulatory surgical (day case) units is continuing to increase. This is due to economic pressures, patient expectation and improvement in surgical and anaesthetic techniques [1]. This drive for expansion in ambulatory surgery has become, in part, politically driven. In the UK, the National Health Service (NHS) plan published in 2000 [2] set an ambitious target of 75% for elective admissions that should be carried out as day cases. Furthermore, the Healthcare Commission in the UK found that at least an extra 74 000 patients each year could be treated as day cases rather than admitted as inpatients, if the least efficient units started employing the practices of the best [3]. The economic benefits of this are obvious and should encourage hospitals to expand their ambulatory surgery centres to accommodate this workload. As diabetes mellitus is also increasing in frequency, currently estimated by the International Diabetes Federation to be 246 million adults worldwide and expected to rise to 380 million by 2025 [4], anaesthetists will face a greater proportion of diabetic patients presenting for day case procedures.

Ambulatory anaesthesia tends to be restricted to mainly healthy individuals undergoing a relatively small list of procedures and is well suited to the application of standard practice protocols as much of the workload is highly predictable [5]. Assessment of patients for day case treatment is frequently done by nurses and, generally, nursing staff are much better at complying with protocols than physicians, who can be unwilling to surrender autonomy. This makes day case procedures ideally suited to quality management methodologies that include assessment, planned intervention and alteration of existing processes, with constant monitoring of outcomes [5]. However, outcomes are also dependent on surgical and anaesthetic skills, technique and surgical setting and so, while guidance can be published based on current research, day case

units still need to develop individual protocols that suit their circumstances.

Children with diabetes mellitus are often excluded from day case management. This is mainly due to difficulty with glycaemic control during the perioperative period, especially during the time of preoperative fasting. With the expansion in the numbers of children with diabetes mellitus in the UK, the general exclusion of children with diabetes for ambulatory surgical procedures will require review.

Preoperative management

Optimal preoperative preparation of outpatients makes ambulatory surgery both safer and more acceptable for patients and staff [6]. The preparation aims to reduce risks inherent in ambulatory surgery, improve patient outcome and make the experience of undergoing surgery more pleasant for patients and their families. The benefits of ambulatory surgery for both the patient and the healthcare provider are lost if the patient requires unplanned admission to hospital or returns to hospital from home following discharge from the day case unit. Little evidence exists on what conditions should be considered predictors of such adverse outcomes after day case surgery but it is generally accepted that non-compensated, poorly-stabilised cardiac and respiratory patients, obstructive sleep apnoea, age > 85 years and preterm infants are at high risk of complications and should not generally be conducted as day cases. In addition, unplanned admission or return to hospital is more frequent after ear, nose and throat (ENT) and urology day procedures.

When assessing diabetic patients for ambulatory procedures, consideration must be given to the patient's understanding of their disease and its management, particularly hypoglycaemia and blood glucose measurement at home. A diabetic patient with a history of repeated hypoglycaemic episodes or

Core Topics in Endocrinology in Anaesthesia and Critical Care, eds. George M. Hall, Jennifer M. Hunter and Mark S. Cooper. Published by Cambridge University Press. © Cambridge University Press 2010.

Table 12.1 Exclusion criteria for diabetic patients as suitable for ambulatory surgery.

Absolute	Repeated hypoglycaemic episodes
	Recurrent hospital admissions with diabetic complications
Relative	Random blood glucose > 13 mmol l⁻¹

recurrent admission to hospital with diabetic complications would generally be unsuitable for ambulatory surgery. Suggested exclusion criteria for diabetic patients as being suitable for ambulatory surgery are given in Table 12.1.

For day case diabetic patients, preoperative investigations should include HbA_{1c} to assess the quality of long-term glycaemic control. An HbA_{1c} greater than 9% indicates poor glycaemic control and might suggest a review of diabetic management before surgery [7]. Random blood glucose concentration does not give an indication of long-term blood glucose control by the patient but it is useful on the day of surgery to help guide perioperative management. A diabetic patient presenting for surgery with a random blood glucose greater than 13 mmol l⁻¹ should be examined for a treatable cause of their hyperglycaemia and the anaesthetist should consider postponing their surgery until normoglycaemia is achieved. However, this recommendation is based on work from critically ill patients which has shown that hyperglycaemia has a detrimental effect on the immune system [8], and so the clinical importance of hyperglycaemia in day surgery patients is not validated and remains laboratory-based.

Anaesthetists will need to become familiar with the pharmacology of the diabetic agents, such as new rapid (insulin glulisine, insulin lispro, insulin aspart) and longer acting (insulin detemir, insulin glargine) insulins, which have therapeutic properties designed to mimic more closely the normal physiological release of insulin. Rapidly acting insulins have an onset time of less than 15 minutes (as a result of recombinant DNA technology with minor amino acid changes that enable these compounds to dissociate rapidly after subcutaneous injection). With a peak activity at one to two hours and a total duration of action of three to four hours, these pharmacokinetic profiles have encouraged the development of insulin pump technology to achieve better serum glucose control with a lower risk of hypoglycaemia. Longer acting insulins (insulin glargine, insulin detemir) have also been developed as a result of amino acid changes that decrease their solubility at physiological pH. Following subcutaneous

injection, insulin glargine precipitates in subcutaneous tissues so delaying absorption and prolonging its action. Insulin glargine has an onset of action of 2–4 hours with no peak and a duration of action of 20–24 hours. While a detailed discussion of these new agents is outside the scope of this chapter (Chapter 8), a policy will need to be developed for patients taking these drugs who present for day case procedures: longer acting insulins should be stopped preoperatively to avoid the risk of undetected intraoperative hypoglycaemia.

Diabetic patients frequently have ischaemic heart disease and other vascular complications and will be prescribed platelet inhibitors and other drug therapies which reduce long-term cardiovascular risk. Ambulatory surgery units should develop a common position, expressed as written guidelines, for patients scheduled for day case surgery who are taking aspirin and/or clopidogrel. It is suggested that aspirin is continued in all cases and possibly clopidogrel as well [9], as day case procedures represent a low bleeding risk. High-risk patients (unstable angina, drug-eluting coronary stents) should not be done as day case procedures [10]. The American College of Cardiology/American Heart Association (ACC/AHA) 2006 Guideline Update on Perioperative Cardiovascular Evaluation for Noncardiac Surgery [11] has a class I recommendation for the continuation of beta-blockers in the perioperative period for patients already receiving them. This guideline suggested that there was insufficient evidence to make any recommendations regarding the introduction of beta-blockers in patients undergoing low-risk surgery (where the probability of a perioperative myocardial infarction is less than 1%), which would include most ambulatory surgery. The recently published POISE (Perioperative Ischemic Evaluation) trial and a meta-analysis of outcome in patients given perioperative beta-blockers before major surgery add to the weight of evidence against starting beta blockade preoperatively solely to reduce risk [12, 13].

Preoperative anaesthetic assessment of diabetic patients should aim to identify any signs and symptoms of delayed gastric emptying to allow the anaesthetic technique to be planned appropriately. However, there is at present no simple mechanism of identifying patients who have an enhanced risk of delayed gastric emptying, so all diabetics should be treated with caution as a delay in gastric emptying has been estimated to be present in as many as 35–50% of those with long-standing type 1 and type 2 diabetes [14]. For most patients this delay is modest in magnitude and there are insufficient data to clarify the clinical relevance for elective surgery and whether fasting guidelines for diabetic patients should be modified from those used for non-diabetic patients.

The rate of gastric emptying in patients with diabetes as a determinant of postprandial glucose control has been investigated in detail [15]. The results showed that gastric emptying of solids in particular, but also of liquids, was frequently delayed in long-standing type 1 and type 2 diabetics. This work also indicated that an acute change in blood glucose concentration can affect gastric emptying, with insulin-induced hypoglycaemia accelerating gastric emptying and marked delays in gastric emptying in type 1 diabetics found with blood glucose concentrations above 15 mmol l^{-1}. This work supports the maintenance of normoglycaemia throughout the perioperative period.

Postoperative insulin resistance increases with the complexity of surgery and has been demonstrated to occur after even minor to moderate surgery [16]. Preoperative fasting contributes to insulin resistance [17] and so adds to perioperative metabolic upset. Recent clinical studies have demonstrated that a preoperative carbohydrate drink may inhibit the postoperative endocrine catabolic responses and reduce insulin resistance [16]. A dose of 800 ml of a carbohydrate-rich beverage (100 g carbohydrates) on the evening before surgery and 400 ml given up to 2 hours before operation has been shown to be safe and to reduce postoperative insulin resistance by about 50% in major colorectal surgery and orthopaedic surgery [16]. This study also demonstrated that well-controlled type 2 diabetics who had an oral carbohydrate-rich drink along with their regular morning medication had gastric emptying similar to healthy controls and a glucose value that had returned to pre-drink levels after three hours. In a recent randomised study involving ASA III–IV patients, including patients with type 2 diabetes mellitus, giving the carbohydrate drink preoperatively reduced inotrope requirements after cardiopulmonary bypass [18]. In orthopaedic surgery, avoiding preoperative fasting was associated with a reduction in immune suppression (as demonstrated by monocyte function) [19], suggesting that maintaining better insulin sensitivity with carbohydrate administration preoperatively is associated with improved immune function postoperatively. However, as yet, evidence for the adoption of this practice in day case surgical patients is lacking.

With further evidence specifically in ambulatory surgical patients, there may be a case for altering preoperative fasting guidelines for diabetics to include clear fluids, optimised glycaemic control and administration of carbohydrate-rich drinks up to two hours preoperatively.

Peroperative management

Advances in day case anaesthesia include the use of anaesthetic agents of short duration and increasing use of regional anaesthetic techniques. Day case procedures are associated with relatively minor surgical trauma and so discharge frequently depends on the speed of recovery from anaesthesia [20]. There are three widely held key principles for the management of diabetic patients:

(1) Diabetic medication omitted on morning of surgery.
(2) Procedure scheduled as early on the list as possible.
(3) Aim to return to usual diet and medication as soon as possible.

Regional techniques whether by epidural, spinal, peripheral nerve blocks or field block techniques provide advantages in diabetic patients as there is some evidence that they provide analgesia without sedation with earlier return to oral intake and earlier discharge [20]. It has been postulated that regional techniques may improve outcome, minimise surgical stress, reduce postoperative pain and allow rapid postoperative recovery [21, 22]. Disappointingly, none of these translate into shorter day surgery unit time and a recent meta-analysis suggested that regional anaesthesia significantly delays home discharge compared with general anaesthesia [23]. Central neuraxial block did not reduce the incidence of nausea and increased the length of stay in the ambulatory unit time by 35 minutes. Peripheral nerve blockade did decrease the incidence of nausea but did not affect the total time spent in the ambulatory unit. Current opinion supports a policy that patients taking clopidogrel and, in particular, those receiving dual therapy with aspirin should not undergo regional anaesthesia.

For patients undergoing general anaesthesia, except for type 2 diabetics having minor surgery, the standard glycaemic management involves administration of intravenous glucose with potassium chloride and a variable insulin infusion regimen. This can be associated with the development of hyponatraemia due to the administration of free water as intravenous glucose [24]. In theory, the best option in the perioperative

Table 12.2 Perioperative glycaemic control regimens for ambulatory surgical patients with diabetes mellitus.

	Type 1 diabetes	Type 2 diabetes
Minor surgical procedure (less than 1-h duration)	Variable intravenous insulin regimen Intravenous glucose and potassium chloride containing fluid	Omit all oral hypoglycaemic agents the morning of surgery
Moderate surgical procedure	Variable intravenous insulin regimen Intravenous glucose and potassium chloride containing fluid	Omit long-acting hypoglycaemic agents the night before surgery Omit all oral hypoglycaemic agents the morning of surgery Variable intravenous insulin regimen Intravenous glucose and potassium chloride containing fluid

period is 5% glucose in 0.45% sodium chloride solution with potassium chloride 20 mmol l⁻¹ but this is not a commercially available fluid in the UK [25]. If a type 2 diabetic is to undergo a minor procedure lasting less than one hour as a day case and their glycaemic control is satisfactory, they may be safely monitored and re-established on their usual diabetic regimen as soon as possible following completion of surgery. Appropriate perioperative glycaemic regimens for ambulatory surgical patients with diabetes mellitus are summarised in Table 12.2.

A recent review by Holte and Kehlet examined the effects of various fluid replacement regimens on postoperative outcomes following minor/moderate surgery [26]. Their conclusion was that compensating for the dehydration induced by preoperative fasting by at least one litre of intravenous fluids perioperatively generally reduced postoperative drowsiness and dizziness. Furthermore, for laparoscopic procedures, the intravenous infusion of one to three litres led to a reduction in postoperative nausea and vomiting (PONV) [26]. So, current evidence shows that all ambulatory patients, not only those with diabetes mellitus, should receive adequate intraoperative intravenous hydration.

There are no studies in the literature specifically evaluating the effect of tight glycaemic control in general surgical patients, even less so in ambulatory surgical populations [27]. The benefits of intensive glucose management reported in studies of critically ill patients or those recovering from major surgery do not necessarily extend to general surgical patients [28, 29]. Moreover, the appropriate blood glucose concentration perioperatively is not clear.

Propofol has been demonstrated to be associated with less PONV in adult patients [30]. This reduction is significant only in the first 12 hours postoperatively and this reduction has not altered admission rates [31, 32]. Total intravenous anaesthesia (TIVA) with propofol reduces the incidence of PONV and is now clearly recommended for the prevention of PONV in high-risk patients [33]. Avoidance of nitrous oxide in at risk patients may also reduce PONV [34].

The majority of day surgery procedures do not require muscle relaxation. However, the possibility of delayed gastric emptying in patients with diabetes mellitus may encourage the use of tracheal intubation for protection of the airway against the risk of aspiration of gastric contents particularly if there are additional risk factors (such as obesity). The ideal neuromuscular blocking agent for day surgery is not yet available and all drugs have some drawbacks. Suxamethonium is associated with myalgia (which may be severe in outpatients). Mivacurium, while a short-acting agent, has the disadvantages of a long onset time and unwanted cardiovascular effects. Atracurium is associated with histamine release and, although cisatracurium has less histamine release, it does have a prolonged onset time. Steroidal agents, such as vecuronium, have recovery profiles modified by hepatic insufficiency and extreme age. Suxamethonium (plus diclofenac or aspirin postoperatively to reduce myalgia) has been recommended for diabetic patients requiring a rapid sequence induction. For those requiring muscle relaxation, but who are at low risk of aspiration, mivacurium or rocuronium (rather than vecuronium, atracurium or cisatracurium) may be the best choices [35]. The main features of general anaesthesia for diabetic patients undergoing ambulatory surgery are listed in Table 12.3.

Sugammadex is a synthetic gamma cyclodextrin that combines with rocuronium irreversibly, allowing rapid reversal of neuromuscular blockade [36]. This may permit the safer use of rocuronium (or vecuronium) for patients undergoing rapid induction therefore avoiding the need for suxamethonium.

Table 12.3 Main features of general anaesthetic technique for diabetic ambulatory surgery patients.

Regular blood glucose monitoring (at least hourly) until return to normal oral intake
Adequate intravenous hydration (at least one litre of appropriate fluid)
Avoidance of nitrous oxide during induction and maintenance of anaesthesia
Suxamethonium or rocuronium if muscle relaxation is required and risk of aspiration
Prophylactic use of ondansetron for prevention of postoperative nausea and vomiting
Re-establishment of normal oral intake as soon as possible postoperatively

Postoperative management

Control of postoperative nausea and vomiting is important in all day surgery patients as it strongly affects patient satisfaction and contributes to prolonged hospital stay [37]. It is of particular importance in patients with diabetes mellitus as PONV will delay return to normal dietary intake and resumption of normal antidiabetic medication. Postoperative nausea and vomiting occurs in approximately 30% of all ambulatory surgical patients with only 36% of patients not experiencing nausea or vomiting before discharge from hospital [38].

Procedure-specific prophylactic management of PONV should be undertaken in all day case patients, but particularly in diabetics. Droperidol, ondansetron and dexamethasone are equally effective in the prevention of PONV in the high-risk patient (patients with four of following: female sex, previous history of PONV or motion sickness, non-smoker and use of perioperative opioids) [39]. Dexamethasone should be generally avoided in diabetics as its administration is associated with an enhanced glycaemic response to surgery. Some ambulatory surgical centres deem that, because of the greater costs of ondansetron, it should be used for the treatment rather than the prevention of PONV [40]. Preventive use of ondansetron at a dose of 4 mg has been shown to reduce post-discharge nausea and vomiting [41] and may be cost-effective in diabetic patients.

Despite the widespread belief that anticholinesterase drugs may be emetic [42], there is no convincing clinical evidence that omitting pharmacological reversal at the end of anaesthesia decreases the risk of PONV [43]. Residual paralysis in the postoperative period is potentially very harmful with hypoventilation, attenuation of the ventilatory response to hypoxia, impaired cough, compromised laryngeal and pharyngeal functions and increased incidence of pulmonary complications [44]. The risks of residual paralysis are amplified in a diabetic patient population because of the likelihood of delayed gastric emptying and these risks outweigh any putative reduction in PONV by the avoidance of anticholinesterase drugs.

Cardiovascular events remain the most common serious intraoperative and postoperative adverse events, occurring at an incidence of 2% during ambulatory surgery [38]. They occur most frequently in patients with pre-existing cardiovascular disease, diabetes and the elderly [45]. The peak incidence of postoperative myocardial infarction in non-cardiac surgery is early in the postoperative period with the highest risk in patients with diabetes mellitus and cardiac disease [46]. Respiratory complications are most likely to occur in patients who are smokers, who are obese and in those with asthma [37]. Diabetes mellitus alone is not a predictor of increased postoperative respiratory complications.

Effective postoperative analgesia is important in diabetic patients as it is in any patient undergoing ambulatory surgical procedures. Paracetamol is useful for patients with mild postoperative pain [47], as well as in combination with codeine to reduce moderate to severe postoperative pain [48]. Furthermore, in patients with no contraindications, non-steroidal anti-inflammatory drugs (NSAIDs), such as ibuprofen or diclofenac when combined with paracetamol, may confer additional analgesic efficacy compared with paracetamol alone [49]. There is conflicting evidence whether the use of NSAIDs increases the risk of bleeding following surgery requiring return to theatre. It should be routine practice to ensure any diabetic patient receiving a NSAID has normal renal function and the NSAID is prescribed for only a short duration postoperatively. The side effects of opioids, in particular PONV, may limit their usefulness in the ambulatory surgical patients.

There are surprisingly few data on the incidence of venous thromboembolism (VTE) in patients undergoing day surgery. The assumption is that earlier resumption of normal physical activities and fewer patient risk factors for VTE means that VTE is less of a problem in day case patients. However, as the scope of patients and procedures for day case expands, it is worth considering that a history of VTE, thrombophilias, cancer, varicose veins, oral contraceptives, obesity and increasing age are all significant risk factors for postoperative VTE [50]. Diabetic patients, particularly type 2, tend to be overweight and so are at higher risk of thromboembolism. Thromboprophylaxis with low molecular weight heparin (LMWH) should be started in every day surgery patient with two or more risk factors (optimal time to start treatment is 6 hours postoperatively and the duration of treatment should be 7–10 days, dose of dalteparin 5000 IU or enoxaparin 40 mg once a day). Compression stockings should be used in every patient with one or more risk factors.

Conclusions

Patients with diabetes mellitus will present in increasing numbers for ambulatory surgical procedures requiring anaesthesia. Such cases require preoperative assessment that includes confirmation of adequate patient understanding of their disease and long-term glucose control. While diabetic patients have a high incidence of delayed gastric emptying which may complicate general anaesthesia, regional anaesthetic techniques have failed consistently to demonstrate any advantage in terms of shorter duration of hospital stay or reduction in complications. The basic principles for day case procedures of good analgesia, adequate fluid administration and the avoidance of postoperative nausea and vomiting hold for diabetic patients. Such practices ensure prompt resumption of oral intake and return to normal antidiabetic medication which enables patients with diabetes mellitus to be treated successfully on an ambulatory basis.

References

1. Bettelli G. High risk patients in day surgery. *Minerva Anestesiol* 2009; **75**: 259–68.

2. Department of Health. The NHS Plan. http://www.dh.gov.uk/PublicationsAndStatistics/Publications/PublicationsPolicyAndGuidance/PublicationPolicyAndGuidanceArticle/fs/en?CONTENT_ID=4002960&chk=07GL5R, accessed 31 December, 2008

3. Healthcare Commission. Acute hospital portfolio review, day surgery, July 2005. http://www.healthcarecommission.org.uk/_db/_documents/04018390.pdf, accessed 31 December, 2008

4. Editorial. The global challenge of diabetes. *Lancet* 2008; **371**: 1723.

5. Merrill D. Management of outcomes in the ambulatory surgery center: the role of standard work

6. White PF, Eng M. Fast-track anesthetic techniques for ambulatory surgery. *Curr Opin Anaesthesiol* 2007; **20**: 545–57.

7. European Diabetes Policy Group. A desktop guide to type 2 diabetes mellitus. *Diabet Med* 1999; **16**: 716–30.

8. Turina M, Fry DE, Polk HC. Acute hyperglycaemia and the innate immune system: clinical, cellular and molecular aspects. *Crit Care Med* 2005; **33**: 1624–33.

9. Llau JV, De Andres J, Gomar C, et al. Anticlotting drugs and regional anaesthetic and analgesia techniques: comparative update of the safety recommendations. *Eur J Anaesthesiol* 2007; **24**: 387–98.

10. Servin F. Low dose aspirin and clopidogrel: how to act in patients scheduled for day surgery. *Curr Opin Anaesthesiol* 2007; **20**: 531–4.

11. Fleisher LA, Beckman JA, Brown KA, et al. ACC/AHA 2006 guideline update on perioperative cardiovascular evaluation for noncardiac surgery: focused update on perioperative beta-blocker therapy: a report of the American College of Cardiology/American Heart Association Task Force on Practice Guidelines. *Circulation* 2006; **113**: 2662–74.

12. POISE Study Group, Devereaux PJ, Yang H, Yusuf S, et al. Effects of extended-release metoprolol succinate in patients undergoing non-cardiac surgery (POISE trial): a randomised controlled trial. *Lancet* 2008; **371**: 1839–47.

13. Bungalore S, Wettersley J, Pranesh S, et al. Perioperative beta blockers in patients having non-cardiac surgery: a meta-analysis. *Lancet* 2008; **372**: 1962–76.

14. Soreide E, Ljungqvist O. Modern preoperative fasting guidelines: a summary of the present recommendations and remaining questions. *Best Pract Res Clin Anaesthesiol* 2006; **20**: 483–91.

15. Horowitz M, O'Donovan D, Jones KL, et al. Gastric emptying in diabetes: clinical significance and treatment. *Diabet Med* 2002; **19**: 177–94.

16. Nygren J. The metabolic effect of fasting and surgery. *Best Pract Res Clin Anaesthesiol* 2006; **20**: 429–38.

17. Svanfeldt M, Thorell A, Hausel J, et al. Effect of 'preoperative' oral carbohydrate treatment in insulin action: a randomised cross-over unblinded study in healthy subjects. *Clin Nutr* 2005; **24**: 815–21.

18. Breuer JP, von Dossow V, van Heymann C, et al. Preoperative oral carbohydrate administration to ASA III–IV patients undergoing elective cardiac surgery. *Anesth Analg* 2006; **103**: 1099–108.

and evidence-based medicine. *Curr Opin Anaesthesiol* 2008; **21**: 1–5.

19. Melis GC, van Leeuwen PA, von Blomberg-van der Flier BM, et al. A carbohydrate-rich beverage prior to surgery prevents surgery-induced immunodepression: a randomized, controlled, clinical trial. *JPEN J Parenter Enteral Nutr* 2006; **30**: 21–6.

20. Rawal N. Analgesia for day-case surgery. *Br J Anaesth* 2001; **87**: 73–87.

21. Kehlet H, White P. Optimizing anesthesia for inguinal herniorraphy: general, regional or local anesthesia? *Anesth Analg* 2001; **93**: 1367–9.

22. Hadzic A, Kerimoglu B, Loreio D, et al. Paravertebral blocks provide superior same-day recovery over general anaesthesia for patients undergoing inguinal hernia repair. *Anesth Analg* 2006; **102**: 1076–81.

23. Liu SS, Strodbeck WM, Richman JM, Wu CL. A comparison of regional versus general anesthesia for ambulatory anesthesia: a meta-analysis of randomized controlled trials. *Anesth Analg* 2005; **101**: 1634–42.

24. Moritz ML, Ayus JC. Hospital-acquired hyponatraemia – why are hypotonic parenteral fluids still being used? *Nat Clin Pract Nephrol* 2007; **3**: 374–82.

25. Simpson AK, Levy N, Hall GM. Peri-operative iv fluids in diabetic patients – don't forget the salt. *Anaesthesia* 2008; **63**: 1043–5.

26. Holte K, Kehlet H. Fluid therapy and surgical outcomes in elective surgery: a need for reassessment in fast-track surgery. *J Am Coll Surg* 2006; **202**: 971–89.

27. Krinsley J. Perioperative glucose control. *Curr Opin Anaesthesiol* 2006; **19**: 111–16.

28. Van den Berghe G, Wouters P, Weekers F, et al. Intensive insulin therapy in the critically ill patients. *N Engl J Med* 2001; **345**: 1359–67.

29. Krinsley JS. Effect of an intensive glucose management protocol on the mortality of critically ill adult patients. *Mayo Clin Proc* 2004; **79**: 992–1000.

30. Eriksson H, Korttila K. Recovery profile after desflurane with or without ondansetron compared with propofol in patients undergoing outpatient gynaecological laparoscopy. *Anesth Analg* 1996; **82**: 533–8.

31. Gurkan Y, Kilickan L, Toker T. Propofol-nitrous oxide versus sevoflurane-nitrous oxide for strabismus surgery in children. *Paediatr Anaesth* 1999; **9**: 495–9.

32. Reimer EJ, Montgomery CJ, Bevan JC, et al. Propofol anaesthesia reduces early post-operative emesis after paediatric strabismus surgery. *Can J Anaesth* 1993; **40**: 927–33.

33. Visser K, Hassink EA, Bonsel GJ, et al. Randomized controlled trial of total intravenous anesthesia with propofol versus inhalation anesthesia with isoflurane-nitrous oxide: postoperative nausea with vomiting and economic analysis. *Anesthesiology* 2001; **95**: 616–26.

34. Baum JA. The carrier gas in anaesthesia: nitrous oxide/oxygen, medical air/oxygen and pure oxygen. *Curr Opin Anaestheisol* 2004; **17**: 513–16.

35. Bettelli G. Which muscle relaxants should be used in day surgery and when. *Curr Opin Anaesthesiol* 2006; **19**: 600–5.

36. De Boer HD, Driessen JJ, Marcus MA, et al. Reversal of rocuronium-induced (1.2 mg/kg) profound neuromuscular block by sugammadex: a multicenter, dose-finding and safety study. *Anesthesiology* 2007; **107**: 239–44.

37. Shnaider I, Chung F. Outcomes in day surgery. *Curr Opin Anaesthesiol* 2006; **19**: 622–9.

38. Chung F, Meizei G. Adverse outcomes in ambulatory anesthesia. *Can J Anaesth* 1999; **46**: R18–R26.

39. Apfel CC, Korttila K, Abdalla M, et al. IMPACT Investigators. A factorial trial of six interventions for the prevention of postoperative nausea and vomiting. *N Engl J Med* 2004; **350**: 2441–51.

40. Hill RP, Lubarsky DA, Phillips-Bute B, et al. Cost-effectiveness of prophylactic antiemetic therapy with ondansetron, droperidol or placebo. *Anesthesiology* 2000; **92**: 958–67.

41. Gupta A, Wu CL, Elkassabany N, et al. Does the routine prophylactic use of antiemetics affect the incidence of postdischarge nausea and vomiting following ambulatory surgery? A systematic review of randomized controlled trials. *Anesthesiology* 2003; **99**: 488–95.

42. Rabey PG, Smith G. Anaesthetic factors contributing to postoperative nausea and vomiting. *Br J Anaesth* 1992; **69** Suppl 1: 40S–45S.

43. Tramer MR, Fuchs-Buder T. Omitting antagonism of neuromuscular block: effect on postoperative nausea and vomiting and risk of residual paralysis. A systematic review. *Br J Anaesth* 1999; **82**: 379–86.

44. Fuchs-Buder T, Mencke T. Use of reversal agents in day care procedures (with special reference to postoperative nausea and vomiting). *Eur J Anaesthesiol* 2001; **18** Suppl 23: 53–9.

45. Chung F, Meizei G, Tong D. Adverse events in ambulatory surgery: a comparison between elderly and younger patients. *Can J Anaesth* 1999; **46**: 309–21.

46. Kikura M, Oikawa F, Yamamoto K, et al. Myocardial infarction and cerebrovascular accident following non-cardiac surgery: differences in postoperative temporal distribution and risk factors. *J Thromb Haemost* 2008; **6**: 742–8.

47. Barden J, Edwards J, Moore A, McQuay H. Single dose oral paracetamol (acetaminophen) for postoperative

pain. *Cochrane Database Syst Rev* 2004;
1: CD 004602.

48. McQuay H, Moore A. Paracetamol with and without codeine in acute pain. In McQuay H, Moore A, eds. *An Evidence-Based Resource for Pain Relief*. Oxford, Oxford University Press, 1998, pp. 58–63.

49. Hyllested M, Jones S, Pedersen JL, Kehlet H. Comparative effect of paracetamol, NSAIDs or their combination in postoperative pain management: a qualitative review. *Br J Anaesth* 2002; **88**:199–214.

50. National Institute for Health and Clinical Excellence (NICE). *Reducing the Risk of Venous Thromboembolism (Deep Vein Thrombosis and Pulmonary Embolism) in Inpatients Undergoing Surgery. NICE CG 46*. London, NICE, 2007. http://www.nice.org.uk/CG046, accessed 31 December, 2008

13

The endocrine response to critical illness

Steven Ball and Simon V. Baudouin

Introduction

The endocrine system functions as a communicator and an effector. It allows 'action at a distance' in response to changes in the external and internal environment: communicating a change and effecting an adaptive response through the actions of hormones. In general, these act at sites distant from the point of release and produce defined responses in a range of target cells through interaction with specific receptors. Release of hormones may be continuous, episodic or follow a periodic pattern. Their action is regulated through complex feedback loops; modulated through protein-binding, receptor modification and the action of functional antagonists; and finally terminated through degradation and/or excretion.

Given that critical illness is associated with profound changes in most if not all physiological systems, it is not surprising that we witness equally marked changes in hormones and hormone action. Through careful observational studies, we are now in a good position to at least describe what the endocrine response to critical illness entails. Taken together with an established knowledge of endocrine physiology, these data should inform our understanding of the role of hormones in this complex pathophysiological process. Moreover, we have now seen the successful completion of a number of important, multicentre trials of endocrine interventions in the critically ill. These include studies on insulin, cortisol, growth hormone and vasopressin. However, the results of these studies have often been contradictory and inconsistent. Thus, while we know a lot more about what happens, we have not made as much progress in understanding why and what, if anything, we should do about it.

It has become clear that the investigation of endocrine changes in the critically ill presents a complex and difficult challenge to the research community. Successful translation of research data in this area into clinical practice is likely to be equally difficult. There remain, therefore, significant challenges to address if we are to maintain progress.

Metabolic changes in the critically ill
Ebb and flow

Over 50 years ago, Cuthbertson described the metabolic consequences of uncomplicated long bone fractures [1]. He found that there was an initial early phase following injury where metabolic rate and oxygen consumption fell below normal levels. He described this as the 'ebb' phase of injury. After 24–48 hours, metabolic rate and oxygen consumption then increased. He described this as the 'flow' phase (Figure 13.1). This period of increased metabolism lasted for several days and subsequently returned to normal. The flow phase was associated with a number of important changes in metabolism which have been interpreted as aiding body defences and promoting recovery from injury. These include changes in protein, glucose and lipid metabolism.

Critical illness is associated with an intense catabolic response, distinct from the response to simple under nutrition [2]. There is increased protein synthesis in the liver and bone marrow, with the release of acute phase proteins (Table 13.1). However, this is more than counteracted by increased protein breakdown, principally from skeletal muscle. Proteolysis leads to increased circulating levels of amino acids. In burn injury, for example, amino acid increases are proportional to the size of the burn. The net result is a profound negative nitrogen balance, with urinary losses of 11–14 g/ 24 hours. This cannot be reversed simply by nutritional support. In prolonged, catabolic critical illness, loss of muscle mass is substantial [3]. It is exacerbated by the process of disuse atrophy, which is a normal response to immobility.

Core Topics in Endocrinology in Anaesthesia and Critical Care, eds. George M. Hall, Jennifer M. Hunter and Mark S. Cooper. Published by Cambridge University Press. © Cambridge University Press 2010.

Table 13.1 Features of the catabolic response to stress.

Increased metabolic rate
Increased oxygen consumption
Increased acute phase protein synthesis
Increased skeletal muscle protein breakdown
Negative nitrogen balance
Hyperglycaemia
Insulin resistance
Increased circulating stress hormone levels

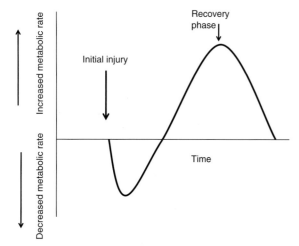

Fig. 13.1 The classic 'ebb and flow' phases of the acute stress response. Metabolic rate initially falls below normal and then increases to supranormal levels before returning once again to normal.

Hyperglycaemia is very common in the severely ill, a result of the combined effects of elevated glucose counter-regulatory hormones, such as cortisol and growth hormone (GH); activation of the sympathetic nervous system; and inflammatory cytokines [4]. The initial phase of critical illness is characterised by alpha-adrenergic inhibition of beta-cell insulin release, despite concurrent hyperglycaemia. In addition, there is both elevated hepatic glucose output and impaired muscle glucose uptake: both features of insulin resistance [5]. There is some evidence that glucose is a preferential fuel for wound healing. In burn patients, for example, there is both increased blood flow and increased tissue glucose uptake in injured limbs compared to non-injured ones. However, in other studies, glucose uptake appears relatively fixed despite increased circulating insulin levels. In prolonged critical illness insulin

resistance may continue, and can result in continued glucose intolerance.

In healthy individuals, body fat stores provide a substantial metabolic reserve. Carbohydrate stores are quickly exhausted in critical illness and lipids rapidly become the primary source of energy. Plasma levels of free fatty acids are elevated with a number of studies reporting a rise in proportion to the magnitude of injury.

Endocrine responses to critical illness: an overview

There is reciprocity in the relationship between the endocrine and metabolic responses to critical illness: the endocrine system driving change while, in turn, the metabolic responses impact on hormone production and action. Understanding this complex relationship is central to developing our views on the contribution of both to the pathophysiological process.

The hypothalamo-pituitary-adrenal axis

Cortisol has a key role in maintaining vascular physiology and mediating acute metabolic responses. The hypothalamo-pituitary-adrenal axis plays a central role in the homeostatic response to severe illness. In acute critical illness, hypothalamic corticotropin releasing factor (CRF) and pituitary adrenocorticotropin (ACTH) drive increases cortisol production by the adrenal cortex. This central drive is further augmented by both vasopressin and inflammatory cytokines. Vasopressin enhances the pituitary ACTH response to CRF while cytokines may act centrally and at the level of the adrenal gland. The increased levels of circulating cortisol stimulate gluconeogenesis; bolster circulating volume; and enhance both vasopressor and inotropic effects of catecholamines. It may also serve to limit inflammatory responses.

While persistent critical illness is associated with continued hypercortisolaemia, ACTH levels are low. This suggests that adrenal glucocorticoid production is, in part, independent of normal physiological feedback mechanisms and driven by alternative agents. Pro-inflammatory cytokines may play a key role in this process [6].

Recently, the concept of relative adrenal insufficiency has been developed to describe a group of patients with persisting critical illness and in whom cortisol levels (basal and/or stimulated) may be inappropriately low [7, 8]. By inference, this serves to highlight a group who may benefit from additional glucocorticoids. However, this area remains controversial. The definition and use of the term lack precision and consistency. Eighty-five to ninety-five per cent of cortisol circulates bound to cortisol binding globulin (CBG) and albumin. The levels of both proteins fall in critical illness. Measures of total plasma cortisol may therefore underestimate the biologically active (free) hormone [9]. There are therefore significant problems defining a normal reference range in the population with critical illness. In addition, incremental cortisol responses to the standard short Synacthen test lack construct validity in this context and must be interpreted with caution.

Etomidate and the cortisol response to stress

Etomidate is a carboxylated imidazole intravenous anaesthetic agent. It has an onset of action within one arm–brain circulation time. It has been widely used as an induction agent in the critically ill because of its relative haemodynamic stability compared with alternative agents. However, this use remains controversial because of evidence that it suppresses the adreno-cortical axis and may contribute to an increased mortality in the critically ill.

Concerns over the use of etomidate in the severely ill were originally raised in the 1980s following its widespread adoption as a continuous infusion for sedation of these patients. An increased mortality was reported in multi-trauma patients who received etomidate infusions [10]. This association was further confirmed by both multifactorial analysis and case matching which found that etomidate appeared to be an independent risk factor for mortality. Investigation into the possible mechanism of this adverse reaction quickly found that cortisol levels were unusually low in patients who had received etomidate. Subsequent studies reported that etomidate inhibited cortisol production in the adrenal gland by inhibition of 11-β-hydroxylase [11].

Even a single induction dose of cortisol will reduce the cortisol response to stimulation for up to 24 hours. This has also been demonstrated in the critically ill. For example in a small study of 35 critically ill patients randomised to induction with either etomidate or thiopentone there was a significant reduction in cortisol stimulation in the etomidate group [12]. A reduction in cortisol stimulation following etomidate was also reported in a retrospective study of 152 patients with septic shock [13]. In neither study were cortisol levels below the normal range.

The key question remains as to whether these biochemical changes, which are essentially 'relative adrenal insufficiency', lead to real changes in patient outcome. This remains a very controversial area [14, 15]. The whole concept of relative adrenal insufficiency has been challenged (see above) and the recent CORTICUS (Corticosteroid Therapy of Septic Shock) study did not report a difference in mortality between responders and non-responders to corticotrophin [16]. In addition there is no high-grade evidence showing that etomidate is harmful, in terms of a randomised controlled trial.

However, there is a substantial body of indirect evidence that supports a cautious approach to the use of etomidate in the critically ill. A retrospective analysis of the CORTICUS database was conducted which found that etomidate increased the odds ratio of dying in hospital significantly (OR 1.53: 95% CI 1.06–2.26) [17]. However, this increased risk was no longer significant in a multivariate analysis suggesting that other co-variables accounted for the higher mortality. In a study of children with meningococcal sepsis, deaths occurred in 1 of 8 (12.5%) intubated without etomidate compared to 7 of 23 (30%) intubated with etomidate [18]. Once again the possibility of other differences in the two groups cannot be excluded.

In summary, there is good evidence that etomidate does reduce the cortisol response to stimulation for up to 24 hours after a single, induction dose. It is less certain that this change translates into any worsening of clinical outcome. It is unlikely that a sufficiently powerful randomised trial will be conducted to give a definitive answer. Critical care practitioners therefore have to decide, on an individual patient basis, as to whether the beneficial haemodynamic profile of etomidate exceeds the possible increased risk of inducing depression of the cortisol response.

The hypothalamo-pituitary-thyroid axis

The thyroid axis response to critical illness is biphasic (Table 13.2). Shortly after the onset, free triiodothyronine (FT_3) levels fall while free thyroxine (FT_4), thyroid stimulating hormone (TSH) and reverse triiodothyronine (rT_3, the inactive product of T_4 inner-ring deiodination) increase. These changes reflect reduced peripheral T_4 to T_3 conversion and reduced degradation of rT_3. These acute changes are followed by a normalisation of TSH and FT_4, but persistent subnormal levels of FT_3 (Chapter 17).

Additional changes can develop over several weeks if critical illness persists. Both FT_4 and FT_3 fall into the subnormal range. Thyroid stimulating hormone values fall into the subnormal or low normal range. Normal

Table 13.2 Key endocrine changes in the acute and chronic phases of critical illness.

Hormone level	Acute phase	Chronic phase
ACTH	↑	↓
CRF	↑	↓
Cortisol	↑	Variable
FT$_3$	↓	↓
FT$_4$	↑	↓
Pulsatile TSH	↑	↔ or ↓
Testosterone	↓	↓↓
Pulsatile LH	↑	↓
Pulsatile GH	↑	↓
GHBP	↓	↑
IGF-1	↓	↓↓
Pulsatile prolactin	↑	↓

ACTH, adrenocorticotrophic hormone; CRF, corticotropin releasing factor; FT$_3$, free triiodothyronine; FT$_4$, free thyroxine; GH, growth hormone; GHBP, GH-binding protein; IGF-1, insulin-like growth factor-1; LH, luteinising hormone; TSH, thyroid stimulating hormone

pulsatile secretion of TSH is lost. This second wave response reflects decreased hypothalamic thyrotropin releasing hormone (TRH) production: effectively part of a resetting of the thyroid neuroendocrine axis. Peripheral thyroid hormone metabolism is also further altered, with down-regulation of hepatic type 1 deiodinase (D$_1$) and up-regulation of type 3 deiodinase (D$_3$). This accentuates changes in the FT$_3$/rT$_3$ ratio, favouring the inactive metabolite [19].

The hypothalamo-pituitary-gonadal axis

The pituitary-gonadal axis also has a biphasic response to critical illness. In the acute phase, testosterone levels are reduced while luteinising hormone (LH) levels are high – indicative of hyperacute suppression at the level of the testes. Prolonged critical illness is associated with progressive hypogonadotrophic hypogonadism. In the male, testosterone levels may become very low. Aromatisation of adrenal androgens may serve to maintain sex hormone levels in the female to some extent.

The growth hormone, insulin-like growth factor (IGF), IGF-binding protein axis

Growth hormone (GH), produced by the anterior pituitary gland, has metabolic functions outwith its role in promotion of linear growth. It is an important regulator of lipid metabolism, promotes positive nitrogen balance and is a key counter-regulatory hormone

in glucose homeostasis. Under normal circumstances, the majority of GH is produced in a series of night-time pulses. Both pulse amplitude and pulse frequency contribute to integrated GH levels. In the acute phase of critical illness, integrated GH production is increased. This reflects an increase in GH pulse amplitude and an elevation in inter-pulse trough values. However, concentrations of the GH-binding protein fall (Table 13.2). As GH-binding protein is derived from the GH receptor, this would suggest the development of a GH-resistant state. This view is further supported by data highlighting reduced levels of the GH-dependent proteins insulin-like growth factor-1 (IGF-1) and insulin-like growth factor binding protein 3 (IGF-BP3).

Persistent critical illness leads to reduced pulsatile GH release. Pulse amplitude is reduced. Inter-pulse trough GH levels are lower than in the acute phase of critical illness, but remain elevated with respect to the normal state. Concentration of GH-binding protein (and by inference GH-receptor expression) returns to normal while IGF-1 and IGF-BP3 remain low. These data are consistent with relative GH insufficiency and normal peripheral GH sensitivity. Given the anabolic effects of GH, they serve to highlight the potential contribution these changes may have to the progressive negative nitrogen balance that characterises this clinical situation.

Metabolic and endocrine response in critical illness: adaptive or part of the problem?

We are complex organisms with an equally complex and highly adaptive physiology which functions to maintain our internal environment. Physiological adaptation is not without limits, however. Critical illness constitutes a severe pathophysiological stressor that elicits a diverse though characteristic pathophysiological response. The metabolic and endocrine components of this response could be considered part of a co-ordinated physiological adaptation to the stressor: directing prioritisation of physiological resources; supporting cardiovascular function; and assisting regenerative responses. In truth, however, this is arguing function from form. More recently, this approach has been challenged on a number of fronts.

First, the metabolic and endocrine responses to critical illness are not uniform and persistent. Rather, as we have seen, acute and persistent critical illness can be associated with responses that are distinct and discordant. Second, specific patterns of metabolic and endocrine response have prognostic value. The lower the FT$_3$ level falls in critical illness, the worse the outcome. Patients with elevated baseline cortisol levels (> 935 nmol l⁻¹) and a relatively small increment following a standard 250 µg ACTH stimulation test (< 250 nmol l⁻¹) also have a worse prognosis [20]. While these data could simply reflect the limits of adaptive physiology, the sickest patients having the most florid endocrine response, they do highlight potential flaws in the adaptive response thesis. Should we simply remain passive in the face of these changes while we support other failing systems?

Recent clinical studies have demonstrated the benefit of interventions targeting specific metabolic and endocrine endpoints that would have previously been considered adaptive. These latter observations certainly challenge the assumption that the metabolic and endocrine responses to critical illness are a positive design feature. Natural selection could have driven adaptive capacity for surviving acute severe illness built, in part, on the physiological responses to other stressors. However, the same process would have struggled to drive adaptation to persisting critical illness – something that has only existed in the modern era of organ support and critical care units. Even if the natural selection thesis held, given the discordant responses to acute and persisting critical illness, we must consider that a process that is adaptive in the short-term may not be thereafter. Could it be these responses go on to form part of the negative pathophysiological cascade that characterises multiple organ failure? Could they be part of the problem rather than an attempt at a partial solution? To address these issues, we need to reflect on the context and the problems inherent in designing, performing and interpreting clinical studies in the critically ill.

The problem of critical illness: if only life were simple

Patients with critical illness are exposed to the very frontier of medical technology. They are assessed thoroughly, progress is monitored closely and outcomes are measured accurately. Yet despite this, studies in the critically ill present unique problems to both the investigators performing them and clinicians who seek to interpret them.

What is critical illness?

The critically ill are a heterogenous group of patients. In medical science, most successful clinical studies are based on specific disease entities or clinico-pathological endpoints that have a common aetiology. For example, the development of thrombolysis for acute myocardial infarction is based on our knowledge of the pathophysiology of coronary artery occlusion following plaque rupture. In contrast, critical illness groups a number of processes which lead to a common pathophysiological end point, one of which is generally based on organ failure. For example, the need to provide respiratory support through mechanical ventilation defines a syndrome of respiratory failure rather than a disease. Many common problems contribute to acute respiratory failure on the critical care unit: community-acquired pneumonia; chronic obstructive pulmonary disease (COPD); hospital-acquired pneumonia; and asthma. It is naïve to think that the syndrome of acute respiratory failure, as defined by the need for artificial respiratory support, is likely to to be associated with a uniform systemic metabolic and endocrine picture. Rather, this heterogeneity of aetiology is likely to be reflected in variable and inconsistent changes in metabolic and endocrine parameters. In turn, interventions that target these parameters and perhaps show benefit in certain subgroups of patients, may not demonstrate benefit to the population with critical illness as a whole.

Critical illness: an evolving process

Patients with critical illness are not simply heterogeneous in the aetiology and degree of multi-organ failure. They vary in their relative position in the time course of the critical illness. In some groups it is possible to define a start point. For example, in those with severe trauma or burn injury the start of the illness is clear. In others, it is impossible to identify the exact point at which their critical illness began. This is particularly the case for those with medical conditions that deteriorate following admission to hospital and in whom multi-organ failure may be a single, continuous process rather than a series of discrete events.

Moreover, critical illness may vary in duration. This is particularly important as the endocrine and metabolic responses to acute and persisting critical illness are distinct and discordant. Over inclusive recruitment and selection criteria for studies in the critically ill may lead to reduced power and resolution because of the varied position of patients in the natural history of their illness. Conversely, limited inclusion threatens bias and lack of generalisability.

Studying dynamic systems in an evolving process: the problem of too many variables

Changes over time are of major importance when studying dynamic and adapting processes such as the endocrine system. Many endocrine changes occur on a cyclical or periodic basis with definite circadian rhythms. When this natural variation is added to the difficult to define time course of critical illness, the possibility of loss of information due to a time-averaging effect becomes significant. This may prevent the recognition of important alterations in the endocrine response to critical illness.

The situation is further complicated by medical intervention. The purpose of critical care is to alter the natural history of the disease process, not simply to observe it. The critically ill will usually receive many parallel and serial interventions. Many of these will have direct and indirect effects on endocrine and metabolic end points. It is not possible to completely adjust for all variables in such a complex and evolving process. Separation of cause and effect becomes difficult.

Variable baselines: confounding co-morbidity

Having established that critical illness is a journey of uncertain duration, taking one of a number of routes to reach a series of similar destinations, there remains an outstanding problem. Not everyone starts from the same point. Many patients who develop a critical illness do so from a base of chronic ill health. Non-insulin-dependent diabetes mellitus, obesity, malnutrition and chronic heart failure are all common co-morbidities. Each of these is associated with changes to baseline endocrine and metabolic status. Patients will therefore start their episode of critical illness with dissimilar characteristics. This will contribute to baseline heterogeneity. Real trends and responses may be masked, while spurious trends and responses may be highlighted.

Understanding sepsis: cellular stress as a model framework for the study of endocrine and metabolic changes in critical illness

Despite the heterogeneity of critical illness, it is clear we must engage with it as a legitimate field of study if we are to resolve our uncertainties over the significance of endocrine and metabolic end points. This is particularly if we are to assess the utility of manipulating these end points. Focusing on a single pathophysiological process leading to critical illness can serve to demonstrate key principles that may help unravel some of the intellectual tangle, and highlight opportunities for moving forward.

Sepsis is one of the commonest problems presenting to critical care. It is the thirteenth most common cause of hospital inpatient mortality in the UK [21]. The incidence of sepsis is also increasing, due to a combination of changes in patient characteristics, the increasing use of intravascular devices and rising treatment expectations.

Sepsis is the result of complex host responses to infection [22]. In the 'standard model' of sepsis, microbial agents and their breakdown products activate both circulating white cells and other target cells, such as endothelial and epithelial cells, by binding to specific surface receptors. This both amplifies and spreads the host response to infection. Cascades of pro- and anti-inflammatory mediators are produced by activated cells with the likely benefit of combating infection, limiting host damage and accelerating recovery. However, this may not be without cost. The global activation of this intense inflammatory response is thought to produce marked 'collateral damage' in some patients, who proceed to develop severe sepsis and septic shock. In this model, it is an excessive and partially mal-regulated inflammatory response which becomes the 'problem rather than the solution'.

A defining feature of severe sepsis is the development of multiple organ failure [23]. Patients commonly require inotropic support, need mechanical ventilation and receive renal replacement therapy. The exact cause of this failure remains controversial, but changes in both the microcirculation and at the cellular levels are well described and likely to be causal. Two fundamental changes occur. First, microvascular control alters and often appears to be maladapted. Microvascular beds should dilate in response to increasing tissue needs for oxygen and nutrients. In sepsis this control appears to malfunction. Tissue beds are in a dynamic and rapidly changing state of vasodilation and constriction which no longer seems directly related to cellular needs. In addition, physical occlusion of these beds, by clot and cellular debris, is often observed.

As well as a failure of distribution of oxygenated blood and nutrients to tissue beds, the relationship between oxygen delivery and consumption is altered in many critically ill patients [24]. In the normal situation, a reduction in the availability of tissue oxygen results in an increased extraction of oxygen from the blood and a fall in mixed venous oxygen tensions. This situation is observed in classic examples of cardiogenic shock. In sepsis there appears to be a failure at the cellular or intracellular level to utilise oxygen efficiently. A variety of mechanisms have been proposed to explain this phenomenon: microvascular changes leading to shunting; thickening of the capillary/cellular barrier causing O_2 diffusion problems; and mitochondrial dysfunction with resulting inefficiencies of the oxidative phosphorylation (OXPHOS) energy transfer system [24].

Cellular stress and critical illness

While critical illness may be characterised by heterogeneity and diversity at a patient level, there is no parallel at the level of the cell. In fact there is a uniformity of response at the cellular level to the acute fall in O_2 delivery/consumption that characterises sepsis and many other conditions producing critical illness [25]. The stress-related induction of a small number of key transcription factors results in a marked alteration in gene expression in most cells studied. In healthy volunteers, for example, injection of small doses of endotoxin produces rapid and reproducible changes in white blood cell gene expression in a number of functional 'groups' [26]. Both up- and down-regulation have been reported. Interestingly, OXPHOS genes are among those that are negatively regulated. Similar changes have been described in 'stressed' endothelial, epithelial and hepatocellular cell lines. This pattern of altered gene expression is initiated by the activation of a group of key stressor-mediating transcription factors including hypoxia inducible factor (HIF) [27].

Ebb and flow revisited: reflections on the past and directions for the future

The classic ebb and flow descriptions were derived from observations of the natural history of unresuscitated patients with moderate, uncomplicated trauma. How applicable are they to the more complex patients admitted to modern critical care units?

A study on early human sepsis reported by Rivers et al. is instructive [28]. They provided data on the pre-and post-resuscitation phases of patients admitted acutely to hospital with severe sepsis. Before volume and inotrope resuscitation, these patients had very reduced mixed venous oxygen tensions. This indicated that a fall in tissue oxygen consumption had occurred due to a failure of global oxygen delivery and is analogous to the ebb phase in Cuthbertson's studies. There, the likely mechanism was hypovolaemia due to blood loss following fracture. In severe sepsis, loss of intravascular volume due to capillary leak results in reduced cardiac output. In Rivers' study, rapid resuscitation was initiated leading to a restoration of cardiac output and tissue oxygen

consumption, usually within a few hours of initial assessment. In fact, cardiac output in post-resuscitation sepsis often rises to 'supra-normal' levels. However, despite the adequate global delivery of oxygen to the tissues, there remains an impairment of O_2 utilisation.

Modern critical care therefore changes the time course and natural history of the flow phase of severe illness (Figure 13.2). Although many critically ill patients rapidly recover, there are a significant number who enter a protracted period of illness. This results in a prolonged catabolic response which typically waxes and wanes. The drivers of the prolonged phase remain poorly understood, but recurrent bouts of infection often appear to contribute. The endocrine system did not evolve to meet such prolonged, and 'man-made', challenges. Endocrine changes in so-called chronic critical illness may therefore not be necessarily beneficial to the host.

In summary, the classic description of the stress response is based on the response to a single, trauma-based, insult which lacks adequate resuscitation and has a natural period of recovery. Critically ill patients are rapidly resuscitated, but often enter a prolonged period of clinical instability. To assume an adaptive function in a series of diverse endocrine and metabolic responses that develop over this period is not inappropriate. However, applying the simple clinical endocrine paradigm of suppression or replacement to normality is probably equally inappropriate given the uncertainties around the utility of normal physiological reference

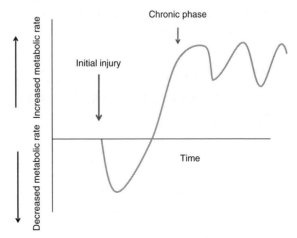

Fig. 13.2 Ebb and flow revisited. In the population of chronically ill patients in critical care the classic ebb and flow pattern is altered. Recurrent bouts of sepsis and other pro-inflammatory stimuli result in a fluctuating metabolic demand which remains chronically elevated.

ranges in the critically ill. Normalising physiology may be neither optimal nor desirable in this context.

We need to develop more sophisticated approaches. Moreover, these approaches need to be firmly based on the cellular and tissue dysfunction common to critical illness. Critical care no longer simply talks about normalising ventilation or increasing PaO_2. Rather, the focus is on multi-modality approaches to optimising tissue oxygen delivery and utilisation. Similarly, we need to move the focus away from simply measuring and interpreting changes in endocrine and metabolic parameters. Combining our current knowledge of the function of endocrine and metabolic regulators; the changes that occur in these regulators with critical illness; and the growing understanding of the cellular dysfunction that underpins multi-organ failure will allow us to develop integrated models of an inherently complex process. These are essential if we are to resolve pathophysiological pathways from epiphenomena; cause from effect; and develop a rational basis for support and intervention. We have come a long way, but there remains a long way to go.

References

1. Cuthbertson D. Observations on the disturbance of metabolism produced by injury to the limbs. *Lancet* 1942; **1**: 433–7.

2. Vincent JL. Metabolic support in sepsis and multiple organ failure: more questions than answers. *Crit Care Med* 2007; **35**: S436–40.

3. Pingleton SK. Nutrition in chronic critical illness. *Clin Chest Med* 2001; **22**: 149–63.

4. Vanhorebeek I, Langouche L, Van den Berghe G. Tight blood glucose control with insulin in the icu: Facts and controversies. *Chest* 2007; **132**: 268–78.

5. Saberi F, Heyland D, Lam M, Rapson D, Jeejeebhoy K. Prevalence, incidence, and clinical resolution of insulin resistance in critically ill patients: An observational study. *JPEN J Parenter Entreal Nutr* 2008; **32**: 227–35.

6. Straub RH, Harle P, Kriegel M, Scholmerich J, Lorenz HM. Adrenal and gonadal hormone variations during a febrile attack in a woman with tumor necrosis factor receptor-associated periodic syndrome. *J Clin Endocrinol Metab* 2005; **90**: 5884–7.

7. Dickstein G. On the term 'relative adrenal insufficiency' – or what do we really measure with adrenal stimulation tests? *J Clin Endocrinol Metab* 2005; **90**: 4973–4.

8. Marik PE. Unraveling the mystery of adrenal failure in the critically ill. *Crit Care Med* 2004; **32**: 596–7.

9. Hamrahian AH, Oseni TS, Arafah BM. Measurements of serum free cortisol in critically ill patients. *N Engl J Med* 2004; **350**: 1629–38.

10. Watt I, Ledingham IM. Mortality amongst multiple trauma patients admitted to an intensive therapy unit. *Anaesthesia* 1984; **39**: 973–81.

11. Wagner RL, White PF, Kan PB, Rosenthal MH, Feldman D. Inhibition of adrenal steroidogenesis by the anesthetic etomidate. *N Engl J Med* 1984; **310**: 1415–21.

12. Absalom A, Pledger D, Kong A. Adrenocortical function in critically ill patients 24 h after a single dose of etomidate. *Anaesthesia* 1999; **54**: 861–7.

13. Mohammad Z, Afessa B, Finkielman JD. The incidence of relative adrenal insufficiency in patients with septic shock after the administration of etomidate. *Crit Care* 2006; **10**: R105.

14. Walls RM, Murphy MF. Clinical controversies: Etomidate as an induction agent for endotracheal intubation in patients with sepsis: Continue to use etomidate for intubation of patients with septic shock. *Ann Emerg Med* 2008; **52**: 13–14.

15. Sacchetti A. Etomidate: Not worth the risk in septic patients. *Ann Emerg Med* 2008; **52**: 14–16.

16. Sprung CL, Annane D, Keh D, et al. Hydrocortisone therapy for patients with septic shock. *N Engl J Med* 2008; **358**: 111–24.

17. Lipiner-Friedman D, Sprung CL, Laterre PF, et al. Adrenal function in sepsis: The retrospective CORTICUS cohort study. *Crit Care Med* 2007; **35**: 1012–18.

18. den Brinker M, Hokken-Koelega AC, Hazelzet JA, de Jong FH, Hop WC, Joosten KF. One single dose of etomidate negatively influences adrenocortical performance for at least 24 h in children with meningococcal sepsis. *Intensive Care Med* 2008; **34**: 163–8.

19. Peeters RP, Wouters PJ, van Toor H, Kaptein E, Visser TJ, Van den Berghe G. Serum 3,3',5'-triiodothyronine (rT3) and 3,5,3'-triiodothyronine/rT3 are prognostic markers in critically ill patients and are associated with postmortem tissue deiodinase activities. *J Clin Endocrinol Metab* 2005; **90**: 4559–65.

20. Annane D, Sebille V, Troche G, Raphael JC, Gajdos P, Bellissant E. A three-level prognostic classification in septic shock based on cortisol levels and cortisol response to corticotropin. *JAMA* 2000; **283**: 1038–45.

21. Jarman B, Aylin P, Bottle A. Trends in admissions and deaths in English NHS hospitals. *BMJ* 2004; **328**: 855.

22. Baudouin SV. Sepsis: introduction and epidemiology. In Baudouin SV, ed. *Sepsis*. London, Springer, 2008, pp. 1–4.

23. Singer M, De Santis V, Vitale D, Jeffcoate W. Multiorgan failure is an adaptive, endocrine-mediated, metabolic response to overwhelming systemic inflammation. *Lancet* 2004; **364**: 545–8.

24. Abraham E, Singer M. Mechanisms of sepsis-induced organ dysfunction. *Crit Care Med* 2007; **35**: 2408–16.

25. Gardner LB, Corn PG. Hypoxic regulation of mRna expression. *Cell Cycle* 2008; **7**: 1916–24.

26. Calvano SE, Xiao W, Richards DR, et al. A network-based analysis of systemic inflammation in humans. *Nature* 2005; **437**: 1032–7.

27. Chavez A, Miranda LF, Pichiule P, Chavez JC. Mitochondria and hypoxia-induced gene expression mediated by hypoxia-inducible factors. *Ann N Y Acad Sci* 2008; **1147**: 312–20.

28. Rivers E, Nguyen B, Havstad S, et al. Early goal-directed therapy in the treatment of severe sepsis and septic shock. *N Engl J Med* 2001; **345**: 1368–77.

Tight glucose control using intensive insulin therapy in the critically ill

Mark E. Seubert, Saheed Khan and A. B. Johan Groeneveld

Introduction

During the past decade, in which the seminal studies by Van den Berghe have been published [1, 2], a series of investigations into glucose homeostasis and insulin therapy in the critically ill have also been reported. This chapter addresses the risks associated with hyperglycaemia; the implementation, efficacy and safety of protocols for tight glucose control (TGC) using intensive insulin therapy (IIT); and measurement of blood glucose in the critically ill.

Glucose values between 4.4 and 6.1 mmol l^{-1} are normal in fasting healthy adults whereas glucose levels of 7.0 mmol l^{-1} or more in this state are considered diagnostic of diabetes mellitus by the World Health Organization. Glucose levels of 11.1 mmol l^{-1} or more at any time are also diagnostic of diabetes. Levels of 4.0–6.1 mmol l^{-1} are aimed for in TGC by IIT in the intensive care unit (ICU) and perioperatively. Hyperglycaemia frequently occurs in critically ill patients particularly if the underlying disease is severe [3, 4]. The incidence varies between 96% on admission to intensive care if the strict threshold of hyperglycaemia is used (6.1 mmol l^{-1}) to between 10 and 40% when 11.0 mmol l^{-1} is used as the hyperglycaemia cut-off value. Risk factors for hyperglycaemia requiring insulin control include advanced age, established diabetes mellitus, obesity, sepsis, use of immunosuppressive drugs (e.g., corticosteroids) or inotropes, hepatic cirrhosis, renal insufficiency, pancreatitis, parenteral nutrition and overfeeding with carbohydrates [3, 4]. All these factors can prolong stay in the ICU. In addition, hyperglycaemia may be the first sign of previously unrecognised diabetes mellitus [3]. A major factor causing hyperglycaemia, however, is the stress response to critical illness, the associated changes in the hormonal environment, and the resultant insulin resistance with increased hepatic gluconeogenesis and impaired glucose uptake in the tissues.

Effects of hyperglycaemia and insulin

Even though potentially protecting body fluid homeostasis when threatened by hypovolaemia, hyperglycaemia is a marker of a worse outcome, particularly in patients with myocardial infarction, those undergoing surgery (cardiac or major), trauma (including brain), stroke, subarachnoid haemorrhage and other life-threatening conditions. Stress hyperglycaemia is at least as detrimental as hyperglycaemia with prior diabetes mellitus, which may be associated with fewer risks [5–7]. The variability of glucose levels may independently contribute to hyperglycaemia-attributable mortality [8, 9]. This may be caused by a plethora of adverse effects that can be ameliorated by insulin [10], including predisposition to infection and an impaired host response (by neutrophils) to overcome microbial infection [11] (Table 14.1). On the one hand, acute hyperglycaemia may have pro-inflammatory actions, including increased endothelial oxidative stress and decreased nitric oxide availability, release of cytokines and adhesion molecules, and increased leukocyte–endothelial interactions with resultant impairment of endothelium-dependent vasodilatation [10, 11]. It may also predispose to supraventricular arrhythmias and increase the incidence of ischaemic events in diabetic coronary artery bypass graft (CABG) patients [12]. Conversely, insulin may have anti-inflammatory and antiapoptotic actions, and may decrease proteolysis and increase anabolism [10]. Insulin may also prevent an impaired (cellular) host response to hyperglycaemia and may thus have some pro-inflammatory effects, perhaps contributing to prevention of postoperative infection [1, 13–18]. Furthermore, TGC may decrease asymmetric dimethylarginine (ADMA), an endogenous and non-selective inhibitor of nitric oxide synthase. It is more likely that potential beneficial effects of TGC are related to control of the

Core Topics in Endocrinology in Anaesthesia and Critical Care, eds. George M. Hall, Jennifer M. Hunter and Mark S. Cooper. Published by Cambridge University Press. © Cambridge University Press 2010.

Table 14.1 Effects of glucose and insulin.

Hyperglycaemia	Insulin
Procoagulant	Anti-inflammatory
Pro-inflammatory	Increases endothelial NO(S) and decreases inducible NO(S)
Decreases endothelial NO(S) and increases ADMA	Variable effect on IGF-1
Proapoptotic	Antiapoptotic
Decreased wound healing	Increased protein synthesis
Increased proteolysis	Increased host defence (by cell responses)
Impaired host defence	Promotes preconditioning; decreased ischaemia/reperfusion injury
Decreased preconditioning; increased ischaemia/reperfusion injury	Vasodilatation and positive inotropy
Impaired vasoreactivity	Decreases hypertriglyceridaemia and increases HDL cholesterol
Decreased fat turnover	Decreases insulin resistance
Risk factor for rhythm disturbance	

Note. Effects of insulin are partly glycaemia-dependent and partly independent.

ADMA, asymmetric dimethylarginine; HDL, high-density lipoprotein; IGF-1, insulin-like growth factor-1; NO(S), nitric oxide synthase

hyperglycaemia rather than to infusion of extra insulin during IIT [19, 20].

Tight glucose control by intensive insulin therapy

The first report on IIT for TGC (glucose values between 4.4 and 6.1 mmol l^{-1}) in critically ill patients was published in 2001 by Van den Berghe et al. from Leuven [1]. This study showed a mortality reduction from 8.0% on conventional treatment to 4.6% in the IIT arm, in adults admitted to the surgical ICU. Furthermore, patients who remained in the ICU for more than 5 days showed a decrease in mortality from 20.2 to 10.6% in the IIT arm. A number of factors were responsible and in the subsequent studies related to this major trial, the effects seemed primarily dependent on the level of control of the glycaemia [19, 20]. The potential mechanisms of decreased morbidity and mortality are manifold and include suppression of inflammation and less mitochondrial damage, organ failure and ventilation days, with the latter being the main contributor to the lower costs from implementing IIT [21]. Many patients had undergone cardiac surgery and were on parenteral nutrition, and the mortality in the control group was relatively high. In a subsequent study of medical patients, albeit less convincingly positive, similar results were obtained [2]. Indeed, a mortality benefit could only be observed in patients staying in the ICU for three days or longer, while IIT in shorter stay patients was associated with increased mortality.

Randomised studies outside Belgium, including the German VISEP (Efficacy of Volume Substitution and Insulin Therapy in Severe Sepsis) study and the Belgium-initiated Glucontrol study failed to reproduce these findings [22–24]. The VISEP studies enrolled 488 patients in 17 German centres and the Glucontrol study 1101 patients across 21 ICU units in 7 European countries. Targets resembled those of the Leuven studies but control may have been less tight, thereby potentially underpowering the studies. Both were prematurely stopped due to the incidence of hypoglycaemia (14–17%) and additional relatively minor reasons. The results of the NICE-SUGAR (Normoglycaemia in Intensive Care Evaluation and Survival Using Glucose Algorithm Regulation) open-label study in 25 Australian, 19 Canadian and 2 American hospitals are negative, showing increased mortality in the strictly controlled arm. This study compared two target ranges for blood glucose (4.5–6.0 mmol l^{-1} vs. < 10.0 mmol l^{-1}) in 6022 patients [25]. Other recent studies [26, 27], also showing no benefit on mortality of IIT, may have been unbalanced and underpowered. In contrast, there are some retrospective and prospective sequential cohort studies in critically ill patients, showing mortality benefits after instituting IIT [14–16, 20, 28, 29], although this was not confirmed in trauma patients [30–32]. Moreover, decreased morbidity may not necessarily translate into mortality benefits. Adopting IIT in a burn unit did not decrease mortality, even though it decreased infections and other complications attributable, in part, to hyperglycaemia [17]. Nevertheless, aiming for control of glucose to values between 6.9 and 11.1 mmol l^{-1} has been confirmed to improve perioperative outcomes and to decrease recurrent episodes of ischaemia, arrhythmias and heart failure in diabetics undergoing coronary artery surgery [12, 18]. During cardiac surgery, however, TGC was associated with increased death and stroke rates [33]. Failure of a glucose-insulin-potassium infusion to benefit the cardiac function of patients with myocardial infarction or those undergoing coronary artery surgery (with or without diabetes) in recent studies may be attributable, in part, to insufficient control of the resultant hyperglycaemia.

Other factors that may be involved in the discrepancy between the Leuven and other studies include the case mix, the use of parenteral nutrition that may predispose to hyperglycaemia, the level and intensity of control, the rate of potentially dangerous hypoglycaemia, the prevalence of prior diabetes, and the number of patients studied and thus the power of the studies. Meta-analyses of major studies did not reach the same conclusions (partly because of different study inclusions), making it impossible to set unambiguous recommendations [34–36]. Surgical, including cardiac, patients and those with acute myocardial infarction or diabetes mellitus may benefit most from targeting euglycaemia with insulin therapy [34, 36].

Intensive insulin treatment protocols

Table 14.2 describes the currently described and reproducible protocols for IIT that have been implemented in ICUs, and Table 14.3 summarises the major differences between these widely varying protocols. There is not a single insulin infusion protocol that fits all patients and units, and the factors, values and calculations required to implement IIT and to judge its efficacy and safety vary among studies [37–39]. Nevertheless, some general conclusions can be drawn. For instance, the time to reach a given target range depends on baseline glycaemia, circadian rhythms, the condition of the patient, and the doses of insulin (bolus vs. continuous). High frequency of glucose measurements (up to hourly), small and consistent insulin dose alterations, and adjustment of IIT according to the degree of change in blood glucose rather than the absolute value, will all contribute to increasing the time that glycaemia is maintained within a target range at an acceptable risk of hypoglycaemia.

Intensive insulin therapy may occasionally result in extremely high insulin requirements because of insulin resistance. The amount of insulin needed to reach normoglycaemia, as prescribed in several protocols, varies between 27 and 115 U within the study time span of 9 hours [38] (Figure 14.1). The lower the target range, the higher the incidence of (possibly unnoticed) hypoglycaemia. Continuous intravenous administration is preferable to intermittent boluses or subcutaneous insulin (using, for instance, so-called sliding scale regimens), since the latter may result in wide fluctuations in blood glucose [40, 41]. Nevertheless, successful combinations have been described [15, 28]. Changes in nutrition, starting continuous venovenous haemofiltration (using bicarbonate solutions), or corticosteroids may all require adjustment of insulin dosage guided by more frequent glucose measurements. The practicality of protocols depends on staffing ratios and their roles (nurse vs. physician), and the use of algorithms/nomograms and automated systems that may increase efficacy and safety (i.e., less hypoglycaemia) [29, 30, 40, 42–52]. An example of an automated system is shown in Figure 14.2, which describes an overview of GRIP (Glucose Regulation for Intensive care Patients), a computer-based algorithm.

Hypoglycaemia

The symptoms of hypoglycaemia are confusion, coma, restlessness and seizures [7]. Tachycardia with other sympathetic manifestations, such as sweating, can also occur. Most commonly, however, hypoglycaemia goes unnoticed and is a coincidental (but alarming) finding during routine monitoring of blood glucose. Depending on definitions and study size, rates of hypoglycaemia on IIT vary between 0 and 32%, with similar to higher rates in medical than in surgical patients for a given protocol [1, 2, 13, 14, 22–28, 30–32, 41, 43, 45–71]. Thus, IIT may lead to more frequent and sometimes severe hypoglycaemia[1, 2, 13, 14, 22, 23, 26–28, 32, 35, 46, 48, 51, 62, 71]. Expressing the number of severe hypoglycaemic episodes (glucose < 2.2–2.5 mmol l^{-1}) per number of blood samples taken for glucose measurement may help to assess quality of control, whereas expression per number of patients treated may be an indicator of safety. Hypoglycaemia warrants intravenous glucose administration which may hamper TGC, for the amount of insulin needed to prevent overshoot is increased. Patients suffering from severe disease, septic shock, liver or renal insufficiency, malnutrition or decreased caloric intake, adrenal

Table 14.2 Insulin protocols in alphabetical order per year of appearance.

Author [Ref]	Number of patients (unless otherwise specified)	Type of insulin protocol	Blood glucose target[1] (mmol l^{-1})	Analyser	Sample frequency (hour or mean/ day)	Hypoglycaemia (BG < 2.2 mmol l^{-1} unless otherwise specified[2])
2001						
Berghe, Van den et al. [1]	765 surgical	Manual	4.0–6.1	BGA	1–4 h	5.1% (P)
Brown and Dodeck [42]	77 mixed	Manual	7–11.5	Lab, GM	14.4	20 times (S) BG < 3.5
2002						
Markovitz et al. [40]	29 surgical	Manual	6.7–11.0		6.4	≥ 1 BG < 3.9 on 1.4% of days 0–4
2004						
Furnary et al. [44]	3896 surgical	Manual, Portand IP	Partly 5.6–8.3	GM	0.5–2.0 h	0.5% (P) BG < 3.3
Goldberg et al. [58]	118 surgical	Manual, Yale IP	5.6–7.7	GM	1 h	0.2% (S) BG < 3.3
Goldberg et al. [43]	52 medical	Manual, Yale IP	5.6–7.7	GM	1–4 h	0.05% (S)
Grey and Perdrizet [13]	34 surgical	Manual	4.4–6.7		4.6	32% (P), 0.8% (S) BG < 3.3
Kanji et al. [59]	50 mixed	Manual	4.4–6.1		11.3	4% (P)
Krinsley [28]	800 mixed	Manual	< 7.8		3 h if insulin s.c., 1 h if i.v.	0.34% (S)
Laver et al. [60]	27 mixed	Manual, Bath IP	4–7	GM	1–2 h	3 times (S)
Orford et al. [61]	148 mixed	Manual	4.4–7.0	BGA	0.5–4.0 h	2.7% (P)
Zimmerman et al. [62]	168 surgical	Manual	4.4–8.3	GM	1–4 h	7.1% (P)
2005						
Bland et al. [47]	5 medical	Manual	4.4–6.1	GM	2–4 h	2 times (S)
Chant et al. [46]	44 mixed	Manual	5–8		7.1	0.2% (S)
Collier et al. [31]	435 surgical	Manual	4.4–6.1		1–4 h	< 5% /day (P) BG < 3.3
Davidson et al. [45]	5080 i.v. insulin runs, mixed	Computer Glu-commander	Most 4.4–6.7		0.3–2 h	2.6% (P)
Dilkhush et al. [63]	30 mixed	Manual	4.4–7.2		1–4 h	50% (P) 0.4% (S)
Ku et al. [64]	50 mixed	Manual	4.4–10	GM	1–4 h	3.8% (P)
Thomas et al. [30]	101 mixed	Computer	4.4–7.1	GM	1–4 h	6% (P)
2006						
Braithwaite et al. [55]	24 surgical	Manual	3.9–6.1	GM	1–2 h	None
Lonergan et al. [65]	11 medical	Manual, Sprint IP	4–6.1	GM	1–2 h	None
Osbourne et al. [53]	20 mixed	Manual	4.4–6.1		1 h	0.9% (S) BG < 3.3
Plank et al. [66]	30 surgical	Computer MPC V1.01.05[3]	4.4–6.1	BGA	1 h	None
Taylor et al. [54]	119 surgical	Manual	4.4–6.1		1–4 h	3.4% (P)

137

continued

Table 14.2 continued

Author [Ref]	Number of patients (unless otherwise specified)	Type of insulin protocol	Blood glucose target[1] (mmol l[-1])	Analyser	Sample frequency (hour or mean/ day)	Hypoglycaemia (BG < 2.2 mmol l[-1] unless otherwise specified[2])
2007						
Balkin et al. [67]	221 mixed	Manual	4.2–6.7	Lab, GM	1–3 h	≤ 0.09% (S)
Barth et al. [48]	366 mixed	Manual	5.6–8.3	Lab, GM	1–2 h	5–7% (P) BG < 3.3
Hovorka et al. [41]	30 surgical	Computer eMPC V1.04.03[3]	4.4–6.1	BGA	1–4 h	None
Laha et al. [68]	661 mixed	Computer	4.5–7.2	GM	0.5–4.0 h	1.7% (P)
McMullin et al. [69]	11 medical	Manual NICE-SUGAR pilot	5–7	GM	0.25–2.0 h	36% (P) BG < 2.5
Meynaar et al. [57]	182 mixed	Computer	4.5–7.5	Lab, GM	0.5–4.0 h	0.5% (P) 0.05% (S)
Shulman et al. [56]	50 mixed	Computer	4.4–6.7	GM, BGA	1–2 h	10% (P) 0.2% (S)
2008						
Alm-Kruse et al. [51]	448 mixed	Manual	4.4–6.1	BGA	1–4 h	8.9 % (P) 0.25% (S)
Arabi et al. [27]	266 mixed	Manual	4.4 – 6.1	GM	0.33–4 h	28.6% (P)
Dortch et al. [50]	552 surgical	A: 309 manual. B:243 computer, based on Boord's IP's	4.4–6.1	GM	2 h	A:15.2% (P) 0.54% (S) B: 9.0% (P) 0.23% (S)
Morris et al. [52]	755 mixed	Computer	4.4–6.1		1–4 h	9.4% (P) 0.33% (S)
Pachler et al. [70]	25 medical	Computer eMPC V1.04.03[3]	4.4–6.1	GM	0.5–4.0 h	4% (P)

[1]If more protocols were used, only the one(s) with the tightest glucose control are implemented here.

[2]In percentage of patients (P) or blood glucose samples (S).

[3](e)MPC$_{version number}$, enhanced-model predictive control algorithm.

BG, blood glucose; BGA, blood gas analyser; GM, glucose meter; Lab, laboratory; IP, insulin protocol.

Table 14.3 Differences in intensive insulin therapy (IIT) protocols.

Dosing by absolute glucose values
Dosing by changes in glucose values
Glucose targets
Type and frequency of glucose measurements
Frequency and dose of insulin adjustments
Computer-based or manual
Nurse-driven with or without physician interference
Bolus and continuous insulin infusion
According to levels of insulin resistance
According to type/level of nutrition

insufficiency or hypopituitarism, are at increased risk of hypoglycaemia [72, 73]. Further risk factors include starting continuous venovenous (bicarbonate) haemofiltration [72], and a decreased response to glucagon, cortisol, growth hormone and/or epinephrine (adrenalin). Hypoglycaemia may be an independent predictor of mortality during IIT [23, 24, 73], suggesting that, under certain circumstances, the benefits of TGC may not outweigh the detriments of hypoglycaemia [35, 73]. In cerebral disorders, cerebral glucose levels may be lower and more sensitive to insulin than blood glucose levels, suggesting a higher threshold of blood glucose is necessary to prevent the adverse neurological effects of hypoglycaemia [7, 74]. Hence, neuroglycopaenia and resultant damage may develop even when TGC seems

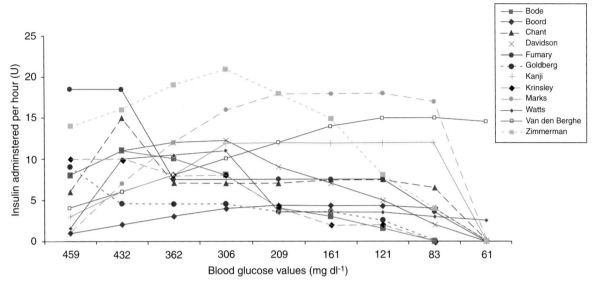

Fig. 14.1 Graphical summary of hourly insulin infusion rates using different insulin protocols to simulate treatment based on laboratory values from a hyperglycaemic patient. From Wilson et al. [38] with permission.

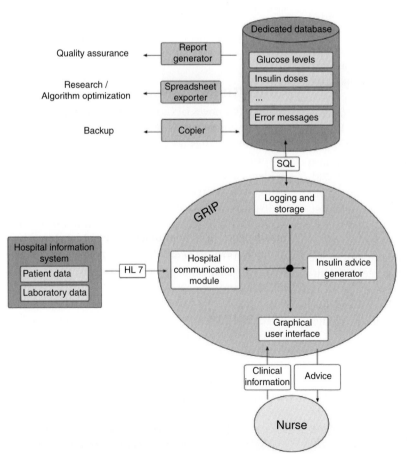

Fig. 14.2 Overview of GRIP (Glucose Regulation for Intensive care Patients). GRIP interaction between an interface with the hospital information system, an interface with the nurse, a component that calculates GRIP's advice, and a component that logs errors and stores all GRIP-generated data. HL 7, Health Level 7 is a communication tool to communicate with the hospital database. SQL, Standard Query Language. From Vogelzang et al. [49] with permission.

effective. Vriesendorp et al. suggested, in contrast, that there were fewer adverse effects of hypoglycaemia in the ICU than had previously been reported [75].

How to measure glucose in the intensive care unit

Frequent blood glucose measurements are needed for implementing safe IIT which warrant accurate point-of-care systems in the ICU, since laboratory measurements are too slow [76–78]. Measurements using hand-held glucose meters utilise enzymes by which glucose is converted to detectable substances. In practice, values from whole blood using these meters are slightly higher than plasma levels partly due to autocorrection by the meter. Falsely elevated levels in point-of-care measurement using glucose meters can result in insulin over treatment [78]. In contrast, whole blood glucose values measured by laboratory techniques and the hexokinase reaction are somewhat lower, at least before correction, than those in plasma, and are dependent on haematocrit, protein levels, pH and temperature. Determinations using finger stick capillary blood should also be avoided since they often vary from measurements taken from arterial or venous blood, or plasma, particularly in hypotensive patients [78]. Determinations in arterial blood are higher than in venous blood by up to 0.6 mmol l^{-1}.

An accurate point-of-care technique utilises arterial blood obtained from indwelling catheters that is then measured in blood gas analysers [76–78]. Point-of-care methods which do not use a blood gas analyser may also dangerously underestimate hypoglycaemia [59, 78]. Fatalities may occur if glucose estimation is carried out from venous blood taken adjacent to a glucose infusion, with subsequent overdosing of insulin. Continuous subcutaneous measurement methods studied mostly in outpatient type 1 diabetics may become useful in the ICU if glucose levels estimated from the interstitial fluids prove to be accurate enough in the critically ill [4, 76, 79]. Due to this difficulty, continuous direct blood measurement methods, i.e., intravascular or through an external circuit, seem more promising.

In search of the right targets

Depending on the efficacy and safety of the IIT protocol and its associated targets, and the frequency of blood glucose measurement, target ranges vary among populations and studies (Table 14.3). Indeed, the cut-off value above which there is a detectable association with increased morbidity and mortality varies among studies, and some observational ones even suggest a target maximum of 8–11.1 mmol l^{-1} that may still benefit patients [12, 20, 26]. Even though Van den Berghe suggests that there is a concentration-morbidity and mortality relationship, arguing in favour of strict control (between 4.4 and 6.1 mmol l^{-1}), more liberal targets (up to 8.3 mmol l^{-1}) may be efficacious and safe [12, 19, 20, 28, 35]. Less strict targets may also be preferable in neurocritical care [74], but this view is not universally supported. Future research is needed to define the most practical, efficacious, cost-effective and safe targets and protocols to be used in the ICU, and these issues may vary between units, glucose measurement methods, patient populations and from country to country [48]. Methods for determining the efficacy and safety of TGC/IIT also vary greatly between studies [39, 80]. Tight glucose control can be expressed as: the time to reach a target; the time spent in a target range; the glycaemic liability, penalty or hyperglycemic indices; the occurrence of hypoglycaemic episodes; the mean glucose levels at various time points and their variability or range; and IIT protocol compliance [39, 80]. The factors that best explain the potential outcome benefits of TGC are the subject of ongoing research.

Conclusions

Many ICUs nowadays practise a form of TGC by IIT and various protocols are in use. Potential benefits should be carefully weighed against the harmful effects of (unnoticed) hypoglycaemia. As there is conflicting evidence as to whether IIT is beneficial, we recommend using computerised protocols to minimise the risk of hypoglycaemia and to target glucose levels below 7.5 mmol l^{-1} in patients expected to stay in the ICU for more than 2 days. Further research is needed to better define the risk to benefit ratios of TGC by IIT, which may be U-shaped, depending on targets, populations, methods and adverse effects.

References

1. Van den Berghe G, Wouters P, Weekers F, et al. Intensive insulin therapy in the critically ill patients. *N Engl J Med* 2001; **345**: 1359–67.

2. Van den Berghe G, Wilmer A, Hermans G, et al. Intensive insulin therapy in the medical ICU. *N Engl J Med* 2006; **354**: 449–61.

3. Cely CM, Arora P, Quartin AA, Kett DH, Schein RMH. Relationship of baseline glucose homeostasis

to hyperglycemia during medical illness. *Chest* 2004; **126**: 879–87.

4. De Block C, van Gaal L, Manuel-y-Keenoy B, Rogiers P. Intensive insulin therapy in the intensive care unit. Assessment by continuous glucose monitoring. *Diabetes Care* 2006; **29**: 1750–6.

5. Corstjens AM, van der Horst ICC, Zijlstra JG, et al. Hyperglycaemia in critically ill patients: marker or mediator of mortality? *Crit Care* 2006; **10**: 216.

6. Egi M, Bellomo R, Stachowski E, et al. Blood glucose concentration and outcome of critical illness: the impact of diabetes. *Crit Care Med* 2008; **36**: 2249–55.

7. Bilotta F, Giovannini F, Caramia R, Rosa G. Glycemia management in neurocritical care patients. A review. *J Neurosurg Anesthesiol* 2009; **21**: 2–9.

8. Ali NA, O'Brien Jr J, Dungan K, et al. Glucose variability and mortality in patients with sepsis. *Crit Care Med* 2008; **36**: 2316–21.

9. Krinsley JS. Glycemic variability: a strong independent predictor of mortality in critically ill patients. *Crit Care Med* 2008; **36**: 3008–13.

10. Groeneveld ABJ, Beishuizen A, Visser FC. Insulin: a wonder drug in the critically ill? *Crit Care* 2002; **6**: 102–5.

11. Turina M, Fry DE, Polk HC. Acute hyperglycemia and the innate immune system: clinical, cellular, and molecular aspects. *Crit Care Med* 2005; **33**: 1624–33.

12. Lazar HL, Chipkin SR, Fitzgerald CA, Bao Y, Carbal H, Apstein CS. Tight glycemic control in diabetic coronary artery bypass graft patients improves perioperative outcomes and decreases recurrent ischemic events. *Circulation* 2004; **109**: 1497–502.

13. Grey NJ, Perdrizet GA. Reduction of nosocomial infections in the surgical intensive-care unit by strict glycemic control. *Endocr Pract* 2004; **10** Suppl 2: 46–52.

14. Reed CC, Stewart RM, Sherman M, et al. Intensive insulin protocol improves glucose control and is associated with a reduction in intensive care unit mortality. *J Am Coll Surg* 2007; **204**: 1048–54.

15. Schmelz LR, DeSantis AJ, Thiyagarajan V, et al. Reduction of surgical mortality and morbidity in diabetic patients undergoing cardiac surgery with a combined intravenous and subcutaneous insulin glucose management strategy. *Diabetes Care* 2007; **30**: 823–8.

16. Scalea TM, Bochicchio GV, Bochicchio KM, Johnson SB, Joshi M, Pyle A. Tight glycemic control in critically injured trauma patients. *Ann Surg* 2007; **246**: 605–12.

17. Hemmila MR, Taddonio MA, Arbabi S, Maggio PM, Wahl WL. Intensive insulin therapy is associated with reduced infectious complications in burn patients. *Surgery* 2008; **144**: 629–35.

18. Kirdemir P, Yildirim V, Kiris I, et al. Does continuous insulin therapy reduce postoperative supraventricular tachycardia incidence after coronary artery bypass operations in diabetic patients? *J Cardiothorac Vasc Anesth* 2008; **22**: 383–7.

19. Van den Berghe G, Wouters PJ, Bouillon R, et al. Outcome benefit of intensive insulin therapy in the critically ill: insulin dose versus glycemic control. *Crit Care Med* 2003; **31**: 359–66.

20. Finney SJ, Zekveld C, Elia A, Evans TW. Glucose control and mortality in critically ill patients. *JAMA* 2003; **290**: 2041–7.

21. Sadhu AR, Martinez DS, Ang AC, Hsueh WA, Ingram-Drake LA, Ettner SL. Economic benefits of intensive insulin therapy in critically ill patients. *Diabetes Care* 2008; **31**: 1556–61.

22. De La Rosa G del C, Donado JH, Restrepo AH, et al. Strict glycaemic control in patients hospitalised in a mixed medical and surgical intensive care unit: a randomised clinical trial. *Crit Care* 2008; **12**: R120.

23. Brunkhorst FM, Engel C, Bloos F, et al. Intensive insulin therapy and pentastarch resuscitation in severe sepsis. *N Engl J Med* 2008; **358**: 125–39.

24. Preiser JC, Devos P, Ruiz-Santane S, et al. A prospective randomized multi-centre controlled trial on tight glucose control by intensive insulin therapy in intensive care units: the Glucontrol study. *Intensive Care Med* 2009; **35**: 1738–48.

25. NICE-SUGAR Study Investigators. Intensive versus conventional glucose control in critically ill patients. *N Engl J Med* 2009; **360**: 1283–97.

26. Oksanen T, Skrifvars MB, Varpula T, et al. Strict versus moderate glucose control after resuscitation from ventricular fibrillation. *Intensive Care Med* 2007; **33**: 2093–100.

27. Arabi YM, Dabbagh OC, Tamim HM, et al. Intensive versus conventional insulin therapy: a randomized controlled trial in medical and surgical critically ill patients. *Crit Care Med* 2008; **36**: 3190–7.

28. Krinsley JS. Effect of an intensive glucose management protocol on the mortality of critically ill adults patients. *Mayo Clin Proc* 2004; **79**: 992–1000.

29. Chase JG, Shaw GM, Le Compte AJ, et al. Implementation and evaluation of the SPRINT protocol for tight glycaemic control in critically ill patients: a clinical practice change. *Crit Care* 2008; **12**: R49.

30. Thomas AN, Marchant AE, Ogden MC, Collin S. Implementation of a tight glycaemia control protocol using a web-based insulin dose calculator. *Anaesthesia* 2005; **60**: 1093–100.

31. Collier B, Diaz J Jr, Forbes R, et al. The impact of a normoglycemic management protocol on clinical outcomes in the trauma intensive care unit. *JPEN J Parenter Enteral Nutr* 2005; **29**: 353–8.

32. Treggiari MM, Karir V, Yanez ND, Weiss NS, Daniel S, Deem SA. Intensive insulin therapy and mortality in critically ill patients. *Crit Care* 2008; **12**: R29.

33. Gandhi GY, Nuttali GA, Abel MD, et al. Intensive intraoperative insulin therapy versus conventional glucose management during cardiac surgery. *Ann Intern Med* 2007; **146**: 233–43.

34. Pittas AG, Siegel RD, Lau J. Insulin therapy and in-hospital mortality in critically ill patients: systematic review and meta-analysis of randomized controlled trials. *JPEN J Parent Enter Nutr* 2006; **30**: 164–72.

35. Wiener RS, Wiener DC, Larson RJ. Benefits and risks of tight glucose control in critically ill adults: a meta-analysis. *JAMA* 2008; **300**: 933–44.

36. Lipshutz AK, Gropper MA. Perioperative glycemic control: an evidence-based review. *Anesthesiology* 2009; **110**: 408–21.

37. Meijering S, Corstjens AM, Tulleken JE, Meertens JHJM, Zijlstra JG, Ligtenberg JJM. Towards a feasible algorithm for tight glycaemic control in critically ill patients: a systematic review of the literature. *Crit Care* 2006; **10**: R19.

38. Wilson M, Weinreb J, Soo Hoo GW. Intensive insulin therapy in critical care: a review of 12 protocols. *Diabetes Care* 2007; **30**: 1005–11.

39. Eslami S, de Keizer NF, de Jonge E, Schultz MJ, Abu-Hanna A. A systematic review on quality indicators for tight glycaemic control in critically ill patients: need for an unambiguous indicator reference subset. *Crit Care* 2008; **12**: R139.

40. Markovitz LJ, Wiechmann RJ, Harris N, et al. Description and evaluation of a glycemic management protocol for patients with diabetes undergoing heart surgery. *Endocr Pract* 2002; **8**: 10–18.

41. Hovorka R, Kremen J, Blaha J, et al. Blood glucose control by a model predictive control algorithm with variable sampling rate versus a routine glucose management protocol in cardiac surgery patients: a randomized controlled trial. *J Clin Endocrinol Metab* 2007; **92**: 2960–4.

42. Brown G, Dodek P. Intravenous insulin nomogram improves blood glucose control in the critically ill. *Crit Care Med* 2001; **29**: 1714–19.

43. Goldberg PA, Siegel MD, Sherwin RS, et al. Implementation of a safe and effective insulin infusion protocol in a medical intensive care unit. *Diabetes Care* 2004; **27**: 461–7.

44. Furnary AP, Wu Y, Bookin SO. Effect of hyperglycemia and continuous intravenous infusions on outcomes of cardiac surgical procedures: the Portland diabetic project. *Endocr Pract* 2004; **10** Suppl 2: 21–33.

45. Davidson PC, Steed RD, Bode BW. Glucommander. *Diabetes Care* 2005; **28**: 2418–22.

46. Chant C, Wilson G, Friedrich JO. Validation of an insulin infusion nomogram for intensive glucose control in critically ill patients. *Pharmacotherapy* 2005; **25**: 352–9.

47. Bland DK, Fankhanel Y, Langford E, et al. Intensive versus modified conventional control of blood glucose level in medical intensive care patients: a pilot study. *Am J Crit Care* 2005; **14**: 370–6.

48. Barth MM, Oyen LJ, Warfield KT, et al. Comparison of a nurse initiated insulin infusion protocol for intensive insulin therapy between adult surgical trauma, medical and coronary care intensive care patients. *BMC Emerg Med* 2007; **7**: 14.

49. Vogelzang M, Zijlstra F, Nijsten MWN. Design and implementation of GRIP: a computerized glucose control system at a surgical intensive care unit. *BMC Med Inform Decis Mak* 2005; **5**: 38.

50. Dortch MJ, Mowery NT, Ozdas A, et al. A computerized insulin infusion titration protocol improves glucose control with less hypoglycemia compared to a manual titration protocol in a trauma intensive care unit. *JPEN J Parent Enter Nutr* 2008; **32**: 18–26.

51. Alm-Kruse K, Bull EM, Laake JH. Nurse-led implementation of an insulin-infusion protocol in a general intensive care unit: improved glycaemic control with increased costs and risk of hypoglycaemia signals need for algorith revision. *BMC Nurs* 2008; **7**: 1–10.

52. Morris AH, Orme J Jr, Truwit JD, et al. A replicable method for blood glucose control in critically ill patients. *Crit Care Med* 2008; **36**: 1787–95.

53. Osbourne RC, Cook CB, Stockton L, et al. Improving hyperglycemia management in the intensive care unit. *Diabetes Educ* 2006; **32**: 394–403.

54. Taylor BE, Schallom ME, Sona CS, et al. Efficacy and safety of an insulin infusion protocol in a surgical ICU. *J Am Coll Surg* 2006; **202**: 1–9.

55. Braithwaite SS, Edkins R, Macgregor KL, et al. Performance of a dose-defining insulin infusion protocol among trauma service intensive care unit admissions. *Diabetes Technol Ther* 2006; **8**: 476–88.

56. Shulman R, Finne SJ, O'Sullivan C, Glynne PA, Greene R. Tight glycaemic control: a prospective observational study of a computerised decision-supported intensive insulin therapy protocol. *Crit Care* 2007; **11**: R75.

57. Meynaar I, Dawson L, Tangkau PL, Salm EF, Rijks L. Introduction and evaluation of a computerised insulin protocol. *Intensive Care Med* 2007; **33**: 591–6.

58. Goldberg PA, Sakharova OV, Barrett PW, et al. Improving glycemic control in the cardiothoracic intensive care unit: clinical experience in two hospital settings. *J Cardiothorac Vasc Anesth* 2004; **18**: 690–7.

59. Kanji S, Buffie J, Hutton B, Bunting PS, et al. Standardization of intravenous insulin therapy improves the efficiency and safety of blood glucose control in critically ill adults. *Intensive Care Med* 2004; **30**: 804–10.

60. Laver S, Preston S, Turner D, McKinstry C, Padkin A. Implementing intensive insulin therapy: development and audit of the Bath protocol. *Anaesth Intensive Care* 2004; **32**: 311–16.

61. Orford N, Stow P, Green D, Corke C. Safety and feasibility of an insulin adjustment protocol to maintain blood glucose concentrations within a narrow range in critically ill patients in an Australian level III adult intensive care unit. *Crit Care Resusc* 2004; **6**: 92–8.

62. Zimmerman CR, Mlynarek ME, Jordan JA, Rajda CA, Horst HM. An insulin infusion protocol in critically ill cardiothoracic surgery patients. *Ann Pharmacother* 2004; **38**: 1123–9.

63. Dilkhush D, Lannigan J, Pedroff T, Riddle A, Tittle M. Insulin infusion protocol for critical care units. *Am J Health Syst Pharm* 2005; **62**: 2260–4.

64. Ku SY, Sayre CA, Hirsch IB, Kelly JL. New insulin infusion protocol improves blood glucose control in hospitalized patients without increasing hypoglycemia. *Jt Comm J Qual Patient Saf* 2005; **31**: 141–7.

65. Lonergan T, Le Compte A, Willacy M, et al. A pilot study of the SPRINT protocol for tight glycemic control in critically ill patients. *Diabetes Technol Ther* 2006; **8**: 449–62.

66. Plank J, Blaha J, Cordingley J, et al. Multicentric, randomized, controlled trial to evaluate blood glucose control by the model predictive control algorithm versus routine glucose management protocols in intensive care unit patients. *Diabetes Care* 2006; **29**: 271–6.

67. Balkin M, Mascioli C, Smith V, et al. Achieving durable glucose control in the intensive care unit without hypoglycaemia: a new practical IV insulin protocol. *Diabetes Metab Res Rev* 2007; **23**: 49–55.

68. Laha SK, Taylor R, Collin SA, Ogden M, Thomas AN. Glucose control in critical illness using a web-based insulin dose calculator. *Med Eng Phys* 2008; **30**: 478–82.

69. McMullin J, Brożek J, McDonald E, et al. Lowering of glucose in critical care: a randomized pilot trial. *J Crit Care* 2007; **22**: 112–18.

70. Pachler C, Plank J, Weinhandl H, et al. Tight glycaemic control by an automated algorithm with time-variant sampling in medical ICU patients. *Intensive Care Med* 2008; **34**: 1224–30.

71. Clayton SB, Mazur JE, Condren S, Hermayer KL, Strange C. Evaluation of an intensive insulin protocol for septic patients in a medical intensive care unit. *Crit Care Med* 2006; **34**: 2974–8.

72. Vriesendorp TM, van Santen S, DeVries JH, et al. Predisposing factors for hypoglycemia in the intensive care unit. *Crit Care Med* 2006; **34**: 96–101.

73. Krinsley JS, Grover A. Severe hypoglycemia in critically ill patients: risk factors and outcomes. *Crit Care Med* 2007; **35**: 2262–7.

74. Oddo M, Schmidt M, Carrera E, et al. Impact of tight glycemic control on cerebral glucose metabolism after severe brain injury: a microdialysis study. *Crit Care Med* 2008 ; **36**: 3233–8.

75. Vriesendorp TM, DeVries JH, van Santen S, et al. Evaluation of short-term consequences of hypoglycemia in an intensive care unit. *Crit Care Med* 2006; **34**: 2714–18.

76. Corstjens Am, Ligtenberg JJM, van der Horst ICC, et al. Accuracy and feasibility of point-of-care and continuous blood glucose analysis in critically ill ICU patients. *Crit Care* 2006; **10**: R135.

77. Dungan K, Chapman J, Braithwaite SS, Buse J. Glucose measurements: confounding issues in setting targets for in patient management. *Diabetes Care* 2007; **30**: 403–9.

78. Hoedemaekers CWE, Klein Gunnewiek JMT, Prinsen MA, Willems JL, van der Hoeven JG. Accuracy of bedside glucose measurement from three glucometers in critically ill patients. *Crit Care Med* 2008; **36**: 3062–6.

79. Ellmerer M, Haluzik M, Blaha J, et al. Clinical evaluation of alternative-site glucose measurements in patients after major cardiac surgery. *Diabetes Care* 2006; **29**: 1275–81.

80. Van Herpe T, De Brabanter J, Beullens M, De Moor B, Van den Berghe G. Glycemic penalty index for adequately assessing and comparing different blood glucose control algorithms. *Crit Care* 2008; **12**: R24.

Chapter 5

Glucocorticoids in the critically ill

Pauline M. O'Neil and Nigel R. Webster

Introduction

Glucocorticoids have been used therapeutically in critical illness for at least 50 years. They are synthetic versions of the physiologically active hormone (cortisol, also known as hydrocortisone), which has a myriad of functions in the body. Glucocorticoids are used in many conditions seen in the critically ill when anti-inflammatory action or immunosuppression is required. We shall consider the rationale for the use of glucocorticoids in sepsis and septic shock, acute respiratory distress syndrome (ARDS), pneumonia, post-extubation stridor, spinal cord injury, meningitis and cerebral oedema.

Pharmacology of glucocorticoids

Synthetic glucocorticoids are administered most commonly to the intensive care unit (ICU) population intravenously, although they may be given by the oral, rectal, intramuscular, inhalational, intra-articular or topical routes. The various glucocorticoids available have subtly different properties, which influences choice in clinical scenarios [1] (Table 15.1).

Glucocorticoids are lipophilic compounds, usually administered as prodrugs. Greater than 70% of the drug is protein-bound in the plasma to cortisol binding globulin (CBG) and albumin [1]. Cortisol binding globulin has a high affinity and low capacity for glucocorticoids, and is saturated at > 1100 nmol l⁻¹, a level achieved by administering hydrocortisone 20 mg [1, 2]. Albumin has low affinity and high capacity for glucocorticoids. Hydrocortisone and prednisolone bind to CBG and albumin and have dose-dependent pharmacokinetics, whereas methylprednisolone and dexamethasone bind only to albumin which results in no dose-dependency [2]. Dose-dependency has the effect of increasing unbound glucocorticoid when drug concentration exceeds a

threshold, through a reduction in protein-binding. It is only the unbound glucocorticoid which has biological activity. This fact has particular relevance in the critically ill where low plasma albumin levels increase unbound, active glucocorticoid concentrations.

Metabolism occurs intracellularly by the enzyme 11β-hydroxysteroid dehydrogenase (11β-HSD). In glucocorticoid target tissues such as the liver, 11β-HSD 1 converts cortisone to the active cortisol. Mineralocorticoid target tissues, such as the kidney, colon, salivary glands and placenta, contain 11β-HSD 2 which converts cortisol to the inactive cortisone [2]. High peak concentrations of glucocorticoids may overwhelm the capacity of this system and cause mineralocorticoid side effects. Once dissociated, the glucocorticoid crosses the cell membrane into the cell cytoplasm.

Within the cytoplasm, the glucocorticoid receptor (GCR) forms an inactive complex with two molecules of heat shock protein (HSP) 90 and other proteins [3]. Binding of glucocorticoid (GC) results in dissociation of GCR from this complex, and translocation to the cell nucleus. Here the GC-GCR complex has a variety of actions both genomic and non-genomic [2]. A homodimer of two GC-GCR complexes acts on glucocorticoid response elements (GRE) on the promoter region of glucocorticoid responsive genes. This results in activation of gene transcription (transactivation) and the formation of anti-inflammatory proteins [3] (Figure 15.1). The GC-GCR complex also acts to inactivate pro-inflammatory gene transcription and inhibit pro-inflammatory transcription factors such as nuclear factor kappa B (NF-κB) and activator protein 1 (AP)-1 (transrepression, Figure 15.1) [3]. Transactivation underlies most of the metabolic actions of the glucocorticoids whereas transrepression is responsible for most of the anti-inflammatory effects.

Core Topics in Endocrinology in Anaesthesia and Critical Care, eds. George M. Hall, Jennifer M. Hunter and Mark S. Cooper. Published by Cambridge University Press. © Cambridge University Press 2010.

Table 15.1 Glucocorticoids commonly used in critical care.

	Glucocorticoid potency	Mineralocorticoid potency	Duration of action (hours)	Comments
Hydrocortisone	1.0	1.0	8	Unwanted mineralocorticoid effects at high doses
Prednisolone	4	0.8	24	Most commonly used oral glucocorticoid
Methylprednisolone	5	0.5	24–36	Better lung penetration than prednisolone. Large volume of distribution; accumulates in alveoli
Dexamethasone	25	0	72	Negligible mineralocorticoid effects. Good CNS penetration

CNS, central nervous system.

From Chin et al. [1] with permission.

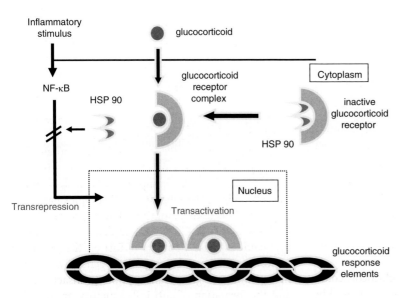

Fig. 15.1 Cellular actions of glucocorticoids. HSP, heat shock protein.

Dissociated steroids are currently in development which target transrepression (thus reducing their metabolic effects) but have little impact on transactivation, in the hope that they will have fewer side effects. Nongenomic mechanisms of glucocorticoid activity have yet to be fully elucidated, but result in the rapid onset of therapeutic effect. The postulated mechanisms include membrane stabilisation, receptor interaction and direct protein interaction [4]. Ultimately, glucocorticoids inhibit pro-inflammatory cytokine synthesis, promote anti-inflammatory cytokine synthesis, stimulate T cell, eosinophil and monocyte apoptosis, and inhibit neutrophil activation [2]. Clearance of glucocorticoids occurs by hepatic metabolism and is affected by enzyme induction and inhibition by other drugs. Clearance is increased by certain drugs including phenytoin, barbiturates and rifampicin [1].

It should also be remembered that glucocorticoids have many side effects, some of which are potentially serious [2] (Table 15.2).

Table 15.2 Side effects of glucocorticoids.

Body system	Side effect
CNS	Depression, mania, psychosis, delirium, cerebral atrophy
CVS	Hypertension, dyslipidaemia
Renal	Hypokalaemia, hypernatraemia, fluid retention
GI	Peptic ulcers, pancreatitis, GI haemorrhage
Metabolic/endocrine	Hyperglycaemia, body fat redistribution, adrenal atrophy
Musculoskeletal	Myopathy, critical illness neuropathy, osteoporosis, bone necrosis
Haematological	Neutropaenia, tumour lysis syndrome
Infection	Recurrent infection, fungal infection, polymicrobial infection
Other	Delayed wound healing, cataracts

CNS, central nervous sytem; CVS, cardiovascular system; GI, gastrointestinal.

From Czock et al. [2] with permission.

Adrenal insufficiency in the critically ill

Primary adrenal insufficiency is rarely seen in the critically ill and it has a prevalence in the general population of between 40 and 110 per million [5, 6]. In primary adrenal insufficiency the adrenal cortex is destroyed by either an autoimmune process, infection, haemorrhage, tumour or thrombosis [7]. Diagnosis is clearly defined as a morning cortisol level of < 83 nmol l^{-1}, with levels > 525 nmol l^{-1} ruling out adrenal insufficiency [7]. All cortisol levels between these values require dynamic testing with the short corticotrophin stimulation test (CST), where a normal result is a basal cortisol or peak of > 500 nmol l^{-1} [7]. Clearly, although rare, a missed diagnosis of primary adrenal insufficiency in a critically ill patient would be catastrophic.

Secondary adrenal insufficiency can result from hypothalamic or pituitary disease, or more commonly from therapy with glucocorticoids. In these situations, ACTH production is inadequate and cortisol secretion correspondingly reduced. In patients with secondary adrenal insufficiency the available diagnostic tests include insulin induced hypoglycaemia, a short metyrapone test, corticotrophin releasing hormone test and the low and high dose corticotrophin stimulation tests [7]. With exogenous glucocorticoid therapy, it has

been suggested that a dose equivalent to < 5 mg day^{-1} of prednisolone will not inhibit hypothalamic-pituitary-adrenal (HPA) axis function [6]. However, some authors believe that development of secondary adrenal insufficiency is dependant on duration of therapy, highest dose and cumulative dose of steroid [8]. Time to full recovery of adrenal function has been quoted as anywhere between two days and one year [9]. Testing of the HPA axis with the short CST would seem prudent in this situation. Glucocorticoid replacement in severe illness should be with hydrocortisone 100–150 mg day^{-1} [9].

Relative (also known as functional) adrenal insufficiency is a widely debated concept with no clearly defined diagnostic criteria, and an incidence which varies between 10 and 71% depending on the definition used [10]. Cortisol levels usually increase in the critically ill patient which reflects an adequate adrenal response to stress, through an increase in corticotrophin releasing hormone [8]. There is increased conversion of cortisone to cortisol, a reduction in hepatic metabolism and renal clearance, an increase in corticotrophin, and a reduction in CBG level which results in an increase in unbound cortisol levels [8, 9, 11]. Interestingly, both high and low levels of cortisol have been shown to correlate with increased mortality in the critically ill [8, 9]. However, the most recent data from the CORTICUS (Corticosteroid Therapy of Septic Shock) study in septic shock found no correlation between mortality and random cortisol but did find a relationship between lower CST increment and mortality [10]. It may be that a low initial cortisol level reflects an inadequate response to stress in the patient, and a persistently raised cortisol indicates continuing inflammatory response to an overwhelming illness.

As can be seen in Table 15.3 [8–14], there is no consensus on the precise level of total plasma cortisol level which reflects an adequate response to critical illness. The short CST increment of < 248 nmol l^{-1} may reflect relative adrenal insufficiency, but this is also problematic as a maximally stimulated HPA axis will not show an adequate increment yet plasma cortisol will be high. This would be inconsistent with a diagnosis of relative adrenal insufficiency.

There is also the issue of the current assessment of total plasma cortisol levels, which does not accurately reflect the physiologically important free cortisol. This is especially relevant in hypoproteinaemic critically ill patients. Therefore, we should be measuring serum free cortisol which can be estimated by either calculated free cortisol, free cortisol index or salivary

Table 15.3 Diagnostic criteria for relative adrenal insufficiency.

Author	Patient group	Plasma cortisol (nmol l⁻¹)	CST peak (nmol l⁻¹)	CST increment (nmol l⁻¹)
Lamberts et al. 1997 [9]	Critically ill	< 275	< 495	
Cooper & Stewart 2003 [8]	Critically ill	< 413 AI likely 413–935 CST		< 248
Cooper & Stewart 2007 [11]	Critically ill	< 413 AI likely 413–688 CST	< 688	
Bouachour et al. 1995 [12]	Sepsis	< 413	< 495	
Annane et al. 2000 [13]	Sepsis			< 248
Marik & Zaloga 2003 [14]	Sepsis	< 688		
Lipiner-Friedman et al. 2007 [10]	Sepsis	< 200 AI 200–700 CST		< 248

AI, adrenal insufficiency; CST, cosyntropin stimulation testing.

cortisol concentration [15]. These tests are not widely available at present.

Of importance in the ICU, adrenal insufficiency will also result from the use of etomidate, as clearly shown by Finlay and Watt in 1983 who reported a mortality increase from 25 to 44% with the use of an etomidate infusion [16]. Even a single dose of etomidate has been shown to cause adrenal suppression for 24 hours [17]. Etomidate should be used with caution in the critically ill and alternative agents considered.

Glucocorticoids in sepsis and septic shock

The history of glucocorticoid use in sepsis and septic shock has waxed and waned. Over the past 50 years, we have seen the use of high doses for short duration, then lower doses for longer durations with tapering of the dose. As new evidence has become available, the indications for the use of glucocorticoids in patients with sepsis have been refined.

In sepsis and septic shock, glucocorticoids are thought to have effects on the immune response and on vascular responsiveness to catecholamines [18]. The immune response is modulated by a reduction in pro-inflammatory cytokine production and a reduction in the inflammatory response without causing immunosuppression [18]. Glucocorticoids enhance vascular endothelial responsiveness to catecholamines by as yet unknown mechanisms [18].

Early studies between 1960 and 1990 used high doses of methylprednisolone, betamethasone and dexamethasone for typically less than 24 hours in patients with sepsis and septic shock. These studies were hampered by a lack of a consensus definition of sepsis and septic shock and poor trial methodology. Work from Schumer in 1976 showed a large mortality benefit from glucocorticoid therapy, which was not replicated in other studies [19]. Two meta-analyses from 1995 found, respectively, 10 and 9 adequate studies of glucocorticoids in sepsis and septic shock [19, 20]. Their conclusions were reassuringly consistent. Lefering and Neugebauer included 10 studies, with a glucocorticoid dose given equivalent to up to 42 times that now routinely used (currently hydrocortisone 200 mg day⁻¹), but 9 of the studies only gave 24 hours of therapy [19]. Overall, there was no mortality benefit in giving glucocorticoids in the treatment of sepsis and septic shock. There was also no difference in adverse events (gastrointestinal bleed, superinfection, hyperglycaemia) in the treatment groups. Of note, the subgroup of patients with gram-negative infection had a 5.6% mortality benefit when given glucocorticoids [19]. Cronin et al.'s meta-analysis from the same year found no statistically significant difference in mortality when glucocorticoids were used to treat sepsis and septic shock [20]. However, their conclusion was that there was a trend to increased mortality when glucocorticoids were used in overwhelming infection and septic shock. This may reflect a slightly higher gastro-intestinal bleed rate in those given glucocorticoids [20]. In 1992, the Infectious Disease Society of North America recommended that glucocorticosteroids should not be used in septic shock [19]. The late 1990s saw a resurgence in interest in glucocorticoid use in septic shock with lower doses of hydrocortisone being used. A meta-analysis in 2004 showed a correlation between higher doses of glucocorticoids and higher mortality [21].

Table 15.4 Post-1997 studies of glucocorticoids in septic shock.

Study	Inclusion criteria	No. of patients	Therapy	CST	Outcome
Bollaert et al. 1998 [22]	Septic shock > 48 h	41	Hydrocortisone 100 mg 3 × day for 5 days	No difference in outcome	Shock reversal at 7 days 68% vs. 21%. 28-day mortality 32 vs. 63% (statistically significant)
Briegel et al. 1999 [23]	Septic shock < 72 h, vasopressor use, cardiac index > 4 l min^{-1} m^2	40	Hydrocortisone 100 mg then 0.18 mg kg^{-1} h^{-1}, then 0.08 mg kg^{-1} h^{-1} for 6 days when shock reversed		Median time to cessation of vasopressors 2 vs. 7 days
Annane et al. 2002 [24]	Septic shock > 1 h, up to 3 h (changed to 8 h during study)	299	Hydrocortisone 50 mg 4 × day & Fludrocortisone 50 µg 1 × day for 7 days	229 non-responders (< 248 nmol l^{-1} increment) 70 responders	Overall 28-day mortality 55 vs. 61% (non-significant) Non-responders 28-day mortality 53 vs. 63% (significant)
Sprung et al. 2008 [25]	Septic shock < 72 h, vasopressors > 1 h	499	Hydrocortisone 50 mg 4 × day for 5 days then tapered over 6 days	233 non-responders, 266 responders (< 248 nmol l^{-1} increment)	No difference in 28-day mortality; CST response had no effect. Median time to shock reversal 3.3 vs. 5.8 days

CST, cosyntropin stimulation testing.

More recent studies are shown in Table 15.4 [22–25]. The study by Annane et al. changed practice in managing the patient with septic shock despite some concerns regarding etomidate use, changes to inclusion criteria during the trial and the fact that the statistically significant results were from a *post hoc* subgroup analysis [24]. Etomidate was used in 24% of the patients in the study, and 68/72 were non-responders to the short CST. These patients would be expected to benefit from receiving glucocorticoid replacement. The CORTICUS study from 2008 has not definitively answered the question, as it was stopped early and had a lower than expected control group mortality and is therefore underpowered [25].

At present, there is convincing evidence that hydrocortisone therapy in septic shock reduces time to reversal of shock, but this has not consistently shown a benefit in survival. The 2008 Surviving Sepsis Campaign guidelines still suggest considering hydrocortisone therapy (≤ 300 mg day^{-1}, tapered once vasopressors have been stopped) in the patient with septic shock if they have hypotension which is poorly responsive to fluids and vasopressors [26]. The evidence is graded as weak and of low quality. The CST does not have a place in assessing suitability for glucocorticoid therapy in septic shock except in the rare patient suspected to have Addison's disease [26].

Glucocorticoids in pulmonary disorders

Glucocorticoids are used in many pulmonary disorders seen in the critically ill. Conditions of most relevance to the critically ill patient population are ARDS, pneumonia and post-extubation stridor. Glucocorticoids also have a role in the management of acute respiratory failure due to asthma, chronic obstructive pulmonary disease, alveolar haemorrhage syndromes, acute lupus pneumonitis, bronchiolitis obliterans organising pneumonia (BOOP), radiation pneumonitis and pulmonary drug toxicity [27]. Although for some of these conditions this is based on limited evidence and is controversial.

Table 15.5 Trials of glucocorticoid therapy in acute respiratory distress syndrome.

Trial	Indication	MP regimen
Meduri et al. 1998 [37]	ARDS not improving at day 7	MP 2 mg kg^{-1} loading dose Day 1–14: 2 mg kg^{-1} day^{-1} Day 15–21: 1 mg kg^{-1} day^{-1} Day 22–28: 0.5 mg kg^{-1} day^{-1} Day 29–30: 0.25 mg kg^{-1} day^{-1} Day 31–32: 0.125 mg kg^{-1} day^{-1} (If extubated, proceed to day 15)
Steinberg et al. 2006 [38]	ARDS > 7 days	MP 2 mg kg^{-1} loading dose 0.5 mg kg^{-1} 6 hourly for 14 days 0.5 mg kg^{-1} 12 hourly for 7 days then taper over 4 days if unable to spontaneously ventilate for 48 h, 2 days if able to spontaneously ventilate for 48 h or disseminated fungal infection
Meduri et al. 2007 [39]	ARDS > 72 h	MP 1 mg kg^{-1} loading dose Day 1–14: 1 mg kg^{-1} day^{-1} Day 15–21: 0.5 mg kg^{-1} day^{-1} Day 22–25: 0.25 mg kg^{-1} day^{-1} Day 26–28: 0.125 mg kg^{-1} day^{-1} (If extubated, proceed to day 15, if no improvement at day 7–9, then MP 2 mg kg^{-1} day^{-1})

ARDS, acute respiratory distress syndrome; MP, methylprednisolone.

Acute respiratory distress syndrome

Acute respiratory distress syndrome (ARDS) is a syndrome of pulmonary inflammation which can develop in response to a variety of precipitants in the critically ill. In 1994 the American–European Consensus Conference Committee recommended the definition of ARDS as a disease of acute onset, with bilateral infiltrates on chest radiography, a pulmonary-artery wedge pressure < 18 mmHg or the absence of clinical evidence of left atrial hypertension and a PaO_2:FiO_2 of < 200 mmHg [28]. Acute respiratory distress syndrome remains an illness with a high mortality rate of 30–50% [29, 30].

Pathologically, ARDS is divided into early exudative and late proliferative phases. During the exudative phase, there is loss of the integrity of the alveolar-capillary barrier and the alveolar spaces fill with an inflammatory exudate composed of neutrophils, macrophages, hyaline membranes and protein-rich fluid [31]. In some patients, ARDS progresses to a late proliferative stage, characterised by progressive pulmonary fibrosis [31]. This can occur as early as 5–7 days into the course of ARDS. Histologically there is fibrosis, new vessel formation, continued inflammation and some resolution of the alveolar oedema.

Corticosteroids are attractive as a therapy in ARDS, as they should theoretically reduce inflammation and therefore prevent late fibrotic lung disease. Table 15.5 shows the recent trials of steroid use in ARDS [37–39].

In unresolving ARDS, Meduri et al. demonstrated that methylprednisolone therapy suppressed the activity of NF-κB, reduced production of the pro-inflammatory cytokines tumour necrosis factor-alpha (TNF-α, interleukin (IL) -1β and IL-6, and increased glucocorticoid receptor mediated activity [32]. The same group found that plasma and bronchoalveolar lavage levels of procollagen aminoterminal propeptide type I and type III were elevated in ARDS, remained elevated at day 7 in patients who did not improve, and reduced rapidly in those non-improvers given methylprednisolone [33].

Use of high dose corticosteroids for a short duration of therapy in early ARDS was studied in the 1980s, with no evidence of a beneficial effect on mortality [34–36]. A small randomised controlled trial by Meduri et al. from 1998 studied the use of lower dose methylprednisolone for a longer duration in 24 patients with unresolving ARDS (> 7 days) [37]. This study used methylprednisolone 2 mg kg^{-1} as a bolus followed by 2 mg kg^{-1} day^{-1} for 14 days then a slowly tapering dose until day 32, as described in Table 15.5. There was an improved PaO_2:FiO_2 ratio, lung injury score, and an ICU mortality reduction from 63 to 13% in the methylprednisolone-treated patients. However, this trial was small and featured a cross-over design which meant that 20 of the 24 patients received corticosteroids.

The 2006 ARDSnet trial studied the use of methylprednisolone in late (> 7 days) ARDS [38]. A total of 180 patients were studied, and there was no difference in mortality at 60 days. The secondary outcomes of ventilator free days, shock free days and ICU free days were lower in the treatment group at 28 days. This was not maintained at 180 days, when there was an increased ICU readmission rate in the treatment group, perhaps related to the increased rate of neuromuscular weakness. The authors also studied the subgroup which commenced methylprednisolone therapy after 14 days of ARDS, and found an increased mortality (35 vs. 8%) in *post hoc* analysis. This *post hoc* analysis is underpowered, so it is not possible to draw any firm conclusions from it.

Meduri et al. has also studied the use of methylprednisolone 1 mg kg^{-1} day^{-1} for up to 28 days in ARDS of less than 72 hours duration [39]. There were 91 patients included in the study, and there was a statistically significant difference in the number of patients with a reduction of one point in the lung injury score in the treatment group. Significantly more patients were ventilator free at 7 days in the treatment group. Limits to this study are the high proportion (66%) of patients who also had septic shock and the small sample size.

Glucocorticoids may have a role in the treatment of ARDS of less than 14 days duration, when it can increase ventilator free days and may reduce mortality [40]. This is at the expense of increased infection rates, which may present without a fever. Indeed, regular surveillance bronchoalveolar lavage should be considered if using glucocorticoids for ARDS.

Pneumonia

It would seem counter-intuitive to prescribe immunosuppressant drugs in an infectious condition, but as with septic shock, glucocorticoids may immunomodulate to prevent excessive inflammation causing damage to the lung. *Pneumocystis jiroveci* pneumonia (PCP) in HIV infected patients had a mortality of below 15% when mechanical ventilation was required [27]. A consensus statement in 1990 recommends the use of prednisolone 40 mg 12 hourly on days 1–5, 40 mg day^{-1} on days 6–10 and 20 mg day^{-1} on days 11–21 when substantial hypoxaemia is present [27]. (Hypoxaemia was defined as $P_aO_2 < 70$ mm Hg or A-a gradient > 35 mm Hg on air). A Cochrane review from 2006 found a reduction in the relative risk of death of 44% at 1 month, most pronounced in patients not treated with antiretroviral therapy [41]. There was also an improvement in mortality at four months and in the need for mechanical ventilation [41].

One study has suggested that a seven-day course of hydrocortisone reduced mortality in severe community acquired pneumonia [42]. Forty-six patients with severe pneumonia were included, and the treatment arm received hydrocortisone 200 mg then 10 mg h^{-1}. There was an improvement in oxygenation, a reduction in multiple organ dysfunction score and a reduction in delayed septic shock by day 8. There were, however, significant discrepancies in the baseline characteristics between the two groups, the study size was small and the study was stopped early. Glucocorticoids do not have a place in the routine management of severe community acquired pneumonia at present.

Post-extubation stridor

In the critically ill patient, post-extubation stridor can result in the need for re-intubation and prolong ICU stay. Glucocorticoids may reduce laryngeal oedema, which may reduce stridor and possibly reduce re-intubation rates. In one study, methylprednisolone 40 mg given 24 hours prior to extubation in patients intubated for greater than 24 hours with a cuff leak volume less than 24% of tidal volume reduced post-extubation stridor [43]. A further large study randomised all patients ventilated for greater than 36 hours to receive methylprednisolone 20 mg every 4 hours until extubation [44]. Laryngeal oedema was reduced from 22 to 3%, and reintubations reduced from 8 to 4%. Methylprednisolone will reduce post-extubation laryngeal oedema in intubated ICU patients, but this has not been shown conclusively to translate into a reduction in re-intubation rate or mortality.

Glucocorticoids in CNS disorders

Cerebral oedema

Glucocorticoids are used in the management of cerebral oedema associated with primary and metastatic tumours, radiotherapy and surgical manipulation [45]. Dexamethasone 10 mg initially, then 4 mg 6 hourly is used, and the dose is tapered slowly. The exact mechanisms of this reduction in vasogenic oedema are not fully understood, but theories include a reduction in endothelial cell permeability, increased extracellular fluid clearance and metabolic changes within the tumour [45]. Response to glucocorticoids is often rapid, so the effects must be mediated through non-genomic actions of glucocorticoids.

Glucocorticoids are not useful in either cytotoxic cerebral oedema due to traumatic brain injury, or in ischaemic or haemorrhagic stroke [45]. The CRASH (corticosteroid randomisation after significant head injury) trial of 10 008 adults with a Glasgow coma scale (GCS) of < 14 following head injury found increased risk of death in the group given glucocorticoids, and was stopped early as a result [46]. In this trial, the treatment group was given methylprednisolone 2 mg kg^{-1} loading dose then 0.4 g h^{-1} for 48 hours. The conclusion from this is that glucocorticoids should not be given to patients with a head injury.

Meningitis

In meningitis, inflammation worsens when antibiotic therapy causes bacterial cell wall breakdown, leading to the release of cytokine and chemokines [45]. These inflammatory mediators facilitate vasogenic oedema by increasing vascular permeability. Glucocorticoids inhibit this inflammation and can improve patient outcome. Initial work from children with meningitis has resulted in the recommendation that dexamethasone 0.15 mg kg^{-1} (with or before the first dose of antibiotic) 6 hourly for 4 days is given to all children over 2 months with meningitis [45]. Dexamethasone given to adult patients with meningitis, before or with the first dose of antibiotic, reduces morbidity and mortality. A trial of 301 patients with bacterial meningitis used dexamethasone 10 mg 6 hourly for 4 days and found a decrease in unfavourable outcome (GCS ≤ 5) from 25 to 15% [47]. Mortality was also reduced from 15 to 7% with the administration of glucocorticoids. Patients with pneumococcal pneumonia demonstrated the most benefit from adjunctive dexamethasone, with unfavourable outcome reducing from 52 to 26% and mortality reducing from 34 to 14%. There is some concern that dexamethasone therapy will reduce CSF penetration by vancomycin through a reduction in permeability of the blood-brain barrier, as has been shown in animal studies [45]. Vancomycin is used in patients with penicillin-resistant *pneumococcus* or *Staphylococcus aureus* meningitis. It has therefore been recommended that patients treated with vancomycin and dexamethasone are carefully observed [47]. Dexamethasone should be administered with or before the first dose of antibiotic in patients with bacterial meningitis, especially if the organism is the pneumococcus.

Spinal cord injury

Spinal cord injury is a devastating condition which results in disability in patients who were previously well. The mechanisms of spinal cord injury can be divided into two phases: primary and secondary. Primary spinal cord injury results from the mechanical force of the trauma, and as such can only be treated by prevention of the trauma. Secondary spinal cord injury occurs up to weeks following the initial insult, and contributes to 10% of the overall pathology [48]. The pathological processes involved include spinal cord hypoxaemia, ischaemia, ion shifts, lipid peroxidation, oedema, free radical and prostaglandin production [48]. Methylprednisolone acts to prevent lipid peroxidation and is a free radical scavenger, which may help prevent secondary spinal cord injury [48].

The National Acute Spinal Cord Injury Studies (NASCIS) I–III were three large randomised studies of the effects of methylprednisolone on neurological recovery following spinal cord injury. Published between 1984 and 1998, their results are summarised in Table 15.6 [48–50]. These studies led to the widespread use of methylprednisolone to manage spinal cord injury. The Cochrane review from 2002 suggested that high dose methylprednisolone would improve functional recovery in patients with spinal cord injury if given within 8 hours of injury, and that for those patients who begin treatment at 3–8 hours following injury a 48-hour course would further improve outcome [49]. Methylprednisolone treatment of spinal cord injury remains controversial, however. There is some concern that the studies all showed no difference in their primary outcome, and that *post hoc* analysis of smaller groups of patients is weaker evidence [48]. Translation of the improved motor scores into meaningful functional recovery is another area which has been questioned by critics [48]. Potentially serious side effects can also occur with the use of methylprednisolone in high doses, and this should be borne in mind when considering using this drug. However, increased side effects did not cause an increase in mortality in the NASCIS trials [49]. Indeed, trauma.org has published an editorial reviewing the evidence for the use of steroids in spinal cord injury [50]. Their recommendations are that 'there is no evidence to support the use of steroids in the management of spinal cord injury' and that 'administration of high dose steroids to trauma patients can have significant adverse effects on patient outcome' [50]. Despite such sentiments, methylprednisolone is still used in spinal cord injury. This may reflect the lack of other treatments which have proven benefit, conviction that steroids can improve patient outcome, the fear of litigation or peer pressure [47].

Conclusions

Glucocorticoids are used in the critically ill either as replacement therapy when the patients' response

Table 15.6 Trials of methylprednisolone (MP) in spinal cord injury.

Trial	Groups	Outcome	Side effects
NASCIS I, 1984	MP 100 mg then MP 25 mg 6 hourly for 10 days, or MP 1000 mg then MP 250 mg 6 hourly for 10 days	No difference in functional recovery at 6 months	High dose MP group had a significantly higher rate of wound infection
NASCIS II, 1990	MP 30 mg kg^{-1} within 1 h, then 5.4 mg kg^{-1} h^{-1} for 23 h, or naloxone 5.4 mg kg^{-1}, then 4.5 mg kg^{-1} h^{-1} for 23 h or placebo	No difference in neurological outcome at 1 year *Post hoc* analysis: MP given < 8 h after injury improved motor and sensory scores at 6 months, improved motor scores at 1 year	Higher rates of infection and pulmonary embolism in MP group
Otani, 1994	MP 30 mg kg^{-1} then 5.4 mg kg^{-1} h^{-1} for 23 h or placebo	No difference in neurological outcome *Post hoc* analysis: improved sensation in MP group	Trend to increased septic complications in MP group
NASCIS III, 1997	MP 30 mg kg^{-1} to all patients then 5.4 mg kg^{-1} h^{-1} for 24 h or 48 h, or Tirilazad 2.5 mg kg^{-1} 6 hourly for 48 hours	No difference in neurological outcome at 1 year *Post hoc* analysis: MP given for 48 h between 3–8 hours after injury improved motor scores at 6 weeks and 6 months	Pneumonia and severe sepsis more common in those given MP for 48 h
Petitjean, Pointillart, 1998, 2000	MP 30 mg kg^{-1} then 5.4 mg kg^{-1} h^{-1} for 23 h, or nimodipine 0.5 mg kg^{-1} h^{-1} for 2 h then 0.03 mg kg^{-1} h^{-1} for 7 days, or MP and nimodipine or placebo	No difference in neurological outcome at 1 year	Trend to increased septic complications in MP group

Data from Hurlbert [48], Bracken [49] and Trauma.org [50].

is inadequate, or for conditions which require their anti-inflammatory or immunomodulatory effects. For absolute adrenal insufficiency, glucocorticoid therapy will be potentially life saving. The central nervous system conditions of vasogenic cerebral oedema and pneumococcal meningitis benefit from glucocorticoid treatment, as does PCP pneumonia. However, in patients with septic shock unresponsive to fluids and vasopressors, ARDS of less than 14 days duration, pneumonia, those at high risk of post-extubation stridor and non-penetrating spinal cord injury, glucocorticoids may be of some use, but the evidence of benefit is not conclusive. For all critically ill patients, we should weigh the risks of using these drugs which have potentially serious side effects against any potential benefits.

References

1. Chin R, Eagerton DC, Salem M. Corticosteroids. In Chernow B, Brater DC, eds. *The Pharmacologic Approach to the Critically Ill Patient*, 3rd edn. Williams and Wilkins, Baltimore, 1994, pp. 715–41.

2. Czock D, Keller F, Rasche FM, et al. Pharmacokinetics and pharmacodynamics of systemically administered glucocorticoids. *Clin Pharmacokinet* 2006; **44**: 61–98.

3. Barnes PJ. How corticosteroids control inflammation: Quintiles prize lecture 2005. *Br J Pharmacol* 2006; **148**: 245–54.

4. Buckingham JC. Glucocorticoids: exemplars of multi-tasking. *Br J Pharmacol* 2006; **147**: S258–68.

5. Rady MY, Johnson DJ, Patel B, et al. Corticosteroids influence the mortality and morbidity of acute critical illness. *Crit Care* 2006; **10**: R101.

6. Coursin DB, Wood KE. Corticosteroid supplementation for adrenal insufficiency. *JAMA* 2002; **287**: 236–40.

7. Oelkers W. Adrenal insufficiency. *N Engl J Med* 1996; **335**: 1206–12.

8. Cooper MS, Stewart PM. Corticosteroid insufficiency in acutely ill patients. *N Engl J Med* 2003; **348**: 727–34.

9. Lamberts SWJ, Bruining HA, De Jong FH. Corticosteroid therapy in severe illness. *N Engl J Med* 1997; **337**: 1285–92.

10. Lipiner-Friedman D, Sprung CL, Laterre PF, et al. Adrenal function in sepsis: The retrospective

CORTICUS cohort study. *Crit Care Med* 2007; **35**: 1012–18.

11. Cooper MS, Stewart PM. Adrenal insufficiency in critical illness. *J Intensive Care Med* 2007; **22**: 348–62.

12. Bouachour G, Tirot P, Gouello JP, et al. Adrenocortical function during septic shock. *Intensive Care Med* 1995; **21**: 57–62.

13. Annane D, Sebille V, Troche G, et al. A three-level prognostic classification in septic shock based on cortisol levels and cortisol response to corticotrophin. *JAMA* 2000; **283**: 1038–45.

14. Marik PE, Zaloga GP. Adrenal insufficiency during septic shock. *Crit Care Med* 2003; **31**: 141–5.

15. Arafah BM. Hypothalamic pituitary adrenal function during critical illness: Limitations of current assessment methods. *J Clin Endocrinol Metab* 2006; **91**: 3725–45.

16. Ledingham IMCA, Watt I. Influence of sedation on mortality in critically ill multiple trauma patients. *Lancet* 1983; **1**: 1270.

17. Absalom A, Pledger D, Kong A. Adrenocortical function in critically ill patients 24h after a single dose of etomidate. *Anaesthesia* 1999; **54**: 861–7.

18. Annane D. Glucocorticoids in the treatment of severe sepsis and septic shock. *Curr Opin Crit Care* 2005; **11**: 449–53.

19. Lefering R, Neugebauer EAM. Steroid controversy in sepsis and septic shock: a meta-analysis. *Crit Care Med* 1995; **23**: 1294–303.

20. Cronin L, Cook DJ, Carlet J, et al. Corticosteroid treatment for sepsis: a critical appraisal and meta-analysis of the literature. *Crit Care Med* 1995; **23**: 1430–9.

21. Minneci PC, Deans KJ, Banks SM, et al. Meta-analysis: The effect of steroids on survival and shock during sepsis depends on the dose. *Ann Intern Med* 2004; **141**: 47–56.

22. Bollaert PE, Charpentier C, Levy B, et al. Reversal of late septic shock with supraphysiological doses of hydrocortisone. *Crit Care Med* 1998; **26**: 645–50.

23. Briegel J, Forst H, Haller M, et al. Stress doses of hydrocortisone reverse hyperdynamic septic shock: A prospective, randomised, double-blind, single center study. *Crit Care Med* 1999; **27**: 723–32.

24. Annane D, Sebille V, Bollaert PE, et al. Effect of treatment with low doses of hydrocortisone and fludrocortisone on mortality in patients with septic shock. *JAMA* 2002; **288**: 862–71.

25. Sprung CL, Annane D, Keh D, et al. Hydrocortisone therapy for patients with septic shock. *N Engl J Med* 2008; **358**: 111–24.

26. Dellinger RP, Levy MM, Carlet J, et al. Surviving sepsis campaign: International guidelines for management of severe sepsis and septic shock: 2008. *Intensive Care Med* 2008; **34**: 17–60.

27. Jantz MA, Sahn SA. Corticosteroids in acute respiratory failure. *Am J Respir Crit Care Med* 1999; **160**: 1079–100.

28. Bernard GR, Artigas A, Brigham KL, et al. The American-European Consensus Conference on ARDS: definitions, mechanisms, relevant outcomes, and clinical trial coordination. *Am J Respir Crit Care Med* 1994; **149**: 818–24.

29. Rubenfeld GD, Caldwell E, Peabody E, et al. Incidence and outcomes of acute lung injury. *N Engl J Med* 2005; **353**: 1685–93.

30. ARDSnet. Ventilation with lower tidal volumes as compared with traditional tidal volumes for acute lung injury and the acute respiratory distress syndrome. *N Engl J Med* 2000; **342**: 1301–8.

31. Ware LB, Matthay MA. The acute respiratory distress syndrome. *N Engl J Med* 2000; **342**: 1334–49.

32. Meduri GU, Tolley EA, Chrousos GP, Stentz F. Prolonged methylprednisolone treatment suppresses systemic inflammation in patients with unresolving acute respiratory distress syndrome. *Am J Respir Crit Care Med* 2002; **165**: 983–91.

33. Meduri GU, Tolley EA, Chinn A, Stentz F, Postlethwaite A. Procollagen types I and III aminoterminal propeptide levels during acute respiratory distress syndrome and in response to methylprednisolone treatment. *Am J Respir Crit Care Med* 1998; **158**: 1432–41.

34. Bone RC, Fisher CJ, Clemmer TP, Slotman GJ, Metz CA. Early methylprednisolone treatment for septic syndrome and the adult respiratory distress syndrome. *Chest* 1987; **92**: 1032–6.

35. Bernard GR, Luce JM, Sprung CL, et al. High dose corticosteroids in patients with the adult respiratory distress syndrome. *N Engl J Med* 1987; **317**: 1565–70.

36. Luce JM, Montgomery AB, Marks JD, Turner J, Metz CA, Murray JF. Ineffectiveness of high-dose methylprednisolone in preventing parenchymal lung injury and improving mortality in patients with septic shock. *Am Rev Respir Dis* 1988; **138**: 62–8.

37. Meduri GU, Headley AS, Golden E, et al. Effect of prolonged methylprednisolone therapy in unresolving acute respiratory distress syndrome. *N Engl J Med* 1998; **280**: 159–65.

38. Steinberg KP, Hudson LD, Goodman RB, et al. Efficacy and safety of corticosteroids for persistent acute respiratory distress syndrome. *N Engl J Med* 2006; **354**: 1671–84.

39. Meduri GU, Golden E, Freire AX, et al. Methylprednisolone infusion in early severe Acute Respiratory Distress Syndrome: Results of a randomised controlled trial. *Chest* 2007; **131**: 954–63.

40. Peter JV, John P, Graham PL, et al. Corticosteroids in the prevention and treatment of acute respiratory distress syndrome (ARDS) in adults: Meta-analysis. *BMJ* 2008; **336**: 1006–9.

41. Briel M, Bucher HC, Boscacci R, et al. Adjunctive corticosteroids for pneumocystis jiroveci pneumonia in patients with HIV infection. *Cochrane Database Syst Rev* 2006; **3**: CD 006150.

42. Confalonieri M, Urbino R, Potena A, et al. Hydrocortisone infusion for severe community-acquired pneumonia. *Am J Respir Crit Care Med* 2005; **171**: 242–8.

43. Cheng KC, Hou CC, Huang HC, et al. Intravenous injection of methylprednisolone reduces the incidence of post-extubation stridor in intensive care unit patients. *Crit Care Med* 2006; **34**: 1345–50.

44. Francois B, Bellisant E, Gissot V, et al. 12-h treatment with methylprednisolone versus placebo for prevention of post-extubation laryngeal oedema: a randomised double-blind trial. *Lancet* 2007; **369**: 1083–9.

45. Rabinstein AA. Treatment of cerebral edema. *Neurologist* 2006; **12**: 59–73.

46. CRASH trial collaborators . Final results of MRC CRASH, a randomised placebo-controlled trial of intravenous corticosteroid in adults with head injury – outcomes at 6 months. *Lancet* 2005; **365**: 1957–9.

47. De Gans J, Van de Beek D. Dexamethasone in adults with bacterial meningitis. *N Engl J Med* 2002; **347**: 1549–56.

48. Hurlbert RJ. Strategies of medical intervention in the management of acute spinal cord injury. *Spine* 2006; **11**: S16–21.

49. Bracken MB. Pharmacological interventions for acute spinal cord injury (Cochrane Review). *The Cochrane Library*, Issue 2, 2002.

50. Trauma.org. Steroids in spinal cord injury, 2005. http://www.trauma.org/index.php/main/article/394, accessed 5 February, 2008.

Chapter 6

Diabetic hyperglycaemic crises

Barbara Philips

Diabetic ketoacidosis (DKA) and hyperglycaemic hyperosmolar state (HHS) are the major hyperglycaemic crises associated with diabetes mellitus. They are frequently considered as separate conditions but as will be shown in the following discussions they really represent two ends of a spectrum of hyperglycaemic and metabolic derangement, and not infrequently exist in combination. As many as 30–33% of all hyperglycaemic crisis admissions can be expected to have a mixed DKA/HHS metabolic picture [1, 2].

Epidemiology

The number of patients admitted to hospital with DKA has remained remarkably unchanged over the past 10 years with approximately 7700 admissions in 1998–1999 and 8400 admissions in 2004–2005 in England alone [3]. In children, 40% (range 26–67% across 24 European centres) with newly diagnosed diabetes mellitus present with DKA [4], and younger age increases this risk. Women are twice as likely as men to be admitted with DKA. If managed in an experienced centre, mortality is reported as < 5% [3], and the majority of deaths occur among the elderly or patients with significant co-morbidities and intercurrent illnesses. However, DKA itself remains a common cause of death in young people with 0.15–0.30% of children with DKA dying of it [5]. The majority of patients with DKA have type 1 diabetes mellitus but it can occur in patients with type 2 diabetes mellitus, even in patients not normally requiring supplemental insulin. Recurrent DKA accounts for 15% of cases and is more common in women [6] and in patients who are socially deprived and poorly educated or those with learning difficulties. Occasionally, recurrent DKA is a manifestation of psychological illness including eating disorders [6].

Hyperglycaemic hyperosmolar state is generally associated with older patients with type 2 diabetes mellitus and significant co-morbidities, and is considered less common than DKA with an incidence of 1 per 1000 person-years in patients with diabetes mellitus (DKA is 4.6–8.0 per 1000 person-years) [7]. However, it is now being observed more often, in young obese patients and in some ethnic groups (e.g., Afro-Caribbean patients) and it is associated with a high mortality (> 15%) [3, 8]. These patients are also more likely to present with a hyperglycaemic crisis which has features of both DKA and HHS. This phenomenon has been given a number of titles, including diabetes type 1B, idiopathic type 1 diabetes, flatbush diabetes, atypical diabetes and ketosis-prone type 2 diabetes. Twenty five to fifty per cent of newly diagnosed diabetics from certain ethnic groups will present with this syndrome, in particular Africans and Hispanic Americans [9]. These patients may or may not require insulin for the management of their diabetes mellitus when not in crisis and in fact may have near normal glycaemic control when well. Obesity and a family history of type 2 diabetes mellitus appear to be significant risk factors [9].

Definitions

There are no universally agreed definitions of DKA or HHS. Both are defined by clinical and biochemical derangements. The biochemical diagnostic criteria are shown in Table 16.1 but these are only guidelines. A mixed picture may occur and the metabolic acid-base imbalance in HHS or indeed DKA may be complicated by concurrent illness or the severity of dehydration with the development of a lactic acidosis. Difficulties may arise if no distinction is made between DKA and HHS.

Pathogenesis (Figure 16.1)

The pathogeneses of these conditions are not fully elucidated but the primary factor is a total or relative deficiency of insulin. The resulting increased circulating concentrations of counter-regulatory hormones (glucagon, cortisol, catecholamines, growth hormone

Table 16.1 Biochemical diagnosis of diabetic hyperglycaemic crises. Patients with a blood glucose concentration greater than 33 mmol l⁻¹ but with ketones in their urine should be considered to have a mixed diabetic ketoacidosis/hyperosmolar state (DKA/HHS).

	DKA	DKA/HHS mixed	HHS
Plasma glucose (mmol l⁻¹)	> 14.0 < 33	> 33	> 33
Arterial pH	< 7.3	< 7.3	> 7.3
Serum bicarbonate (mmol l⁻¹)	< 18	< 18	> 15
Plasma ketones	+++	+/++	Negative
Urine ketones	++/+++	++/+++	Negative
Effective serum osmolality (mOsm kg⁻¹)	Variable	> 320	> 320
Anion gap	> 10	> 10	< 12
Conscious level	Variable	Confusion	Depressed/coma

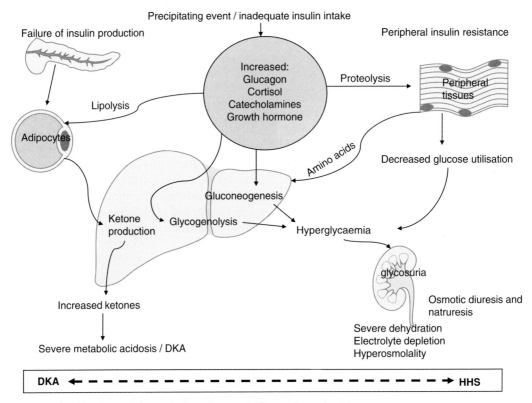

Fig. 16.1 Hormonal and biochemical changes in the pathogenesis of hyperglycaemic crisis.

and cytokines) augment the hyperglycaemia [10–12]. Diabetic ketoacidosis and HHS are the two ends of a continuum from the total deficiency of insulin causing DKA to the relative lack and insulin resistance which causes HHS.

Insulin

Deficiency of insulin prevents the entry of glucose, potassium and some amino acids into many tissues (e.g.,

muscle, liver, adipocytes). Glycogen synthesis is decreased from the lack of substrate and glycogen synthase is inhibited. Glycogenolysis is increased and gluconeogenesis is unopposed. In adipocytes, hormone-sensitive lipase is activated and lipoprotein lipase inhibited. Lipogenesis is thus decreased and lipolysis increased [1]. Lipolysis increases the availability of glycerol for gluconeogenesis and free fatty acids (FFA) are released which are oxidised within mitochondria to ketones (acetoacetate and β-hydroxybutyrate). The deficiency of insulin also prevents the uptake of ketones into insulin dependent cells, further aggravating the ketonaemia. Protein catabolism is unopposed, protein synthesis is decreased, and gluconeogenic amino acids are released into the circulation.

Insulin may have anti-inflammatory properties through the inhibition of the synthesis of pro-inflammatory cytokines, and therefore insulin deficiency may be associated with increased circulating concentrations of tumour necrosis factor-alpha (TNF-α), interleukin (IL) -1β, IL-6 and IL-8 [13, 14]. Whether this is primarily an effect of insulin or secondary to hyperglycaemia rather than insulin deficiency per se is uncertain.

Glucagon

Despite the absence of hypoglycaemia to stimulate glucagon secretion, the plasma glucagon concentration is increased in DKA secondary to a variety of stressors including cortisol, catecholamines (beta-adrenergic effect), infection and failure of inhibition by insulin. Glucagon is gluconeogenic, glycogenolytic, lipolytic and ketogenic. The ratio of glucagon to insulin may determine the severity of ketosis. This ratio determines the concentration of malonyl coenzyme A (malonyl CoA) [15]. Malonyl CoA inhibits carnitine palmitoyl acyltransferase (CPT1), a facilitator of FFA transport across mitochondrial membranes and the rate limiting step in the generation of ketones. In the absence of malonyl CoA, CPT1 is uninhibited [1, 16, 17].

Catecholamines

Insulin deficiency causes increased secretion of epinephrine (adrenaline) and norepinephrine (noradrenaline) via a number of mechanisms and in response to stressors including ketoacidosis, lactic acidosis, hyperosmolality and infection. Catecholamines augment glycogenolysis in both muscle and liver and increase gluconeogenesis in liver and kidney. They also directly increase the activity of hormone-sensitive lipase, aggravating lipolysis [1].

Cortisol

Glucocorticoid secretion is similarly increased by stressors and cortisol has a marked effect on intermediary metabolism. Many, although not all, effects are mediated via the promotion of increased DNA transcription leading to enzyme synthesis. Peripheral insulin resistance is increased secondary to an inhibition of glucose phosphorylation and glucocorticoids directly increase protein catabolism and increased gluconeogenesis.

However, much of the diabetogenic effects of cortisol are permissive; notably, steroids have to be present in order for glucagon and the catecholamines to exert their effects. Insulin effects are enhanced in the absence of corticosteroids.

Growth hormone

Growth hormone mobilises FFA from adipocytes and is a potent promoter of ketogenesis [18]. It decreases glucose uptake into some tissues, increases hepatic glucose output and decreases tissue insulin binding. The actions of glucagon, cortisol and growth hormone cause insulin resistance in the peripheries and are important in the pathogenesis of HHS [1, 10].

Water deficit

Both DKA and HHS are characterised by severe electrolyte and fluid derangements. All patients are severely dehydrated secondary to an osmotic diuresis. Glucose is a highly effective osmotic agent and increased plasma concentrations increase the osmolality of blood and the urine. Glucose is freely filtered and once the renal threshold for reabsorption of glucose is exceeded (approximately 12 mmol l⁻¹) glucose accumulates within the renal tubules and causes an osmotic diuresis with loss of water and electrolytes, including sodium, potassium and magnesium.

Patients with DKA tend to present to hospital earlier than patients with HHS possibly because of the ketoacidosis and the rapidity with which intolerable symptoms develop. Hyperglycaemic hyperosmolar state has a more insidious onset: patients are less severely acidotic, but plasma glucose concentrations are markedly greater. Consequently, patients with HHS are likely to be much more dehydrated than patients with DKA. Typical water deficits in adults are 100 mg kg⁻¹ (7 litres for a 70 kg man) in patients with DKA, and 100–200 mg kg⁻¹ (average 10.5 litres for a 70 kg man) in patients with HHS (Table 16.2). As will be discussed later, patients with HHS, despite being more dehydrated, need to be resuscitated more cautiously than patients with DKA.

Sodium

On admission the patient should be assumed to be sodium deplete in the order of 7–10 mmol kg⁻¹ (490–700 mmol per 70 kg man) for DKA and 5–13 mmol kg⁻¹ (350–910 mmol per 70 kg man) for HHS [7]. Patients frequently present with hyponatraemia, although normal or even high sodium concentrations at presentation may be observed. The interpretation of

Table 16.2 Total body deficits for water and electrolytes with typical values for a 70 kg man.

Deficits per kg body weight	DKA	HHS
Water (ml kg^{-1})	100 (7 litres)	100–200 (7–14 litres)
Na$^+$ (mmol kg^{-1})	7–10 (490–700)	5–13 (350–910)
K$^+$ (mmol kg^{-1})	3–5 (210–350)	4–6 (280–420)
Cl$^-$ (mmol l^{-1})	3–5 (210–350)	5–15 (350–1050)
Mg^{2+} (mmol kg^{-1})	0.5–1.0 (35–70)	0.5–1.0 (35–70)
Ca^{2+} (mmol kg^{-1})	0.5–1.0 (35–70)	0.5–1.0 (35–70)
PO$_4^{2-}$ (mmol kg^{-1})	0.5–1.0 (35–70)	0.5–1.0 (35–70)

From Kitabchi et al. [10] with permission.

sodium concentrations is complex; it is dependent on the duration and severity of the presenting condition and probably best considered in terms of the movement of water rather than sodium ions per se (Figure 16.2). The osmotic force generated by the increasing plasma glucose concentration initially draws water out of the intracellular compartment, diluting the plasma sodium concentration (Figure 16.2a). Glucose in the renal tubules increases renal water and sodium loss exacerbating the effect of increased plasma glucose concentrations and cells become profoundly dehydrated. If allowed to continue, the water content of the extracellular compartment, after initially expanding will contract as the severity of the dehydration worsens. Eventually, the patient may present with normal or increased sodium concentration, despite total body sodium deficiency. Indeed, normal or high sodium at presentation, prior to any treatment may be indicative of a prolonged and severe hyperglycaemia. Other signs of severe dehydration may be evident, including shock, a raised urea and acute kidney injury.

On the initiation of treatment with insulin, cells immediately take up glucose (Figure 16.2b). As the plasma glucose concentration decreases, the osmotic forces within the extracellular compartment diminish and the net movement of water is no longer out of the cells. In the period of dehydration it is thought that cells may accumulate osmotically active molecules (idiogenic osmoles, since their identity is uncertain) and become osmotically charged and the net movement of water changes, favouring movement of water into the cells. This rehydration of cells may be desirable but if excessive may cause serious complications, including cerebral oedema. It is possible that patients with HHS and children with DKA are particularly vulnerable to rapid and excessive movement of water: first, because of the high plasma glucose concentrations observed; second, because of the profound dehydration; and, third, because of the damage caused to the regulatory mechanisms of cells by the period of stress and inflammation [19].

The movement of water from the extracellular compartment is too rapid for the adaptation of ion concentrations and hypernatraemia is observed which may be severe (> 165 mmol l^{-1}) despite the large total body sodium deficit (Figure 16.2b). Although it is recommended that active steps are taken to correct the sodium concentration once it exceeds 155 mmol l^{-1} [12], there is emerging evidence that hypernatraemia is protective against the development of cerebral oedema [20]. Hypernatraemia may be of benefit by conferring a maintained osmotic potential. This would counter the movement of water out of the extracellular compartment into cells. The key to the successful management of these patients is the slow correction of glucose and sodium. There is no indication for the use of hypotonic solutions to correct hypernatraemia.

Diabetic patients with DKA may develop a severe hyperlipidaemia. This can interfere with indirect sodium assays (frequently found in automated laboratories) and factitiously low sodium concentrations may be reported. Blood gas analysers use a direct method of sodium measurement and are unaffected by hyperlipidaemia. If a means of direct measurement is not available or in the presence of excess triglycerides, the true sodium concentration can be calculated using the following formula:

$$[Na^+]_{corrected}\ mmol\ l^{-1} = [Na^+]_{measured}\ mmol\ l^{-1}$$
$$+\ ((1.6 \times ([glucose]_{plasma} - 5.6)/5.6))\ [5].$$

Potassium

Diabetic ketoacidosis and HHS are associated with a total body potassium deficit ranging from 3 to 15 mmol kg^{-1}

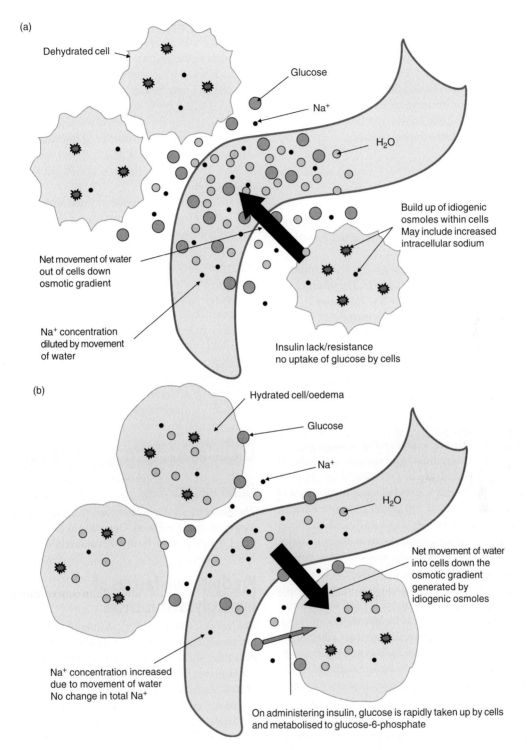

Fig. 16.2 (a) Hyperglycaemia draws water into the extracellular fluid compartment, dehydrating the intracellular space. Glycosuria causes an osmotic diuresis and natriuresis but the initial hyponatraemia observed is primarily caused by the movement of water. Dehydrated cells become osmotically charged with an increase in intracellular idiogenic osmoles. (b) Glucose is rapidly taken up by cells after the administration of insulin. The osmotic potential of the extracellular compartment decreases and water moves into cells down a reversed osmotic gradient. The plasma concentration of sodium increases but total sodium does not change; the change in concentration is secondary to the movement of water and may be protective against the development of cerebral oedema.

(210–1050 mmol per 70 kg man) [7]. Potassium moves with water from the intracellular space to the extracellular space and patients may appear hyperkalaemic when first presenting to hospital. Potassium is, however, lost with the osmotic diuresis and initial insulin therapy can cause a precipitous decrease in serum potassium as it is moved back into cells. Losses may be exacerbated by secondary hyperaldosteronism, vomiting and poor oral intake.

Osmolality

In healthy individuals, intracellular and extracellular osmolality are equal, approximating between 280 and 295 mOsm kg^{-1} H_2O and can be measured directly or calculated.

Calculated osmolality $(Osm_c) = 2 \times [Na^+]$ mmol l^{-1} + [urea] mmol l^{-1} + [glucose] mmol l^{-1}. For instance, for a normal healthy person with a Na 140 mmol l^{-1}, urea 5 mmol l^{-1} and glucose 5 mmol l^{-1}, osmolality is equal to 290 mOsm kg^{-1} H_2O. Although urea is an osmotically active solute, it is described as an ineffective solute because it is freely soluble across cell membranes. The effective osmolality of plasma (or tonicity) is determined by solutes unable to move freely, i.e., sodium, chloride and glucose. The effective osmolality (tonicity) is calculated as $2 \times [Na^+] \times$ mmol l^{-1} + [glucose] mmol l^{-1}.

A patient with DKA presenting with a glucose concentration of 30 mmol l^{-1} and sodium 130 mmol l^{-1} would have an osmolality of 290 mOsm kg^{-1} H_2O. A patient with HHS with a blood glucose of 80 mmol l^{-1} and an initial sodium of 130 mmol l^{-1} would have an osmolality of 340 mOsm kg^{-1} H_2O. As described above, on the initiation of treatment the movement of water as glucose is taken up into cells may cause the patient to develop hypernatraemia (e.g., sodium of 160 mmol l^{-1}). The glucose concentration will have decreased with fluid and insulin (e.g., to 40 mmol l^{-1}) and the effective osmolality will have increased to 360 mOsm kg^{-1} H_2O. Although on first inspection this appears alarming it may well be protective against sudden and rapid movement of water into cells. Hypernatraemia should not be actively corrected in the early stages of resuscitation.

Acid-base balance

Both DKA and HHS are associated with a metabolic acidosis (Table 16.1). The acidosis associated with DKA is more severe and is the probable cause of its earlier presentation. Ketogenesis is the precipitating factor. Acetoacetic acid and β-hydroxybutyric acid are the two ketones generated and these dissociate at physiological pH. Bicarbonate is lost in the buffering of the hydrogen ions generated and β-hydroxybutyrate and acetoacetate circulate as the anions. The result is a severe metabolic acidosis with an increased anion gap (AG).

The AG may be calculated as AG = $[Na^+] + [K^+]$ – $[Cl^-] - [HCO_3]$ and is normally 8–12 mmol l^{-1}. In critical care, calculating the corrected anion gap (AGc) is useful for identifying the presence of unusual anions [21], and can be calculated as AGc = $([Na^+] + [K^+] - [Cl^-] - [HCO_3])$ – (albumin (g l^{-1}) + 1.5 $[PO_4^{2-}]$ (mmol l^{-1}) + [lactate] (mmol l^{-1})).

DKA is one condition associated with an increased AG, others include, uraemia, lactic acidosis and poisoning from methanol, salicylates and ethylene glycol.

Hyperglycaemic hyperosmolar state is not characterised by a metabolic acidosis generated by ketones but patients frequently present with a lactic acidosis. Profound dehydration and circulatory compromise increase tissue lactate production causing a metabolic acidosis. In keeping with the greater dehydration, this is usually more severe in HHS than DKA, although this may not be apparent from the initial pH. Patients with a ketoacidosis tend to be more acidotic than those with a lactic acidosis. However, whereas recovery from ketoacidosis may be rapid as the biochemical abnormality is reversed by insulin, recovery from lactic acidosis may be more protracted requiring the restoration of an adequate circulation and correction of biochemistry.

Other electrolytes

The osmotic diuresis also causes loss of phosphate, magnesium and calcium. Deficits may be in the order of 0.5–1.0 mmol kg^{-1} in both DKA and HHS (Table 16.2).

Precipitating factors of hyperglycaemic crises

The most common precipitating factor for hyperglycaemia crisis is infection (19–25%) [6, 7, 13, 22], including pneumonia, urinary tract infection and sepsis. However, for a substantial number of patients, up to 20% of adults [10] and 40% of children [23], a hyperglycaemic crisis is the presenting feature of diabetes mellitus and the lack of a prior history should not influence the diagnosis. Other precipitants include: insulin error (omission or inadequate dosing), acute pancreatitis, myocardial infarction, cerebrovascular accident, acute intestinal obstruction, certain drugs (e.g., corticosteroids, thiazide diuretics, beta-adrenergic blockers, chlorpromazine and phenytoin), heat stroke, acromegaly, thyrotoxicosis, Cushing's syndrome and excessive ingestion of high glucose containing drinks. This list is not exhaustive and the precipitating factor may not always be clearly identified [10]. It may also be difficult to distinguish between a precipitating factor and a complication of the crisis.

Clinical presentation

Diabetic ketoacidosis

Diabetic ketoacidosis occurs most frequently in younger patients with type 1 diabetes mellitus, but 13% of cases in the USA are patients over the age of 60 years and a small proportion of patients will have type 2 diabetes mellitus [12]. Normally DKA has a rapid onset (1–3 days) and patients present with polyuria, polydipsia, weight loss and weakness. On examination, patients will exhibit the signs of dehydration: dry mucosa, lax skin turgor, tachycardia and tachypnoea, progressing to hypotension or even shock. Kussmaul–Kien respiration (rapid and deep breathing) is classical in DKA and exhaled breath may have the typical sweet fruity odour of ketones, although not everyone is capable of detecting this smell. Other signs and symptoms associated with underlying conditions (e.g., infection) or co-morbidities may occur.

One of the more difficult symptoms to manage is severe abdominal pain. The risk and severity of acute abdominal pain appears to be related to the severity of the acidosis and indeed may indicate impaired mesenteric perfusion [7, 17]. The difficulty is that the signs and symptoms including nausea, vomiting, absent bowel sounds and peritonitis do not distinguish DKA from a surgical cause. Furthermore, an acute abdominal crisis requiring urgent surgery may precipitate DKA [24–26]. Blood tests are not particularly helpful; an increased amylase may indicate pancreatitis, but it is also increased in bowel perforation and by DKA itself. Similarly, markers of infection (e.g., white cell counts [wcc] and C-reactive protein [CRP]) may be raised by a variety of factors, and serum lactate may not distinguish between life-threatening causes and DKA. Consequently, these patients require urgent surgical review, close observation during resuscitation of the DKA and possibly further imaging, including CT scanning of the abdomen.

Hyperglycaemic hyperosmolar syndrome

Hyperglycaemic hyperosmolar syndrome (HHS) usually occurs in older patients with type 2 diabetes mellitus and has traditionally been discounted in young patients presenting in hyperglycaemic crisis. However, HHS is increasing in frequency in all age groups and this has been attributed to the increasing prevalence of type 2 diabetes associated with obesity [2, 5, 27]. Hyperglycaemic hyperosmolar syndrome presents with a longer history than DKA (typically 7–10 days) but symptoms are similar. Most patients present complaining of polyuria, polydipsia and lethargy but as the severity of HHS increases the patient may present with confusion and even coma. Given the usual age of the patients, co-morbidities and concurrent illnesses are common, and signs and symptoms may vary considerably due to the many potential precipitating factors. Important precipitants include: cerebrovascular accidents (CVAs), myocardial infarction (MI) and serious infection. Occasionally and particularly in the previously undiagnosed patient, HHS may be precipitated by a high intake, in response to thirst, of glucose-rich fluids. Medications that predispose to the development of HHS include corticosteroids and thiazide diuretics.

Patients with HHS are profoundly dehydrated. They present with tachycardia, hypotension, cool peripheries, dry mucous membranes and decreased skin turgor. The dehydration and osmolality may be so severe that HHS causes myocardial infarction or limb or gut ischaemia. Severe hyperosmolality (e.g., > 330 mOsm kg^{-1}) is associated with deteriorating mental status and 30% of patients with HHS present in coma. Patients may alternatively present with focal neurology or seizures [17]. Coma is rare if the osmolality is < 320 mOsm kg^{-1}. However, the risk of severe mental deterioration is not isolated to presentation. Patients with HHS are at a serious risk of cerebral complications during treatment, particularly cerebral oedema and even death.

Investigations

The aim of any immediate investigations is to ascertain the severity of the metabolic derangement and to identify underlying treatable causes. It is important to distinguish between DKA and HHS as the initial management is different. Any patients with a blood glucose concentration > 33 mmol l^{-1} or a serum osmolality > 315 mOsm kg^{-1} should be treated as having HHS regardless of whether they have ketones in their urine or not.

Immediate management

The immediate management of DKA and HHS are similar but not the same. If in doubt, treat the patient as if they have HHS. The most important difference is in

Table 16.3 Investigations.

Investigations required		Comments
Blood	Glucose	Greater than 33 mmol l⁻¹ implies HHS or HHS/DKA
	Full blood count	White cell count may be increased or decreased in sepsis
	Electrolytes	Patients are both sodium and potassium deplete. This may not be obvious in the initial blood test
	Urea and creatinine	Urea may be increased secondary to dehydration or AKI. Creatinine is increased in cases of AKI.
	LFTs	LFTs may be impaired, particularly if dehydration is profound.
	C-reactive protein	Increased in cases precipitated or complicated by infection
	Amylase	May be mildly increased in DKA and HHS secondary to dehydration, impaired gut perfusion and even non-pancreatic sources (e.g., parotid gland). Moderately increased secondary to bowel perforation. Markedly increased if the crisis secondary to pancreatitis
	Osmolality	Markedly increased in HHS, may be increased in DKA
	Arterial blood gas	Severe metabolic acidosis in DKA with normal/mildly increased lactate Less severe metabolic acidosis in HHS but more likely to have a marked increase in lactate $PaCO_2 < 4.5$ kPa secondary to hyperventilation caused by metabolic acidosis. PaO_2 normal unless crisis precipitated by lung infection or if crisis causes a thromboembolic complication, e.g., pulmonary embolus
	Lactate	May be increased in DKA Increased in HHS
	Blood cultures	Blood cultures should be taken, even if patient is not pyrexial. Severe dehydration can cause hypothermia, therefore pyrexia may not be evident, even if patient is severely septic
Urine	Dipstick	Ketones will be strongly positive in DKA and absent in HHS. Presence of ketones in a patient with a glucose > 33 mmol l⁻¹ suggests mixed DKA/HHS picture. Blood and protein may indicate a unrinary tract infection
	Microscopy and culture	For identifying urinary tract infection
CXR		A CXR may confirm pneumonia as the cause of the hyperglycaemic crisis. If an acute abdomen is suspected, the CXR should be performed as erect as possible to look for air under the diaphragm
ECG		An acute myocardial infarction may precipitate a diabetic crisis or may be precipitated by hyperosmolar conditions
CT	Head	Presentation in coma or progression to coma may occur in hyperglycaemic crises, especially HHS. Either DKA or HHS may be precipitated by a cerebrovascular accident in vulnerable patients. A CT scan of the head will: (1) exclude a haemorrhagic event; (2) indicate an ischaemic event (imaging may be too early for definite diagnosis); and (3) reveal cerebral oedema (BUT the absence of CT signs does not exclude cerebral oedema as a complication)
	Abdomen	May be required if the diagnosis of an acute abdomen is uncertain

AKI, acute kidney injury; CXR, chest X-ray; DKA, diabetic ketoacidosis; HHS, hyperglycaemic hyperosmolar state; LFTs, liver function tests.

the speed with which it is safe to correct the metabolic and fluid derangements. Diabetic ketoacidosis has a rapid onset and can be corrected relatively quickly. Hyperglycaemic hyperosmolar syndrome develops much more slowly, the intracellular compartment is much more profoundly affected, and correction must be gradual to avoid severe, even fatal complications. Hyperglycaemic hyperosmolar syndrome and severe DKA must always be managed in a high dependency area or intensive care unit.

The principles of treating both are to correct the dehydration, hyperglycaemia and electrolyte imbalances, to identify the precipitating factors (Table 16.3), and to closely monitor the patient. The priority is to fluid resuscitate the patients sufficiently to ensure adequate organ perfusion but without causing harm.

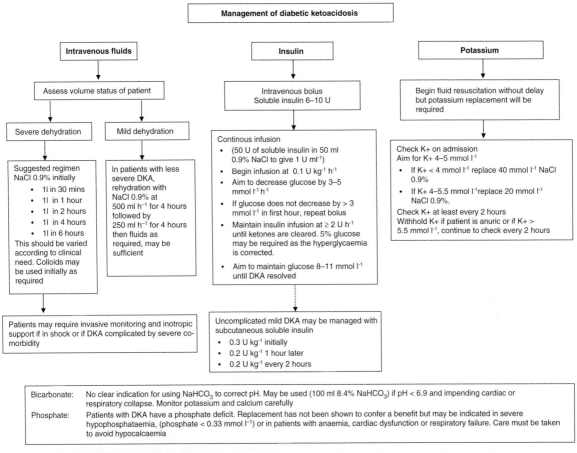

Fig 16.3 Treatment algorithm for patients with diabetic ketoacidosis (DKA).

This can be achieved rapidly in patients with DKA, assuming no significant co-morbidities (e.g., heart failure), but needs to be done with great care in patients with HHS or mixed HHS/DKA.

Fluid management

Resuscitation should begin with an isotonic, sodium-based fluid. Usually this is sodium chloride 0.9% (NaCl 0.9%) but may be a sodium containing colloid if the patient is in shock. The rate of administration is dependent on the nature of the hyperglycaemic crisis and guidance is given in the algorithms for management (Figures 16.3 and 16.4). Sodium poor fluids should not be used in the initial stages of resuscitation to avoid a precipitous decrease in plasma osmolality. Potassium (see below) should be added to most if not all bags of fluid.

Advice regarding the choice of fluid in patients who have hypernatraemia is conflicting. European and American opinions differ particularly on when to use NaCl 0.45%. The American consensus is that NaCl 0.45% should be started if the corrected plasma sodium concentration is high [12]. The Europeans are more circumspect about the use of hypotonic solutions and only suggest using NaCl 0.45% if the sodium plasma concentration is > 155 mmol l^{-1} after 2 litres of NaCl 0.9% [6]. More recent evidence suggests that NaCl 0.45% is contraindicated. The metabolic chaos in HHS is secondary to the osmotic diuresis causing water and sodium depletion via the kidneys and a marked increase in the osmolality of the plasma causing movement of water from the intracellular compartment to the extracellular fluid compartments. As described previously, the hyperosmolality of the extracellular compartment is thought to cause cells, including cells within the brain, to accumulate intracellular osmotically active molecules in an attempt to maintain cellular fluid volume. This may be aggravated by intracellular acidosis which favours the movement of sodium into cells and

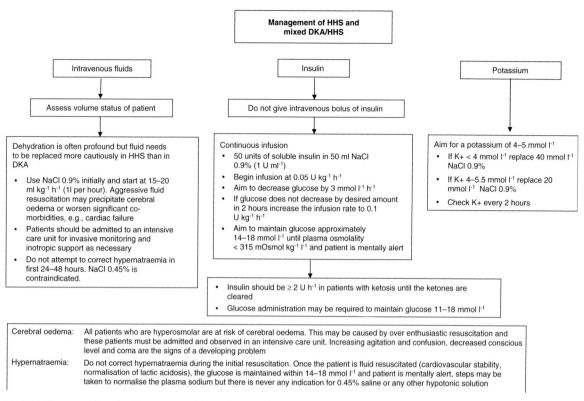

Fig 16.4 Treatment algorithm for patients with hyperglycaemic hyperosmolar state (HHS) or mixed diabetic ketoacidosis/hyperglycaemic hyperosmolar state (DKA/HHS).

over time the cells become osmotically charged [6, 28–30] (Figure 16.2). Immediately insulin is administered, extracellular glucose concentrations decrease, decreasing extracellular osmolality. Water moves by osmosis back into the profoundly dehydrated, osmotically charged cells. In patients with HHS this movement may be rapid and extreme and cerebral oedema may be profound, causing deterioration in the mental status and even death. Although patients may present with confusion or even coma in HHS, the mental status is often observed to deteriorate once therapy has started and may be related to the rapidity with which the glucose and therefore osmolality is corrected [20]. Patients with HHS ultimately require more fluid resuscitation than patients with DKA but it has to be given more slowly, the glucose should be corrected more slowly and the raised plasma sodium should not be corrected until fluid resuscitation is well established. Hypernatraemia may be protective and should not be actively corrected.

Cerebral oedema is rare in DKA except in children in whom it is a recognised cause of death from DKA [31]. It occurs in approximately 1% of childhood DKA cases

and has a mortality of 20–90%. A recent retrospective analysis of children with cerebral oedema suggested that outcome was worse if they received a bolus of insulin and better if they developed hypernatraemia [20]. It is not universally accepted that treatment may be causal in the development of cerebral oedema [32], and it is likely that many factors are contributory, but the prospective studies do not exist. This may be an example of where our desire to normalise biochemistry is harmful.

Insulin

Most recommended insulin regimens are based on continuous intravenous infusions of rapidly-acting soluble insulin, (this does not include the new human insulin analogues which have not yet been evaluated for intravenous management of diabetic hyperglycaemia crisis). Suggested regimens are given in the algorithms (Figures 16.3 and 16.4). For DKA (but not HHS), an initial bolus of 6–10 U of soluble insulin may be given to patients once severe hypokalaemia has been excluded although there is no evidence to show that this is of definite benefit [7, 13]. The aim is to decrease the blood glucose concentration by up to 5 mmol l^{-1} h^{-1} and the rate of infusion should be titrated to achieve this (normally 6–10 U h^{-1}). Once the blood glucose concentration has decreased to < 14 mmol l^{-1} in DKA, the insulin infusion should be decreased to 2–3 U h^{-1} and intravenous glucose solution (5% glucose at 100 ml h^{-1}) administered to prevent hypoglycaemia. Sufficient insulin is required to clear a ketosis, and if the insulin infusion rate is inadequate ketones will re-accumulate and worsen the metabolic acidosis. There is therefore no point in decreasing the rate of the insulin infusion to < 2 U h^{-1} until ketones are no longer detectable in the urine.

Regimens using subcutaneous insulin administration for the management of DKA have been shown to be effective [33–35], but can only be recommended if the DKA is mild. Severe DKA is associated with marked dehydration and therefore the reliability of absorption of subcutaneous insulin may be in doubt.

Insulin should be given more cautiously to patients with HHS [7]. Rapid correction of glucose may precipitate cerebral oedema and insulin should be administered in order to decrease the glucose concentration by approximately 3 mmol l^{-1} h^{-1}. An initial bolus of insulin is contraindicated and glucose 5% should be started once the blood glucose concentration is < 18 mmol l^{-1}. The aim is to maintain the blood glucose 14–18 mmol l^{-1} until the plasma osmolality is < 315 mOsmol kg^{-1} and the patient is mentally alert.

Potassium

Patients with DKA and HHS are potassium deplete even if the initial measured serum potassium concentration is normal or raised. Almost all patients will require significant potassium replacement once fluid resuscitation and insulin therapy are started. The rare exception is patients with severe renal dysfunction. The serum potassium should be checked as soon as possible after admission. Administration of insulin to a patient with a low potassium (e.g., < 3.3 mmol l^{-1}) may precipitate serious cardiac dysrhythmias and potassium replacement at 40 mmol h^{-1} via central venous access should be commenced prior to giving the insulin. The serum potassium will require frequent and regular checking (at least every 2 hours). Suggested rates of potassium replacement are given in the treatment algorithms (Figures 16.3 and 16.4).

Phosphate

Patients with DKA and HHS are phosphate deplete and theoretically replacement of phosphate may benefit respiratory function, restore 2,3-diphosphoglycerate concentrations and improve oxygen delivery to tissues. Studies have failed to show a treatment benefit from the routine administration of phosphate and its use is therefore only recommended in patients who are severely hypophosphataemic (phosphate < 0.33 mmol l^{-1}), anaemic or who have severe cardiac or respiratory disease [6, 13, 36]. Calcium should be closely monitored in any replacement regimen. Hypophosphataemia has been implicated in the development of hyperglycaemic-related rhabdomyolysis [37, 38].

Bicarbonate

The American consensus for the management of diabetic emergencies recommends that bicarbonate is given to patients with a pH < 6.9 [12]. There is, however, no direct evidence for this advice and indeed there are potential risks [39]. Administration of bicarbonate may: aggravate intracellular acidosis [40], particularly if oxygen delivery to cells has been compromised; worsen central nervous system acidosis; increase the risk of hypokalaemia; and delay the resolution of ketosis [41]. The rationale of administering bicarbonate to patients with a severe metabolic acidosis is that it may improve cardiac function and enhance resuscitation in the short term but this remains controversial [42]. There is no proven role for bicarbonate administration in patients with pH > 6.9.

Additional measures

The underlying precipitating cause should be treated and patients managed to minimise complications. All patients should be given high flow oxygen to optimise oxygen delivery and if obtunded or in shock, they may require intubation and artificial ventilation. If this is necessary, vigilance is needed in case of developing cerebral oedema. A nasogastric tube should be passed to prevent gastric dilation, decrease the risk of aspiration and allow the administration of oral medications. Broad spectrum antibiotics should be given and for all but mild cases of DKA a urinary catheter should be inserted. Central venous access is indicated in patients with moderate/severe DKA, all patients with HHS and in patients with significant co-morbidities. Patients should receive high-risk thromboprophylaxis (unfractionated or low molecular weight heparin), and may require formal anticoagulation.

Complications

Complications may occur secondary to the hyperglycaemic crisis or the treatment.

Hypoglycaemia and hypokalaemia

Patients with HHS and DKA require frequent and regular review during management (Table 16.3, Figures 16.3 and 16.4). Hypoglycaemia is not common but may occur if there is failure to monitor patients closely and the insulin infusion is continued without the introduction of a dextrose solution to maintain the blood glucose (< 12 mmol l^{-1} in patients with DKA, < 14–18 mmol l^{-1} for patients with HHS, Figures 16.3 and 16.4). Hypokalaemia will occur if insulin is started without consideration of the plasma potassium concentration or if replacement is inadequate. Plasma potassium should be checked at least every 2 hours.

Cerebral oedema

Cerebral oedema is the leading cause of death in HHS and in children with DKA. Controversy persists on whether cerebral oedema is caused by the conditions or their treatment. The studies to resolve this do not exist but it is clear that cerebral complications may occur before and during treatment, and are in some way related to the severity of hyperosmolality. These patients must be managed in a critical care area with the means of managing cerebral oedema, although traditional methods may not be useful. Mannitol therapy is unproven and hyperventilation to decrease the arterial partial pressure of carbon dioxide is detrimental causing impaired cerebral perfusion [31]. Factors which appear to worsen outcome include: a failure of sodium to increase during treatment, boluses of insulin, rapid decreases in plasma glucose, the administration of bicarbonate and severe hypocapnia [20, 29, 31].

Rhabdomyolysis

Overt rhabdomyolysis resulting in acute kidney injury is a rare but serious complication of hyperglycaemia causing increased morbidity and mortality [32, 37, 38]. Subclinical rhabdomyolysis may be quite common, particularly in hyperosmolar conditions complicated by hypokalaemia and hypophosphataemia.

Adult respiratory distress syndrome

A rare but serious complication of hyperglycaemic crises is acute lung injury progressing to adult respiratory syndrome. The aetiology is uncertain but thought to be related to the pro-inflammatory state caused by the metabolic chaos.

Vascular thrombosis

Patients with hyperglycaemia are pro-coagulant, and dehydration and hyperosmolality increase the viscosity of blood. Various thrombotic complications are reported including myocardial infarction, cerebral vascular accidents, venous thrombosis, including cerebral vein thrombosis and pulmonary embolism, and limb ischaemia. Many authors advocate anticoagulation, either formally or as high-risk thromboprophylaxis, but no studies are available to support or contradict this advice [2, 7, 13, 17, 32].

Prognosis

In experienced centres, mortality from DKA should be < 5%, but mortality from HHS is higher, between 10 and 50%. Although HHS is more difficult to manage, the excess mortality for this condition is largely accounted for by the age of the patients and the co-morbidities prevalent in the older age group [2]. In children with DKA, the prognosis is good, unless the child is one of the 0.9% of children who develop cerebral oedema. Mortality in this group is very high (40–90%) [31].

References

1. Magee MF, Bhatt BA. Management of decompensated diabetes. Diabetic ketoacidosis and hyperglycemic hyperosmolar syndrome. *Crit Care Clin* 2001; **17**: 75–106.

2. MacIsaac RJ, Lee LY, McNeil KJ, et al. Influence of age on the presentation and outcome of acidotic and hyperosmolar diabetic emergencies. *Intern Med J* 2002; **32**: 379–85.

3. Kearney T, Dang C. Diabetic and endocrine emergencies. *Postgrad Med J* 2007; **83**: 79–86.

4. Levy-Marchal C, Patterson CC, Green A. Geographical variation of presentation at diagnosis of type 1 diabetes in children: the EURODIAB study. European and Diabetes. *Diabetologia* 2001; **44 Suppl 3**: B75–80.

5. Wolfsdorf J, Craig ME, Daneman D, et al. Diabetic ketoacidosis. *Pediatr Diabetes* 2007; **8**: 28–43.

6. English P, Williams G. Hyperglycaemic crises and lactic acidosis in diabetes mellitus. *Postgrad Med J* 2004; **80**: 253–61.

7. Chiasson JL, Aris-Jilwan N, Belanger R, et al. Diagnosis and treatment of diabetic ketoacidosis and the hyperglycemic hyperosmolar state. *CMAJ* 2003; **168**: 859–66.

8. Koul PB, Diabetic ketoacidosis: a current appraisal of pathophysiology and management. *Clin Pediatr (Phila)* 2008; **20**: 1–10.

9. Umpierrez GE, Smiley D, Kitabchi AE. Narrative review: ketosis-prone type 2 diabetes mellitus. *Ann Intern Med* 2006; **144**: 350–7.

10. Kitabchi AE, Umpierrez GE, Murphy MB, et al. Management of hyperglycemic crises in patients with diabetes. *Diabetes Care* 2001; **24**: 131–53.

11. Wachtel TJ, Tetu-Mouradjian LM, Goldman DL, et al. Hyperosmolarity and acidosis in diabetes mellitus: a three-year experience in Rhode Island. *J Gen Intern Med* 1991; **6**: 495–502.

12. Kitabchi AE, Umpierrez GE, Murphy MB, et al. Hyperglycemic crises in adult patients with diabetes: a consensus statement from the American Diabetes Association. *Diabetes Care* 2006; **29**: 2739–48.

13. Kitabchi AE, Umpierrez GE, Fisher JN, et al. Thirty years of personal experience in hyperglycemic crises: diabetic ketoacidosis and hyperglycemic hyperosmolar state. *J Clin Endocrinol Metab* 2008; **93**: 1541–52.

14. Stentz FB, Umpierrez GE, Cuervo R, et al. Proinflammatory cytokines, markers of cardiovascular risks, oxidative stress, and lipid peroxidation in patients with hyperglycemic crises. *Diabetes* 2004; **53**: 2079–86.

15. McGarry JD, Woeltje KF, Kuwajima M, et al. Regulation of ketogenesis and the renaissance of carnitine palmitoyltransferase. *Diabetes Metab Rev* 1989; **5**: 271–84.

16. Unger RH, Orci L. Glucagon and the A cell: physiology and pathophysiology (first two parts). *N Engl J Med* 1981; **304**: 1518–24.

17. Kitabchi AE, Nyenwe EA. Hyperglycemic crises in diabetes mellitus: diabetic ketoacidosis and hyperglycemic hyperosmolar state. *Endocrinol Metab Clin North Am* 2006; **35**: 725–51.

18. Moller N, Schmitz O, Porksen N, et al. Dose-response studies on the metabolic effects of a growth hormone pulse in humans. *Metabolism* 1992; **41**: 172–5.

19. Hoffman WH, Stamatovic SM, Andjelkovic AV. Inflammatory mediators and blood brain barrier disruption in fatal brain edema of diabetic ketoacidosis. *Brain Res* 2009; **1254**: 138–48.

20. Hoorn EJ, Carlotti APCP, Costa LAA, et al. Preventing a drop in effective plasma osmolality to minimise the likelihood of cerebral edema during treatment of children with diabetic ketoacidosis. *J Pediatr* 2007; **150**: 467–73.

21. Kellum JA. Determinants of blood pH in health and disease. *Crit Care* 2000; **4**: 6–14.

22. Kitabchi AE, Umpierrez GE, Murphy MB, et al. Hyperglycemic crises in diabetes. *Diabetes Care* 2004; **27** Suppl 1: S94–102.

23. Cardella F. Insulin therapy during diabetic ketoacidosis in children. *Acta Biomed* 2005; **76** Suppl 3: 49–54.

24. Umpierrez G, Freire AX. Abdominal pain in patients with hyperglycemic crises. *J Crit Care* 2002; **17**: 63–7.

25. Campbell IW, Duncan LJ, Munro JF. Acute diabetic abdomen. *BMJ* 1976; **2**: 1074.

26. Campbell IW, Duncan LJ, Innes JA, et al. Abdominal pain in diabetic metabolic decompensation. Clinical significance. *JAMA* 1975; **233**: 166–8.

27. Kershaw MJ, Newton T, Barrett TG, et al. Childhood diabetes presenting with hyperosmolar dehydration but without ketoacidosis: a report of three cases. *Diabet Med* 2005; **22**: 645–7.

28. Edge JA. Cerebral oedema during treatment of diabetic ketoacidosis: are we any nearer finding a cause? *Diabetes Metab Res Rev* 2000; **16**: 316–24.

29. Dunger DB, Edge JA. Predicting cerebral edema during diabetic ketoacidosis. *N Engl J Med* 2001; **344**: 302–3.

30. Edge JA, Hawkins MM, Winter DL, et al. The risk and outcome of cerebral oedema developing during diabetic ketoacidosis. *Arch Dis Child*, 2001; **85**: 16–22.

31. Glaser N, Barnett P, McCaslin I, et al. Risk factors for cerebral edema in children with diabetic ketoacidosis. *N Engl J Med* 2001; **344**: 264–9.

32. Rosenbloom AL. Hyperglycemic crises and their complications in children. *J Pediatr Endocrinol Metab* 2007; **20**: 5–18.

33. Umpierrez GE, Lati, K, Stoever J, et al. Efficacy of subcutaneous insulin lispro versus continuous intravenous regular insulin for the treatment of patients with diabetic ketoacidosis. *Am J Med* 2004; **117**: 291–6.

34. Umpierrez GE Cuervo R, Karabell A, et al. Treatment of diabetic ketoacidosis with subcutaneous insulin aspart. *Diabetes Care* 2004; **27**: 1873–8.

35. Della Manna T, Steinmetz L, Campos PR, et al. Subcutaneous use of a fast-acting insulin analog: an alternative treatment for pediatric patients with diabetic ketoacidosis. *Diabetes Care* 2005; **28**: 1856–61.

36. Fisher JN, Kitabchi AE. A randomized study of phosphate therapy in the treatment of diabetic ketoacidosis. *J Clin Endocrinol Metab* 1983; **57**: 177–80.

37. Singhal PC, Abramovici M, Ayer S, et al. Determinants of rhabdomyolysis in the diabetic state. *Am J Nephrol* 1991; **11**: 447–50.

38. Singhal PC, Abramovici M, Venkatesan J. Rhabdomyolysis in the hyperosmolal state. *Am J Med* 1990; **88**: 9–12.

39. Viallon A, Zeni F, Lafond P, et al. Does bicarbonate therapy improve the management of severe diabetic ketoacidosis? *Crit Care Med* 1999; **27**: 2690–3.

40. Johnson BA, Weil MH, Tang W, et al. Mechanisms of myocardial hypercarbic acidosis during cardiac arrest. *J Appl Physiol* 1995; **78**: 1579–84.

41. Okuda Y, Adrogue HJ, Field JB, et al. Counterproductive effects of sodium bicarbonate in diabetic ketoacidosis. *J Clin Endocrinol Metab* 1996; **81**: 314–20.

42. Kraut JA, Kurtz I. Use of base in the treatment of severe acidemic states. *Am J Kidney Dis* 2001; **38**: 703–27.

Chapter 7

Thyroid dysfunction and critical care

Brian Mullan

Introduction

Thyroid hormone is essential for the regulation of tissue metabolism. The thyroid axis is comprised of thyrotropin releasing hormone (TRH) at the hypothalamic level; thyrotropin or thyroid stimulating hormone (TSH) at the pituitary level; and thyroxine (T_4), triiodothyronine (T_3) and reverse T_3 (rT_3) at the peripheral level. Abnormalities in thyroid function can have a major impact on physiological processes throughout the body. During critical illness multiple and complex alterations occur to the central and peripheral parts of the thyroid axis (Figure 17.1). This chapter will review the mechanisms behind these changes and also the critical care management of hypo- and hyperthyroidism.

The thyroid axis during critical illness

Thyrotropin releasing hormone is a tripeptide which is produced in the parvocellular region of the paraventricular nuclei of the hypothalamus. It is released into the hypothalamic-pituitary portal plexus and controls the secretion of TSH from the thyrotrophs of the anterior pituitary. Thyrotropin releasing hormone is a glycoprotein. It is released in secretory bursts superimposed on non-pulsatile secretion. It is also the major regulator of the morphological and functional states of the thyroid gland. Both TRH and TSH secretion are controlled in a typical negative feedback manner by the availability of the thyroid hormones. Although the thyroid gland predominantly produces T_4, the biological activity of thyroid hormones is exerted largely by T_3. Different types of deiodinases are responsible for the peripheral conversion of T_4 to either T_3 or to the biologically inactive rT_3. These processes require the presence of specific thyroid hormone transporters.

Changes within the thyroid axis during critical illness have been described as the euthyroid sick syndrome (ESS), non-thyroidal illness syndrome (NTIS)

or the low-T_3 syndrome [1]. The response of the thyroid axis is dependent on the duration and severity of the critical illness [2]. The acute phase consists of a rapid decline in the circulating levels of T_3 and an increase in the levels of rT_3 (Table 17.1). Levels of T_4 and TSH rise briefly and then normalise. These acute phase changes are probably secondary to disturbances in deiodination. There are three selenodeiodinases – D1, D2 and D3. D1 is expressed in the thyroid, liver and kidney and plays a key role in the production of circulating T_3 from T_4 and in the breakdown of rT_3. D2 is expressed in the brain, thyroid and skeletal muscle. This enzyme is important for local T_3 production but may also contribute to circulating T_3. D3 is present in the brain, skin, placenta and fetal tissues. It is an inactivating enzyme which catalyses the conversion of T_4 into rT_3 and of T_3 into diiodothyronine (T_2). In critical illness, liver D1 activity is down-regulated and liver and skeletal muscle D3 activity, not present in healthy individuals, is induced [3]. These alterations in D1 and D3 activity may be responsible for the changes in plasma T_3 and rT_3 (Figure 17.1).

In the prolonged phase of critical illness, central effects on the thyroid axis become important (Figure 17.1 and Table 17.1). Initially the set-point for feedback inhibition is altered and the nocturnal TSH surge seen in healthy individuals is absent. Eventually pulsatile TSH secretion is reduced secondary to reduced TRH availability. Up-regulation of D2 activity in the hypothalamus may be important in the pathophysiology of the central neuroendocrine effects. Theoretically, an increase in local hypothalamic levels of T_3, secondary to D2 induction, would result in the suppression of TRH [4]. Patients in the chronic phase of critical illness have reduced circulating levels of T_4, T_3 and TSH. The reduction in T_4 may mean that the increased rT_3 levels seen during the acute phase may now be no longer evident.

Core Topics in Endocrinology in Anaesthesia and Critical Care, eds. George M. Hall, Jennifer M. Hunter and Mark S. Cooper. Published by Cambridge University Press. © Cambridge University Press 2010.

Changes during critical illness

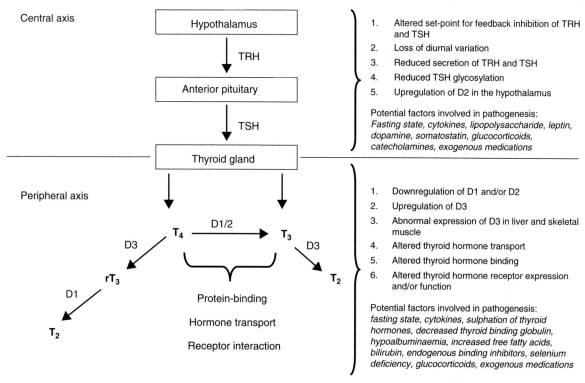

Central axis

Hypothalamus

↓ TRH

Anterior pituitary

↓ TSH

Thyroid gland

Peripheral axis

T_4 — D1/2 → T_3

D3 ↙   ↘ D3

rT_3 T_2

D1 ↙

T_2

Protein-binding

Hormone transport

Receptor interaction

1. Altered set-point for feedback inhibition of TRH and TSH
2. Loss of diurnal variation
3. Reduced secretion of TRH and TSH
4. Reduced TSH glycosylation
5. Upregulation of D2 in the hypothalamus

Potential factors involved in pathogenesis: *Fasting state, cytokines, lipopolysaccharide, leptin, dopamine, somatostatin, glucocorticoids, catecholamines, exogenous medications*

1. Downregulation of D1 and/or D2
2. Upregulation of D3
3. Abnormal expression of D3 in liver and skeletal muscle
4. Altered thyroid hormone transport
5. Altered thyroid hormone binding
6. Altered thyroid hormone receptor expression and/or function

Potential factors involved in pathogenesis: *fasting state, cytokines, sulphation of thyroid hormones, decreased thyroid binding globulin, hypoalbuminaemia, increased free fatty acids, bilirubin, endogenous binding inhibitors, selenium deficiency, glucocorticoids, exogenous medications*

Fig. 17.1 Response of the thyroid axis to critical illness. The biological activity of triiodothyronine (T_3) is eightfold greater than that of thyroxine (T_4). Diiodothyronine (T_2) and reverse T_3 (rT_3) are biologically inactive. The selenodeiodinases are abbreviated D1, D2 and D3 for type 1, 2 and 3 respectively. TRH, thyroid releasing hormone; TSH, thyroid stimulating hormone.

Table 17.1 The temporal changes to thyroid function during critical illness.

	Acute phase	Chronic phase	Recovery
TSH	↑ / N	↓	↑
T_4	↑ / N	↓	N
T_3	↓	↓↓	N
rT_3	↑	↑ / N	N

↑, increased; ↓, decreased; N, normal; TSH, thyroid stimulating hormone; rT_3, reverse triiodothyronine; T_4, thyroxine.

This abnormality can be difficult to distinguish from a variant of central or secondary hypothyroidism.

Critical illness may affect additional aspects of thyroid hormone physiology. These include abnormalities in thyroid hormone transport [5], inhibition of thyroid hormone binding [6], elevation of thyroid hormone sulphation [7] and alterations in thyroid hormone receptor expression and/or function [8]. The pathogenesis of these changes may be related to other systemic factors associated with critical illness. Potential pathogenic factors include cytokines, elevated stress hormones (i.e., glucocorticoids, catecholamines), elevated free fatty acids and other acute phase reactants. Furthermore, some of the pharmacological agents used in the treatment of the critically ill may also affect thyroid hormone bioavailability (see below).

As critical illness resolves, so do the alterations in thyroid hormone concentrations. This stage may be characterised by TSH levels above the upper limit of the normal range (Table 17.1). This abnormality may persist for several months and may be mistaken for sub-clinical primary hypothyroidism. Alteration in the thyroid axis is associated with higher mortality in critically ill patients. All of T_4, T_3, TSH, and rT_3 have been shown to be prognostic for survival [6, 9–11]. Both the absolute values of these variables and the time course of their changes are completely different between survivors and non-survivors. However, it remains controversial whether exogenous administration of TRH, T_4 or T_3 to raise circulating T_3 levels have beneficial effects in critical illness [1, 2, 12, 13]. There is no evidence that replacement in critically ill patients is disadvantageous but also no clear proof that it

Table 17.2 Medications used in the intensive care unit that may affect thyroid function.

Thyroid disturbance	Medication
Inhibition of TSH secretion	Dopamine and dopamine agonists, glucocorticoids, octreotide, phenytoin
Increase in thyroid hormone synthesis: Jod–Basedow effect[1]	Iodinated contrast agents, amiodarone
Increase in thyroid hormone release: destructive thyroiditis	Amiodarone
Decrease in thyroid hormone synthesis: Wolff–Chaikoff effect[2]	Iodinated contrast agents, amiodarone
Decrease in thyroid hormone release	Iodinated contrast agents
Displacement of thyroid hormone from binding proteins	Furosemide, salicylates, NSAIDs, carbamazepine, phenytoin, heparin
Impairment of T_4 to T_3 deiodination	Beta-blockers, glucocorticoids, amiodarone, contrast agents
Decrease in thyroid-binding globulin	Glucocorticoids
Increase in thyroid hormone clearance	Phenytoin, carbamazepine, barbiturates, rifampicin
Modification of thyroid hormone action	Amiodarone, phenytoin
Impairment of enteral thyroxine absorption	Sucralfate, proton pump inhibitors, aluminium hydroxide

[1] Occurs in patients with absent thyroid autoregulation (e.g., underlying autonomous nodules, latent Graves' disease or euthyroid iodine deficient goitre).
[2] In patients with defective thyroid autoregulation (e.g., underlying Hashimoto's disease) 'escape' from the Wolff–Chaikoff effect may not occur and hypothyroidism can develop.

NSAIDS, non-steroidal anti-inflammatory drugs; TSH, thyroid stimulating hormone; T_3, triiodothyronine; T_4, thyroxine.

is advantageous. Further studies are required to answer this important clinical question.

Effects of medication on the thyroid axis

A wide variety of medications which may be used during critical illness can affect thyroid hormone physiology and the interpretation of thyroid function tests (Table 17.2). Drugs may interfere with TSH secretion or the production, secretion, transport and metabolism of thyroid hormones [14].

The antiarrhythmic drug amiodarone is probably the most complex drug to affect thyroid function [15]. It is a benzofuran which contains iodine (about 37% of its mass) and it is structurally similar to T_4 and T_3. The effects of amiodarone on the thyroid gland and thyroid hormone metabolism can be divided into intrinsic drug effects and iodine-induced effects. The intrinsic drug effects include: D1/D2 deiodinase inhibition; blockade of T_4 entry into cells; direct antagonism of T_3 with the thyroid hormone receptor; and thyroid gland cytotoxicity, which can result in a destructive thyroiditis. The iodine-induced effects can lead to either hypothyroidism or hyperthyroidism.

Amiodarone-induced hypothyroidism (AIH) is more prevalent in iodine-replete regions. The inability to escape from the Wolff–Chaikoff effect may be the most likely pathogenic mechanism for AIH. The Wolff–Chaikoff effect is an autoregulatory mechanism within the thyroid gland which inhibits organification when iodine is present in excessive quantities [16]. The Wolff–Chaikoff effect is an effective means of rejecting large quantities of iodine and therefore preventing the thyroid from synthesising large amounts of thyroid hormones. The acute Wolff–Chaikoff effect lasts for a few days and then, through the so-called 'escape' phenomenon, normal synthesis of T_4 and T_3 returns. However, in subjects with underlying thyroid disease, such as Hashimoto's autoimmune thyroiditis, the escape from the inhibitory effect of large doses of iodine does not occur and clinical or sub-clinical hypothyroidism can develop. Forty per cent of patients who develop AIH have positive thyroid antibodies. This suggests that iodide excess from amiodarone administration can unmask pre-existent subclinical thyroid disease to produce overt thyroid failure [17].

Amiodarone-induced thyrotoxicosis (AIT) can occur via two mechanisms. One is related to excess iodine. This condition is an iodine-induced thyrotoxicosis or type I AIT. The other mechanism is due to the amiodarone inducing destruction of the thyroid follicles with release of preformed hormones. This condition is called amiodarone-induced destructive thyroiditis or type II AIT. Patients developing type I AIT in general have

Table 17.3 Potential clinical features of thyroid storm and myxoedema coma.

	Thyroid storm	Myxoedema coma
Central nervous system	Delerium Psychosis Coma Seizures Brisk reflexes	Somnolence Coma Seizures Delayed reflexes
Respiratory system		Reduced ventilatory drive Pleural effusions
Cardiovascular system	Sinus tachycardia Atrial tachyarrhythmias Hypertension Widened pulse pressure Systolic flow murmur Congestive cardiac failure	Sinus bradycardia Hypotension Narrowed pulse pressure Pericardial effusion Congestive cardiac failure
Renal system		Acute renal impairment Bladder atony
Hepatobiliary system	Elevated liver enzymes Jaundice Liver failure	Ascites
Gastrointestinal system	Nausea Vomiting Diarrhoea	Constipation Paralytic ileus
Musculoskeletal system	Muscle weakness Tremor Hyperkinesia	Muscle weakness
Body temperature	Hyperthermia	Hypothermia
Biochemistry	Hypercalcaemia Hyperglycaemia	Hyponatraemia (euvolaemic) Hypoglycaemia Dyslipideamia Elevated creatinine kinase
Haematology	Leucocytosis	Anaemia

pre-existing thyroid disease (e.g., multinodular goitre or latent Graves' disease) with absent thyroid autoregulation i.e., no Wolff–Chaikoff effect. The provision of excess iodine in this situation results in unregulated hormone synthesis (Jod–Basedow effect) [18]. Patients with type II AIT do not have pre-existing thyroid disease but may develop permanent hypothyroidism after recovery as a consequence of fibrosis of the thyroid gland.

Acute administration of amiodarone to euthyroid patients results almost immediately in a decrease in T_3 and an increase in T_4, rT_3 and TSH. These changes are due to inhibition of the D1 and D2 deiodinases, impairment of intracellular thyroid hormone uptake and antagonism of intranuclear thyroid receptor binding. The change in thyroid function is not that dissimilar to that observed during the very early phase of critical illness (Table 17.1). Acute administration of amiodarone can therefore potentiate the fall in T_3 and the increase in rT_3 in critically ill patients.

Hyperthyroidism and thyroid storm

Hyperthyroidism is the consequence of excessive thyroid hormone action. The causes of hyperthyroidism are:

- Antibody-mediated stimulation of thyroid tissue
- Autonomously functioning thyroid tissue
- Autonomously functioning heterotopic thyroid tissue
- Thyroiditis
- Iodine-induced hyperthyroidism
- Excessive TSH secretion
- Exogenous administration of thyroid hormone.

The classic signs and symptoms of hyperthyroidism are well described in standard medical textbooks (also see Chapter 2). A thyroid storm is the abrupt and severe exacerbation of hyperthyroidism. It is extremely rare and life-threatening [19]. The clinical features of thyroid storm are summarised in Table 17.3. It occurs in untreated or partially treated thyrotoxic patients. Precipitating factors include stress from other acute illnesses, trauma, anaesthesia, surgery, parturition, sepsis, diabetic ketoacidosis, radioiodine therapy, administration of iodinated contrast agents, amiodarone therapy and withdrawal or discontinuation of antithyroid medications. The cardinal features of thyroid storm are hyperthermia (temperature > 38.5°C) and tachycardia out of proportion to the temperature. Differential diagnoses might include malignant hyperthermia, neuroleptic malignant syndrome or the serotonin syndrome. These conditions, however, are usually associated with neuromuscular rigidity, which would be an unusual feature for thyroid storm. Thyroid function abnormalities are similar to those seen in uncomplicated hyperthyroidism, i.e., undetectable TSH levels and elevated T_4 and T_3 levels. In patients with critical illness the T_3 levels may not be as high as expected and may only be in the 'high–normal' range. Thyroid storm is primarily a clinical diagnosis.

The treatment of thyroid storm is best provided within a critical care facility and involves general physiological supportive measures, treatment of the precipitating factor and suppression of the thyroid axis. Patients may require neurological support with sedation, airway protection and mechanical ventilation. Invasive cardiovascular monitoring is essential to guide fluid therapy and treatment for any associated cardiac compromise. Beta-blockers, magnesium, digoxin or calcium antagonists can be used to treat atrial tachyarrhythmias. Temperature control is achieved with the use of paracetamol (provided there is no hepatic derangement) and active cooling measures. If normothermia is difficult to achieve then the administration of dantrolene should be considered [20]. Other investigations may be required to identify the factor which precipitated the thyroid crisis. As leucocytosis may be a feature of thyroid storm, patients should have a full sepsis screen to exclude underlying infection. If sepsis is suspected then empirical antimicrobial therapy should be commenced prior to obtaining microbiological confirmation.

Suppression of the thyroid axis is achieved via a combination of strategies. Propylthiouracil or carbimazole block iodide organification and the formation of thyroid hormone. Propylthiouracil may have the additional benefit of also blocking the conversion of T_4 to T_3. There are no intravenous preparations so it must be administered either orally, via a nasogastric tube, or rectally (200 mg, 4 hourly). Lugol's iodine (0.3 ml diluted to 50 ml, 8 hourly) or lithium carbonate (300 mg, 6 hourly) can be used to block the release of preformed hormone from the thyroid gland. Lithium carbonate requires plasma monitoring. The target range is 1 mmol l^{-1}. Lugol's iodine should only be given 2–3 hours after the administration of carbimazole or propylthiouracil. If iodine-containing medications are given first, thyrotoxicosis may worsen (Jod–Basedow effect) [18]. Beta-blockers (especially propranolol) and high dose glucocorticoids (hydrocortisone, 100 mg, 6 hourly) are useful adjuncts to further block peripheral thyroid hormone conversion. Hydrocortisone is also indicated as there is a high incidence of concomitant adrenal insufficiency in patients with Graves' disease. In rare situations, haemodialysis or haemoperfusion have been used to enhance thyroid hormone clearance [21]. Once the acute crisis is over, consideration must then be given to the long-term management of the hyperthyroidism.

Hypothyroidism and myxoedema coma

Hypothyroidism results from under secretion of thyroid hormone from the thyroid gland. It can be classified as primary (thyroid gland abnormality), secondary (insufficient TSH) and tertiary (insufficient TRH). The most common cause of primary hypothyroidism is chronic autoimmune thyroiditis (Hashimoto's disease). Other causes include surgical removal of the thyroid gland, thyroid gland ablation with radioactive iodine, infiltrative diseases, iodine deficiency, congenital enzymatic defects which affect thyroid hormone synthesis and drug-induced effects. Secondary and tertiary hypothyroidism are usually due to pituitary and hypothalamic disorders respectively. The symptoms of hypothyroidism are related to the duration and severity of the disease, and the rapidity with which hypothyroidism occurs. The most severe form of untreated hypothyroidism is myxoedema coma. The clinical features of this condition are summarised in Table 17.3. It is most frequently encountered in winter months after exposure to the cold [22]. Extremely cold weather seems to lower the threshold for vulnerability. As with thyroid storm, myxoedema coma may be triggered by other acute medical illnesses, trauma, sepsis, anaesthesia and various medications. The cardinal features of myxoedema coma are hypothermia, respiratory depression and unconsciousness. It is a medical emergency and even with early diagnosis and treatment, the mortality can be high. The clues to making a diagnosis may come from identifying other telltale signs of hypothyroidism, such as skin, hair and nail changes.

The diagnosis should be considered in all comatose patients with a history of hypothyroidism or in patients with one or more manifestations of the triad of hypothermia, hyponatraemia and hypercapnia. Thyroid function tests in myxoedema coma include an elevated TSH concentration with low or undetectable levels of T_4 and T_3. Critical illness may reduce the degree of TSH elevation. In secondary or tertiary hypothyroidism the TSH levels will be low.

Treatment of myxoedema coma requires replacement of thyroid hormone, treatment of any precipitating condition and correction of the physiological abnormalities. There are no clinical trials to suggest the best method of replacing the thyroid hormone. As the activity of the deiodinases may be reduced in hypothyroidism there is an argument for using T_3 (liothyronine) over T_4 (levothyroxine) as T_3 has a more rapid effect and it can be given intravenously. However, T_3 therapy is not without risk. Excess T_3 administration has been associated with increased mortality in myxoedema coma [23, 24]. High dose thyroid hormone therapy can induce atrial tachyarrhythmias and myocardial ischaemia or infarction. Thyroxine has a much longer half life and is converted to T_3 endogenously, resulting in a slower but steadier rise in T_3 levels. Different thyroid hormone replacement strategies have been described for myxoedema coma [22, 25, 26]. Both T_3 or T_4 can be given alone or in combination. As it is such a rare condition, there is not sufficient evidence available to objectively recommend the most effective dosing regimen. One method of managing unconscious patients is to give T_3 (liodothyronine) intravenously (25–50 µg initially and then 10–25 µg 8 hourly). Once consciousness improves, therapy can be switched to oral or nasogastric T_4 (levothyroxine, 100 µg daily). Adjustment of the T_4 dose is based on subsequent clinical and laboratory results, as in any hypothyroid patient. In patients with known severe cardiovascular disease, it may be more appropriate to initiate therapy with T_4 only (200–500 µg loading dose). No general guide to treatment can take into account all the factors that might affect sensitivity to thyroid hormone, such as age and co-morbidities. Patients should be monitored closely before each dose of thyroid hormone is administered.

The amelioration of hypothermia by thyroid hormone may take several days. Patients will therefore require active warming. This should be done cautiously because of the risk of hypotension secondary to vasodilatation. The susceptibility to hypotension is further aggravated by impaired cardiac function. This is due to underlying bradycardia, impaired cardiac contractility and the possibility of underlying pericardial effusion. Vasopressors and intravenous fluids must be used carefully with full invasive cardiovascular monitoring as the risk of fluid overload and congestive cardiac failure is high. Of important note, co-existent primary or secondary adrenal insufficiency has a high association with thyroid failure. Thus all patients with myxoedema coma should be treated with stress-dose corticosteroids (hydrocortisone 100 mg, 8 hourly). Ideally, a Synacthen test should be performed prior to the administration of the steroids, but this is not always possible in the emergency situation. The hydrocortisone dose is tapered over the following days as the patient's condition improves. Pituitary-adrenal function can be checked subsequently after full recovery.

The hyponatraemia observed in myxoedema coma falls under the euvolaemic classification (Chapter 18) [27]. Fluid resuscitation for hypotension makes management of the hyponatraemia difficult, since fluid restriction would normally be indicated for this abnormality. In patients with symptomatic hyponatraemia, hypertonic saline may need to be given (initially 200 ml of 2.7% as an intravenous bolus). The serum sodium should not be increased by more than 12 mmol l^{-1} in a 24-hour period.

The mechanism of hypoglycaemia in myxoedema coma is not fully understood. It is likely to be multifactorial in origin and may be due to decreased gluconeogenesis. Blood glucose need to be monitored frequently in these patients and intravenous dextrose given as required.

Patients should only be weaned from mechanical ventilation and extubated once fully conscious. This may take a number of days and in some cases several weeks [28]. Myxoedema patients have a decreased response to hypoxia and hypercapnia. The decrease in hypoxic ventilatory drive reverses after thyroid hormone replacement but the depression in hypercapnic ventilatory drive remains [29]. Other physical factors which may make weaning from ventilation difficult include obesity, macroglossia, oedema of the pharynx and larynx, muscle weakness, pleural effusions and ascites. Some individuals may require a tracheostomy to assist recovery.

Finally, as with thyroid storm, the underlying precipitating cause for the acute decompensation must be identified and treated. Empirical antimicrobial therapy may be indicated if sepsis cannot be excluded. Early diagnosis and a multifaceted approach are essential prerequisites for a good outcome.

References

1. Alder SM, Wartofsky L. The nonthyroidal illness syndrome. *Endocrinol Metab Clin North Am* 2007; **36**: 657–72.

2. Mebis L, Debaveye Y, Visser TJ, et al. Changes within the thyroid axis during the course of critical illness. *Endocrinol Metab Clin North Am* 2006; **35**: 807–21.

3. Peeters RP, Wouters PJ, Kaptein E, et al. Reduced activation and increased inactivation of thyroid hormone in tissues of critically ill patients. *J Clin Endocrinol Metab* 2003; **88**: 3202–11.

4. Fekete C, Sarkar S, Christoffolete MA, et al. Bacterial lipopolysaccharide (LPS)-induced type 2 iodothyronine deiodinase (D2) activation in the mediobasal hypothalamus (MBH) is independent of the LPS-induced fall in serum thyroid hormone levels. *Brain Res* 2005; **1056**: 97–9.

5. Lim CF, Docter R, Visser TJ, et al. Inhibition of thyroxine transport into cultured rat hepatocytes by serum of nonuremic critically ill patients: effects of bilirubin and nonesterified fatty acids. *J Clin Endocrinol Metab* 1993; **76**: 1165–72.

6. den Brinker M, Joosten KF, Visser TJ, et al. Euthyroid sick syndrome in meningococcal sepsis: the impact of peripheral thyroid hormone metabolism and binding proteins. *J Clin Endocrinol Metab* 2005; **90**: 5613–20.

7. Peeters RP, Kester MHA, Wouters PJ, et al. Increased thyroxine sulphate levels in critically ill patients as a result of a decreased hepatic type I deiodinase activity. *J Clin Endocrinol Metab* 2005; **90**: 6460–5.

8. Thijssen-Timmer DC, Peeters RP, Wouters P, et al. Thyroid hormone receptor isoform expression in livers of critically ill patients. *Thyroid* 2007; **17**: 105–12.

9. Chinga-Alayo E, Villena J, Evans AT, et al. Thyroid hormone levels improve the prediction of mortality among patients admitted to the intensive care unit. *Intensive Care Med* 2005; **31**: 1356–61.

10. Peeters RP, Wouters PJ, van Toor H, et al. Serum 3,3',5'-triiodothyronine (rT3) and 3,5,3'-triiodothyronine/rT3 are prognostic markers in critically ill patients and are associated with post-mortem tissue deiodinase activities. *J Clin Endocrinol Metab* 2005; **90**: 4559–65.

11. Plikat K, Langgartner J, Buettner R, et al. Frequency and outcome of patients with nonthyroidal illness syndrome in a medical intensive care unit. *Metabolism* 2007; **56**: 239–44.

12. De Groot LJ. Non-thyroidal illness syndrome is a manifestation of hypothalamic-pituitary dysfunction, and in view of current evidence, should be treated with appropriate replacement therapies. *Crit Care Clin* 2006; **22**: 57–86.

13. Dulawa A, Buldak L, Krysiak R, et al. Hormonal supplementation in endocrine dysfunction in critically ill patients. *Pharmacol Rep* 2007; **59**: 139–49.

14. Surks MI, Sievert R. Drugs and thyroid function. *N Engl J Med* 1995; **333**: 1688–94.

15. Basaria S, Cooper DS. Amiodarone and the thyroid. *Am J Med* 2005; **118**: 706–14.

16. Vagenakis AG, Downs P, Braverman LE, et al. Control of thyroid hormone secretion in normal subjects receiving iodides. *J Clin Invest* 1973; **52**: 528–32.

17. Loh K-C. Amiodarone-induced thyroid disorders: a clinical review. *Postgrad Med J* 2000; **76**: 133–40.

18. Woeber KA. Iodine and thyroid disease. *Med Clin North Am* 1991; **75**: 169–78.

19. Burch HB, Wartofsky L. Life-threatening thyrotoxicosis. Thyroid storm. *Endocrinol Metab Clin North Am* 1993; **22**: 263–77.

20. Ebert RJ. Dantrolene and thyroid crisis. *Anaesthesia* 1994; **49**: 924.

21. Sebe A, Satar S, Sari A. Thyroid storm induced by aspirin intoxication and the effect of hemodialysis: a case report. *Adv Ther* 2004; **21**: 173–7.

22. Wartofsky L. Myxedema Coma. *Endocrinol Metab Clin North Am* 2006; **35**: 687–98.

23. Hylander B, Rosenqvist U. Treatment of myxoedema coma: factors associated with fatal outcome. *Acta Endocrinol* 1985; **108**: 65–71.

24. Yamamoto T, Fukuyama J, Fujiyoshi A. Factors associated with mortality of myxedema coma: report of eight cases and literature survey. *Thyroid* 1999; **9**: 1167–74.

25. Ringel MD. Endocrine and metabolic dysfunction syndromes in the critically ill. *Crit Care Clin* 2001; **17**: 59–74.

26. Kwaku MP, Burman KD. Myxedema Coma. *J Intensive Care Med* 2007; **22**: 224–31.

27. Reynolds RM, Padfield PL, Seckl JR. Disorders of sodium balance. *BMJ* 2006; **332**: 702–5.

28. Yamamoto T. Delayed respiratory failure during the treatment of myxedema coma. *Endocrinol Jpn* 1984; **31**: 769–75.

29. Zwillich, CW, Pierson DJ, Hofeldt FD, et al. Ventilatory control in myxedema and hypothyroidism. *N Engl J Med* 1975; **292**: 662–5.

Chapter 8

Disorders of sodium balance

Martin Smith

Disturbance of sodium balance is a frequent finding in the hospital inpatient population and is particularly common in critically ill patients and after brain injury [1]. It can lead to serious complications and adverse outcomes, including neurological damage and death. An understanding of the normal physiology of sodium homeostasis allows a systematic approach to the diagnosis and treatment of dysnatraemia.

Normal physiology of salt and water regulation

Sodium and water homeostasis are inextricably linked. Sodium is the major extracellular cation and with its accompanying anions, principally chloride and bicarbonate, is the major determinant of plasma osmolality. The extracellular to intracellular sodium concentration gradient is maintained by cell membrane Na-K-ATPase and total body sodium is controlled by the kidneys. Sodium is freely filtered at the glomerulus and the majority is reabsorbed at the proximal tubule under the control of sympathetic nerves and atrial (ANP) and brain (BNP) natriuretic peptides, which result in natriuresis by a direct effect on the inner medullary collecting duct and by inhibition of renin and aldosterone release [2]. C-type (CNP) and dendroaspis (DNP) natriuretic peptides are also implicated in sodium regulation and reduce sympathetic outflow from the brainstem and inhibit thirst and salt appetite [3]. Water, which constitutes 60% of body mass, moves freely between intra- and extracellular compartments along concentration gradients. The extracellular fluid (ECF) water content is the principle determinant of plasma sodium concentration (Na^+) and is controlled by balancing water intake and urinary dilution via thirst, arginine vasopressin (AVP) and the kidneys.

Urinary dilution is determined by the circulating level of AVP, also called antidiuretic hormone. It is synthetised in the supraoptic and paraventricular nuclei and transported to, and released from, the posterior lobe of the pituitary gland. Arginine vasopressin binds to type 2 vasopressin (V2) receptors in the renal collecting ducts and initiates phosphorylation of aquaporin-2 water channels resulting in increased reabsorption of water and urinary concentration [4]. Arginine vasopressin release is stimulated in response to activation of osmoreceptors in the hypothalamus when plasma osmolality reaches 280 mOsm kg^{-1}. Thirst is stimulated at slightly higher osmolality (295 mOsm kg^{-1}), prompting increased water intake in conscious patients. Decreases in blood pressure and intravascular volume, detected by low pressure baroreceptors in the right atrium/great veins and high pressure receptors in the carotid sinus, result in non-osmotic release of AVP. Hypovolaemia and hypotension also increase sympathetic activity and activate the renin-angiotensin-aldosterone system. Normal plasma Na^+ is maintained between 135 and 145 mmol l^{-1} and osmolality between 285 and 295 mOsm kg^{-1}.

Pain, nausea and smoking also stimulate AVP release whereas caffeine and alcohol inhibit its release, explaining the latter's mild diuretic effects.

Hyponatraemia

Epidemiology

Hyponatraemia is defined as plasma $Na^+ < 135$ mmol l^{-1}. It is the most common electrolyte disorder with an incidence of 15–30% depending on the diagnostic threshold [4]. It is associated with substantially increased mortality rates.

Classification of hyponatraemia

Hyponatraemia is often classified into hypovolaemic, euvolaemic or hypervolaemic types depending on the

Table 18.1 Causes of hyponatraemia.

Hypovolaemic hyponatraemia	Normovolaemic hyponatraemia	Hypervolaemic hyponatraemia
Intrarenal sodium losses	SIADH	Congestive cardiac failure
CSWS	CNS pathology	Cirrhosis
loop diuretics	drugs	Nephrotic syndrome
osmotic diuretics	pulmonary pathology	Acute renal failure
adrenal insufficiency	Thiazides	Iatrogenic
ketonuria	Glucocorticoid deficiency	
Extrarenal sodium losses	Hypothyroidism	
vomiting	Iatrogenic	
diarrhoea		
excessive sweating		

CNS, central nervous system; CSWS, cerebral salt wasting syndrome; SIADH, syndrome of inappropriate antidiuretic hormone secretion.

associated volume disturbance. However, it can be difficult to distinguish between them in clinical practice and several causes of hyponatraemia can be associated with more than one volume state [5].

Causes of hyponatraemia

Hyponatraemia reflects an excess of water relative to sodium either because of dilution of sodium by increases in total body water or depletion of total body sodium in excess of simultaneous water losses [6]. The causes of hyponatremia are numerous (Table 18.1).

Normovolaemic hyponatraemia

Normovolaemic hyponatraemia is the most common and most heterogeneous dysnatraemia.

Syndrome of inappropriate antidiuretic hormone secretion

The syndrome of inappropriate antidiuretic hormone secretion (SIADH) is one of the most commonly encountered causes of hyponatraemia in hospital inpatients and in the critically ill. It was first described by Schwartz et al. in 1957 in patients with bronchial carcinoma [7]. Although the pathophysiology of SIADH is not fully understood, there appears to be a lower thirst threshold for AVP release in patients with SIADH and associated loss of control of AVP, with levels being unchanged by drinking or by osmotic stimulus [8]. The inappropriate elevations of AVP that occur in SIADH result in water retention and dilutional hyponatraemia. The SIADH is a common complication of a wide range of clinical disorders, including malignancy, benign pulmonary disease and neurological disorders, and is a side effect of many drugs (Table 18.2).

Table 18.2 Causes of the syndrome of inappropriate antidiuretic hormone secretion (SIADH).

Central nervous system
Traumatic brain injury
Subarachoid haemorrhage
Brain tumour
Stroke
Infections
Drugs
Carbamazepine
Chlorpropamide
Oxcarbazepine
Phenothiazines
Serotonin re-uptake inhibitors
Tricyclic antidepressants
Vincristine
Pulmonary conditions
Infection
Neoplasia
Acute lung injury

Endocrine disorders

Hyponatraemia occurs in around 10% of patients with hypothyroidism, although it is usually mild [9]. Secondary adrenal failure, including that related to high dose therapeutic glucocorticoids, causes hyponatraemia with features that can be indistinguishable from SIADH. Since glucocorticoid deficiency is the likely cause, it has been suggested that small doses of hydrocortisone should be administered empirically to patients with hyponatraemia of unknown aetiology [10]. If in doubt, an adrenocorticotrophic hormone (Synacthen) test should be performed to confirm or exclude cortisol deficiency.

Hypovolaemic hyponatraemia

Hypovolaemic hyponatraemia occurs in situations of extracellular fluid (ECF) depletion when sodium losses exceed those of water. As volume status is low, it is usually associated with non-osmotic release of AVP.

Diuretic therapy

Thiazide diuretic use is one of the most common causes of hypovolaemic hyponatraemia, although thiazides can also be associated with normovolaemic hyponatraemia [4]. They block the renal reabsorption of sodium and prevent the formation of maximally dilute urine. Unlike loop diuretics, they do not interfere with urine concentrating capacity and urinary Na^+ is therefore normal or high [11].

Cerebral salt wasting syndrome

The cerebral salt wasting syndrome (CSWS) is characterised by hyponatremia and hypovolaemia in patients with intracranial disease [12]. While the pathophysiology of CSWS is not fully understood, it is believed that the natriuretic peptides are implicated and BNP appears to be the most likely candidate [12]. Substantial increases in BNP levels are associated with hyponatraemia, cerebral vasospasm and worsened neurological outcome in patients with subarachnoid hemorrhage (SAH) [13]. In addition to the effects of natriuretic peptides, down-regulation of transporters of sodium reabsorption and catecholamine-induced pressure natriuresis might also contribute to CSWS.

Gastrointestinal losses

Gastrointestinal losses causing hypovolaemic hyponatraemia are usually associated with renal retention of sodium, and urinary sodium is therefore low (< 10 mmol l^{-1}).

Adrenal insufficiency

In primary adrenal failure, mineralocorticoid deficiency causes hyponatraemia because of urinary sodium loss, resulting in a high urinary sodium (> 20 mmol l^{-1}). Glucocorticoid deficiency impairs the ability to excrete a water load appropriately because of increased AVP secretion and direct renal effects.

Hypervolaemic hyponatraemia

Hypervolaemic hyponatraemia occurs in situations of fluid overload associated with congestive cardiac failure (CCF), cirrhosis and the nephrotic syndrome. Total body sodium is increased but total body water is increased more, resulting in hyponatraemia and oedema. In CCF, a fall in cardiac output and blood pressure triggers AVP release and a simultaneous reduction in renal blood flow stimulates the renin-angiotensin-aldosterone system, causing sodium and water reabsorption [14]. In addition, the hyponatraemia of CCF is likely to be complicated by concurrent diuretic therapy.

Miscellaneous

Iatrogenic hyponatraemia

Iatrogenic hyponatraemia is not uncommon, particularly in the perioperative period and in critically ill patients, because of administration of hypotonic intravenous fluids. It may also occur in patients receiving isotonic saline because of stress-related AVP release [15]. The absorption of large quantities of irrigation solution during transurethral resection of the prostate can also lead to hyponatraemia.

Water intoxication

Water intoxication results in hyponatraemia when renal water control mechanisms become overwhelmed, most usually in psychiatric patients because of the large volumes that must be ingested. This is more likely if the urine continues to be inappropriately concentrated because of concurrent diuretic therapy or AVP release secondary to smoking or nausea.

Exercise-induced hyponatraemia

Significant hyponatraemia can occur in healthy individuals during high-endurance exercise. Plasma sodium < 135 mmol l^{-1} has been found in 13% of marathon runners and a small proportion (0.6%) develop a critically low plasma sodium concentration (< 120 mmol l^{-1}) [16].

Assessment and investigation of the hyponatraemic patient

Sodium measuring devices that determine the amount of sodium in a given volume can produce spuriously low plasma sodium concentrations in hyperlipidaemia or hyperproteinaemia. This is often referred to as pseudohyponatraemia [4]. Hyponatraemia is diagnosed by confirmation of plasma Na^+ < 135 mmol l^{-1} after the exclusion of pseudohyponatraemia. Clinical evaluation should note any symptoms of the hyponatraemia, assess volume status and identify underlying causes. This should be supplemented by measurement of plasma and urine Na+ and osmolality [1, 12]. A practical algorithm for the assessment of hyponatremia is shown in Figure 18.1.

The SIADH is essentially a diagnosis of exclusion in the presence of hyponatraemia in association with a low serum osmolality (< 270 mOsmol l^{-1}) and inappropriately high urine osmolality (usually > 100 mOsmol l^{-1}) in a normovolaemic patient with normal pituitary, adrenal, thyroid and renal function who is not taking diuretics [11]. The general diagnostic criteria for CSWS, which are often inconclusive, include low or normal serum Na+ in the presence of high or normal plasma osmolality, a high or normal urine osmolality and hypovolaemia-related increases in haematocrit, urea, bicarbonate and albumin as a consequence of hypovolaemia.

In patients with neurological disease, it is important to differentiate between SIADH and CSWS because the management of these two conditions is diametrically opposed [1]. Urine biochemistry will confirm whether the urine is dilute or concentrated and should be reviewed with simultaneous measurements of plasma Na+ and osmolality (Table 18.3). However, biochemical criteria may fail to differentiate CSWS from SIADH and the diagnosis is confirmed by a careful clinical examination, with the key difference being the presence of volume depletion in CSWS [1, 12]. Central venous pressure, interpreted alongside fluid balance charts and daily weight change offer additional information [4]. Measurement of AVP levels is not particularly helpful because they can be raised in both SIADH and CSWS, although in the latter the elevated AVP is an appropriate response to hypovolaemia [17]. The availability of this assay is in any case limited and the results not available rapidly. Attempts have been made to identify derived parameters of sodium and water homeostasis for the differentiation of SIADH and CSWS in order to avoid the need to measure total body water and circulating blood volume [18].

Cerebral effects of hyponatraemia

The brain is the organ most susceptible to sudden changes in plasma sodium concentration and the symptoms of dysnatraemia are therefore primarily neurological (Table 18.4). A reduction in plasma sodium creates an osmotic gradient between extra- and intracellular compartments causing water to move into brain cells, leading to cerebral oedema and raised intracranial pressure. Cerebral oedema accounts for the serious and potentially fatal complications of hyponatraemia and, in an attempt to minimise brain swelling, hyponatraemia activates a protective mechanism called regulatory volume decrease [19]. This begins with an immediate extrusion of electrolytes, including sodium, potassium and chloride, from

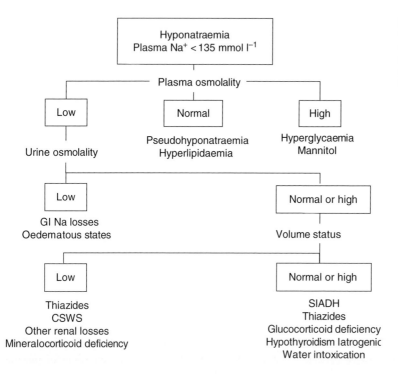

Fig. 18.1 Algorithm for assessment of the hyponatraemic patient. Na+, sodium concentration; CSWS, cerebral salt wasting syndrome; GI, gastrointestinal; SIADH, syndrome of inappropriate antidiuretic hormone secretion.

Table 18.3 Clinical and biochemical features of syndrome of inappropriate antidiuretic hormone secretion (SIADH) and cerebral salt wasting syndrome (CSWS).

Feature	SIADH	CSWS
Clinical		
Central venous pressure	Normal/increased	Decreased
Orthostatic hypotension	Absent	Present
Fluid balance	Positive	Negative
Volume status	Increased	Decreased
Body weight	Increased	Decreased
Biochemical		
Plasma Na⁺	Low	Low
Plasma osmolality	Low	Normal/increased
Urine Na⁺	High	High
Urine osmolality	High	Normal/high
Sodium balance	Equal	Negative
Haematocrit	Decreased/normal	Decreased
Urea	Decreased/normal	Decreased

Na⁺, sodium concentration.

Table 18.4 Symptoms and signs of hypo- and hypernatraemia.

	Moderate	Severe
Hyponatraemia	Lethargy	Drowsiness/confusion
	Nausea/vomiting	Depressed reflexes
	Irritability	Seizures
	Headache	Coma
	Muscle weakness/cramps	Death
Hypernatraemia	Lethargy	Hyperreflexia
	Thirst	Ataxia
	Irritability	Seizures
		Coma

brain cells and concomitant loss of intracellular water. Regulatory volume decrease is maintained by movement of osmotically active organic molecules from the intracellular to extracellular compartment over 48–72 hours. The ability of the brain to adapt to hyponatraemia is therefore related to the rate of change in plasma Na⁺ [20]. In chronic hyponatraemia, developing over a period of 48 hours or more, the slow and gradual reduction in Na⁺ provides sufficient time for the completion of regulatory volume decrease, and cerebral swelling is limited. Patients with chronic hyponatraemia may therefore be asymptomatic even when the reduction in Na⁺ is large [3]. In acute onset hyponatraemia however, the rapid decline in plasma Na⁺ may overwhelm adaptive mechanisms and symptoms are likely to occur even in the presence of only modest reductions in Na⁺ [21].

Symptoms of hyponatraemia

Mild hyponatraemia (130–135 mmol l⁻¹) is almost always asymptomatic. Plasma sodium concentrations between 125 and 130 mmol l⁻¹ are associated with non-specific symptoms, such as nausea, vomiting, dizziness and ataxia, whereas more severe hyponatraemia (< 125 mmol l⁻¹) usually causes more serious symptoms, including agitation and confusion (Table 18.4). When serum sodium concentration falls below 115 mmol l⁻¹, the arbitrary definition of severe hyponatraemia, there is a risk of cerebral oedema and the development of irreversible neurological complications including seizures, coma and death [22].

Treatment of hyponatremia

Except in life-threatening disturbances, the initial finding of low plasma Na$^+$ should prompt investigation into the aetiology of the hyponatraemia before management is initiated. Symptomatic acute hyponatraemia, on the other hand, is a medical emergency and prompt treatment is required to reduce the risk of complications, including brain damage and death. The correction of hyponatraemia can itself lead to neurological sequelae and these risks can be minimised by gradual correction of sodium deficits (see below) [19].

Specific treatment of SIADH

Fluid restriction, initially to 800–1000 ml day^{-1}, forms the mainstay of treatment of SIADH and usually results in a slow rise in plasma sodium of 1.5 mmol l^{-1} day^{-1} [23, 24]. The SIADH is often self-limiting in patients with brain injury and treatment is only indicated in the presence of symptoms or if the Na$^+$ is significantly low or falling rapidly [1]. If supplemental intravenous fluid is required, 0.9% saline is the usual choice, particularly after SAH when fluid restriction is associated with an increased incidence of cerebral ischaemia [24]. The use of hypertonic saline should be restricted to symptomatic acute hyponatraemia. It should be discontinued when plasma Na$^+$ reaches 120–125 mmol l^{-1} and further management continued with fluid restriction whenever possible.

Pharmacological treatment is an option when the diagnosis of SIADH is certain. Diuretics, such as furosemide, increase water excretion, although simultaneous saline or salt supplementation is required to replace the associated sodium loss. Demeclocycline and lithium inhibit the renal responses of AVP. Demeclocycline is the least toxic and an initial daily dose of 900–1200 mg should be reduced to 600–900 mg per day after therapeutic effect is achieved, usually by 3 days to 3 weeks. Arginine vasopressin-receptor antagonists, such as conivaptan and lixivaptan, inhibit the binding of AVP to renal receptors and have been shown to be effective in small clinical trials [25].

Specific treatment of CSWS

The primary treatment of CSWS is volume and sodium resuscitation, although the saline solution used is more controversial. In the first instance, 0.9% saline is generally recommended [1–3] but in acute symptomatic hyponatraemia, hypertonic (1.8% or 3%) saline is indicated, with the co-administration of furosemide if there is a risk of fluid overload [12–23]. Administration of 3% saline requires central venous access and 1.8% saline, which can be administered peripherally in the short term, is equally effective in many circumstances [3]. In some patients with CSWS, administration of sodium may actually increase the natriuresis and associated water loss, thereby worsening the clinical status. Once normovolaemia and normonatraemia have been restored, ongoing losses should be replaced with either intravenous 0.9% saline or oral water and sodium tablets until there is resolution of the CSWS. The CSWS may rarely be refractory to standard therapy and fludrocortisone (0.1–0.4 mg daily) can limit the sodium loss by increasing reabsorption from the renal tubule.

Challenges in the treatment of hyponatraemia

The treatment of symptomatic hyponatraemia poses a considerable challenge for several reasons. First, hyponatraemia often has a multifactorial aetiology, with more than one mechanism identified in an individual patient [26]. Second, in the acute setting, treatment may have to be initiated before the underlying diagnosis can be confirmed. Finally both under treatment and over-correction can have devastating and irreversible effects on the brain [1, 20].

The normalisation of plasma Na$^+$ that occurs during the treatment of hyponatraemia causes an increase in the previously depressed plasma osmolality. The osmotic gradient now drives water out of brain cells and restoration of intracellular osmolality by reaccumulation of solutes lost during regulatory volume decrease is necessary to prevent brain dehydration [20]. The movement of electrolytes again occurs rapidly but the reaccumulation of organic osmolytes may take several days. Rapid correction of hyponatraemia, before the reversal of regulatory volume decrease, can therefore lead to brain cell dehydration and the syndromes of central pontine and extrapontine myelinolysis [19, 20]. These are associated with a wide spectrum of symptoms and clinical outcomes, ranging from lethargy and dysarthria to severe disabilities, coma and death. The risk of myelinolysis can be minimised by gradual correction of sodium deficit at a rate of no more than 0.5 mmol l^{-1} h^{-1} or 8–10 mmol l^{-1} day^{-1} [1–6]. Treatment should be targeted to the point of alleviation of symptoms rather than to an arbitrary serum sodium value. Sodium replacement therapy can be guided using simple formulae (Figure 18.2) [6]. Close monitoring is mandatory during

$$\text{Change in plasma Na}^+ = \frac{\text{Infusate Na}^+ - \text{plasma Na}^+}{\text{Total body water} + 1} \qquad \text{eqn. 1}$$

$$\text{Change in plasma Na}^+ = \frac{(\text{Infusate Na}^+ + \text{infusate K}^+) - \text{plasma Na}^+}{\text{Total body water} + 1} \qquad \text{eqn. 2}$$

Fig. 18.2 Calculation of sodium replacement regimens in hyponatraemia. From Adrogue and Madias [6] with permission.

Note:
Equation 1 estimates the effect of one litre of a sodium containing fluid on plasma Na$^+$ and equation 2 the effect of replacement of one litre of fluid containing sodium and potassium.
Total body water is estimated as a fraction of body weight, being 0.6 and 0.5 in adult men and women respectively.

Na$^+$, sodium concentration

correction and, if over-rapid correction is suspected, reversal using desmopressin and water may be appropriate, but this is not without risk [27]. Although the treatment of symptomatic hyponatraemia must balance the risks of the low sodium against the risks of treatment, it is important to remember that patients with severe acute hyponatraemia are always at risk of the development of neurological complications from cerebral oedema, but rarely of myelinolysis from overcorrection [11, 22]. Not treating symptomatic patients is therefore never an option.

Hyponatraemia is frequently associated with hypokalaemia and, because potassium is the major intracellular cation, hypokalaemia reflects a significant deficit in total body potassium. The majority of the replaced potassium therefore moves from the ECF to restore intracellular stores and, as the cells become replete with potassium, water also moves intracellularly. This has the effect of increasing plasma Na$^+$, irrespective of sodium administration and must be accounted for in the calculation of sodium replacement regimens (Figure 18.2) [6].

Hypernatraemia

Epidemiology

Hypernatraemia is defined as plasma Na$^+$ > 145 mmol l^{-1}. It is much less common than hyponatraemia with an incidence of around 1% across the spectrum of all hospital patients. It is relatively more common in critically ill and neurological patients [1]. Water depletion is especially common in the intensive care setting, where a 9% incidence of Na > 150 mmol l^{-1} has been reported [28]. Hypernatraemia is often a paraphenomenon, being an indicator of the severity of the underlying disease process.

Except in cases of uncontrollable diabetes insipidus (DI), a hypernatraemic state can only be maintained when thirst is impaired or access to free water is restricted. Patients with an altered mental state or decreased level of consciousness are therefore particularly susceptible [6].

Classification

Hypernatraemia reflects a net loss of water or hypertonic sodium gain, with inevitable hyperosmolality. It can also be categorised on the basis of the associated ECF volume status. There is much overlap between eu- and hypovolaemic hypernatraemic states which are generated when water losses exceed those of salt in the context of an inability to replace water. Acute hypervolaemic hypernatraemia may result from ingestion of large amounts of salt without associated water intake or the infusion of large volumes of hypertonic saline solutions. Chronic hypervolaemic hypernatraemia can be associated with over diuresis in oedematous patients when loop diuretics cause proportionately greater loss of water than salt.

Causes

Causes of hypernatraemia are shown in Table 18.5. Hypernatraemia is usually related to water deficiency and only rarely does it represent salt excess. After brain injury, hypernatraemia is most commonly related to the development of central DI (CDI), although other causes of high urine volume, such as the use of mannitol or hypertonic saline for control of raised intracranial pressure and triple-H therapy to treat cerebral vasospasm, should be considered in this patient group. Nephrogenic DI (NDI) is a relatively rare cause of hypernatraemia in which the kidney is unresponsive to the water-retaining effects of AVP [29]. Nephrogenic DI can be acquired or congenital. The common causes of acquired NDI are

Table 18.5 Causes of hypernatremia.

Hypo/normovolaemic hypernatraemia	Hypervolaemic hypernatraemia
Poor thirst/reduced water intake	Excess salt intake
Intrarenal water loss	Iatrogenic: administration of hypertonic fluids
central diabetes insipidus	Mineralocorticoid excess
nephrogenic diabetes insipidus	hyperaldosteronism
osmotic diuresis	Cushing's syndrome
Extrarenal water loss	exogenous
gastrointestinal tract	
fever	

lithium therapy, hypercalcaemia, hypokalaemia, low protein diets and malnutrition. Congenital NDI results from genetic abnormalities resulting in mutations of V2 or aquaporin-2 water channels leading to a clinical syndrome characterised by hypernatraemia, hyperthermia, mental retardation and repeated episodes of dehydration [30]. Therapy to prevent dehydration permits many children with NDI to survive into adulthood and develop without mental retardation.

Central diabetes insipidus

Central DI occurs when there is failure of the homeostatic release of AVP from the hypothalamo-pituitary axis. The ability to concentrate urine is impaired resulting in the production of large volumes of dilute urine. This inappropriate loss of water leads to an increase in plasma Na^+ and osmolality and a state of clinical dehydration. Damage or compromise of the hypothalamus above the median eminence may lead to permanent DI, whereas damage below this level, or disturbance of the posterior lobe of the pituitary gland, leads to transient DI because AVP can subsequently be released from nerve fibres ending in the median eminence. This explains why DI is transitory in some patients but not in others.

Central DI is particularly common in neurological patients where it is associated with pituitary surgery, traumatic brain injury (TBI) and aneurysmal SAH [1]. The incidence of CDI can be as high as 35% after TBI and it is associated with more severe injury and increased mortality [31]. Patients who become brain dead often develop severe CDI and this can lead to challenges in the diagnosis of brainstem death and in the management of potential organ donors [32].

Symptoms

Non-specific symptoms, such as anorexia, muscle weakness, nausea and vomiting, occur first and, as the Na^+ continue to rise, are followed by lethargy, irritability and coma (Table 18.4). Severe symptoms are usually only evident with acute and large increases in plasma $Na^+ > 160$ mmol l^{-1} [5]. Rapid onset hyperatraemia does not allow sufficient time for organic osmolytes to accumulate in brain cells, thereby rendering patients susceptible to potentially fatal cerebral dehydration. The subsequent brain shrinkage can lead to rupture of bridging vessels between periosteum and brain, and result in subarachnoid and intracerebral haemorrhage.

Investigation

In awake patients, the classic symptoms of polyuria, polydipsia and thirst makes CDI relatively easy to diagnose. Hyperglycaemia has similar symptomatology and should be excluded. Clinical examination allows differentiation between hypovolaemic hyponatraemia and the rarer hypervolaemic type, although assessment of plasma and urine osmolality and Na+ is necessary to confirm the clinical suspicion. It is also necessary to differentiate between simple dehydration and CDI, bearing in mind that, in brain-injured patients, thirst is often an unreliable or absent sign. Dehydration is associated with low urine volume (in the absence of renal failure), whereas CDI results in high urine output. Central DI and NDI may be differentiated by desmopressin-induced concentration of urine in patients with CDI.

In the context of brain injury, the diagnosis of CDI is made in the presence of:

- increased urine volume (usually > 3000 ml/24 hours)
- high plasma Na^+ (> 145 mmol l^{-1})
- high plasma osmolality (> 305 mmol kg^{-1})
- abnormally low urine osmolality (< 350 mmol kg^{-1}).

The results of laboratory tests may not be available for some time and measurement of urine specific gravity (SG) is a useful adjunct to diagnosis when urgent treatment is required [1]. A urine SG of less than 1.005, in association with elevated plasma Na^+, strongly suggests a diagnosis of CDI. This simple bedside test can produce a false-negative test result when the plasma Na^+ is grossly raised and the diagnosis should always be confirmed by formal laboratory measurement of urine and plasma osmolality. An algorithm for assessment of the hypernatraemic patient is shown in Figure 18.3.

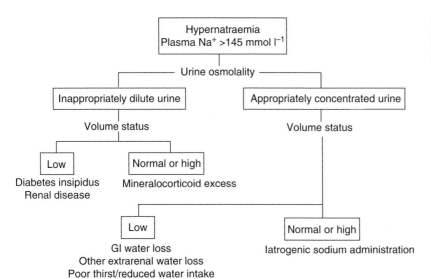

Fig. 18.3 Algorithm for assessment of the hypernatraemic patient. Na+, sodium concentration; GI, gastrointestinal.

Management of hypernatraemia

Hypernatraemia secondary to excessive sodium ingestion responds to normalisation of intake and, similarly, iatrogenic causes are relatively easy to recognise and usually respond to normalisation of sodium intake. The current therapeutic options for NDI are limited and only partially effective. Ensuring adequate water intake is the most important aspect of treatment. A very low sodium diet, thiazide diuretic or indomethacin may partially decrease urine volume. In acquired NDI, removing or treating the underlying cause may be beneficial but prolonged lithium therapy can lead to irreversible NDI.

Central diabetes insipidus

There are two aims in the management of CDI-related hypernatraemia – replacement and retention of water and, if necessary, replacement of AVP. Conscious patients with CDI are able to increase oral intake and often this is sufficient treatment. In unconscious patients, electrolyte-free water should be replaced via the nasogastric route wherever possible but, in those unable to absorb water, fluid replacement should be given as intravenous dextrose 5% in water. Careful monitoring is required to avoid water intoxication from excessive fluid administration and accurate clinical assessment of volume status and laboratory monitoring of urine and plasma biochemistry are required to guide treatment.

If fluid replacement alone fails, or if urine output is greater than 250 ml h^{-1}, synthetic AVP should be administered. Titrated doses of 1-deamino-8-D-arginine vasopressin (DDAVP) that can be given intranasally (100–200 μg) or intravenously (0.4 μg) is the best option. Small doses minimise the risk of an over prolonged action but can be repeated as required, dependent on clinical effect [1].

Rehydration must replace ongoing losses as well as deficits but, if the losses are large, as in CDI, treatment with dextrose 5% can lead to complications. Administration of > 500 ml of dextrose 5% per hour may result in hyperglycaemia, glycosuria and further dehydration and, if urine output remains high, DDAVP should always be administered.

Over-rapid correction of hypernatraemia may have serious consequences, most notably pulmonary and cerebral oedema. In patients in whom hypernatraemia has developed over only a few hours, rapid correction of plasma Na+ (reducing by 1 mmol l^{-1} h^{-1}) is safe and improves outcome without the risk of rebound cerebral oedema and neurological complications [33]. In patients with chronic hypernatraemia, or that of unknown duration, plasma Na+ should be reduced more slowly (10 mmol l^{-1} day^{-1}) in order to minimise the risk of neurological complications [1, 5].

Conclusions

Disturbances of sodium balance are common in the general hospital population but more so in critically ill and brain-injured patients. Patients are at risk not only from the dysnatraemia but also from the consequences of over treatment. Asymptomatic patients can often be managed successfully with a 'wait and see' approach because the dysnatraemia may be transitory. Urgent treatment is required in acute symptomatic patients in whom the risks of the dysnatraemia far outweigh the potential side effects of treatment.

References

1. Tisdall M, Crocker M, Watkiss J, Smith M. Disturbances of sodium in critically ill adult neurologic patients: a clinical review. *J Neurosurg Anesthesiol* 2006; **18**: 57–63.

2. Levin ER, Gardner DG, Samson WK. Natriuretic peptides. *N Engl J Med* 1998; **339**: 321–8.

3. Rabinstein AA, Wijdicks EF. Hyponatremia in critically ill neurological patients. *Neurologist* 2003; **9**: 290–300.

4. Reynolds RM, Seckl JR : Hyponatraemia for the clinical endocrinologist. *Clin Endocrinol (Oxf)* 2005; **63**: 366–74.

5. Reynolds RM, Padfield PL, Seckl JR. Disorders of sodium balance. *BMJ* 2006; **332**: 702–5.

6. Adrogue HJ, Madias NE. Hyponatremia. *N Engl J Med* 2000; **342**: 1581–9.

7. Schwartz WB, Bennett W, Curelop S, Bartter FC. A syndrome of renal sodium loss and hyponatremia probably resulting from inappropriate secretion of antidiuretic hormone. 1957. *J Am Soc Nephrol* 2001; **12**: 2860–70.

8. Smith D, Moore K, Tormey W, et al. Downward resetting of the osmotic threshold for thirst in patients with SIADH. *Am J Physiol Endocrinol Metab* 2004; **287**: E1019–23.

9. Montenegro J, Gonzalez O, Saracho R, et al. Changes in renal function in primary hypothyroidism. *Am J Kidney Dis* 1996; **27**: 195–8.

10. Bahr V, Franzen NF, Pfeiffer AF, et al. Vasopressin excess and hyponatremia: hydrocortisone treatment should be considered. *Am J Kidney Dis* 2006; **48**: 339–40.

11. Biswas M, Davies JS. Hyponatraemia in clinical practice. *Postgrad Med J* 2007; **83**: 373–8.

12. Cerda-Esteve M, Cuadrado-Godia E, Chillaron JJ, et al. Cerebral salt wasting syndrome: review. *Eur J Intern Med* 2008; **19**: 249–54.

13. McGirt MJ, Blessing R, Nimjee SM, et al. Correlation of serum brain natriuretic peptide with hyponatremia and delayed ischemic neurological deficits after subarachnoid hemorrhage. *Neurosurgery* 2004; **54**: 1369–73.

14. Oren RM. Hyponatremia in congestive heart failure. *Am J Cardiol* 2005; **95**: 2B–7B.

15. Steele A, Gowrishankar M, Abrahamson S, et al. Postoperative hyponatremia despite near-isotonic saline infusion: a phenomenon of desalination. *Ann Intern Med* 1997; **126**: 20–5.

16. Almond CS, Shin AY, Fortescue EB, et al. Hyponatremia among runners in the Boston Marathon. *N Engl J Med* 2005; **352**: 1550–6.

17. Nelson PB, Seif SM, Maroon JC, Robinson AG. Hyponatremia in intracranial disease: perhaps not the syndrome of inappropriate secretion of antidiuretic hormone (SIADH). *J Neurosurgery* 1981; **55**: 938–41.

18. Lolin Y, Jackowski A. Hyponatraemia in neurosurgical patients: diagnosis using derived parameters of sodium and water homeostasis. *Br J Neurosurg* 1992; **6**: 457–66.

19. Martin RJ. Central pontine and extrapontine myelinolysis: the osmotic demyelination syndromes. *J Neurol Neurosurg Psychiatry* 2004; **75 Suppl 3**: iii22–iii28.

20. Nathan BR. Cerebral correlates of hyponatremia. *Neurocrit Care* 2007; **6**: 72–8.

21. Palmer BF, Gates JR, Lader M. Causes and management of hyponatremia. *Ann Pharmacother* 2003; **37**: 1694–702.

22. Vachharajani TJ, Zaman F, Abreo KD. Hyponatremia in critically ill patients. *J Intensive Care Med* 2003; **18**: 3–8.

23. Arieff AI. Management of hyponatraemia. *BMJ* 1993; **307**: 305–8.

24. Diringer MN, Zazulia AR. Hyponatremia in neurologic patients: consequences and approaches to treatment. *Neurologist* 2006; **12**: 117–26.

25. Gross P. Treatment of hyponatremia. *Intern Med* 2008; **47**: 885–91.

26. Lien YH, Shapiro JI. Hyponatremia: clinical diagnosis and management. *Am J Med* 2007; **120**: 653–8.

27. Soupart A, Ngassa M, Decaux G. Therapeutic relowering of the serum sodium in a patient after excessive correction of hyponatremia. *Clin Nephrol* 1999; **51**: 383–6.

28. Polderman KH, Schreuder WO, Strack van Schijndel RJ, Thijs LG. Hypernatremia in the intensive care unit: an indicator of quality of care? *Crit Care Med* 1999; **27**: 1105–8.

29. Sands JM, Bichet DG. Nephrogenic diabetes insipidus. *Ann Intern Med* 2006; **144**: 186–94.

30. Knoers NV, Deen PM. Molecular and cellular defects in nephrogenic diabetes insipidus. *Pediatr Nephrol* 2001; **16**: 1146–52.

31. Powner DJ, Boccalandro C, Alp MS, Vollmer DG. Endocrine failure after traumatic brain injury in adults. *Neurocrit Care* 2006; **5**: 61–70.

32. Smith M. Physiologic changes during brain stem death – lessons for management of the organ donor. *J Heart Lung Transplant* 2004; **23**: S217–22.

33. Weiss-Guillet EM, Takala J, Jakob SM. Diagnosis and management of electrolyte emergencies. *Best Pract Res Clin Endocrinol Metab* 2003; **17**: 623–51.

Index